T0293403

Androgen Deficiency and Testosterone Replacement: Current Controversies and Strategies

Androgen Deficiency and Testosterone Replacement: Current Controversies and Strategies

Editor: Adeline Branson

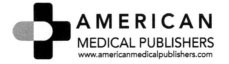

AMERICAN
MEDICAL PUBLISHERS
www.americanmedicalpublishers.com

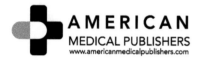

AMERICAN
MEDICAL PUBLISHERS
www.americanmedicalpublishers.com

Cataloging-in-Publication Data

Androgen deficiency and testosterone replacement : current controversies and strategies / edited by Adeline Branson.
   p. cm.
Includes bibliographical references and index.
ISBN 978-1-63927-872-5
1. Androgens. 2. Testosterone--Therapeutic use. 3. Infertility, Male. 4. Androgens--Physiological effect.
5. Testosterone--Physiological effect. 6. Hormones, Sex. I. Branson, Adeline.
RM296.5.T47 A53 2023
615.366--dc23

© American Medical Publishers, 2023

American Medical Publishers,
41 Flatbush Avenue,
1st Floor, New York,
NY 11217, USA

ISBN 978-1-63927-872-5 (Hardback)

This book contains information obtained from authentic and highly regarded sources. Copyright for all individual chapters remain with the respective authors as indicated. All chapters are published with permission under the Creative Commons Attribution License or equivalent. A wide variety of references are listed. Permission and sources are indicated; for detailed attributions, please refer to the permissions page and list of contributors. Reasonable efforts have been made to publish reliable data and information, but the authors, editors and publisher cannot assume any responsibility for the validity of all materials or the consequences of their use.

Trademark Notice: Registered trademark of products or corporate names are used only for explanation and identification without intent to infringe.

Contents

Permissions

List of Contributors

Index

Preface

Androgen deficiency refers to a type of medical condition characterized by low levels of androgenic activity in the human body. It indicates that the level of male sex hormones, specifically testosterone, is lower than the requirement in a healthy adult. There are various signs and symptoms of androgen deficiency, such as exhaustion and lethargy, loss of body hair, diminished sex drive, melancholy, decreased ejaculate production, etc. It can be caused by impairments in testicles, hypothalamus or pituitary gland. The diagnosis of androgen deficiency is done by utilizing a variety of evaluations, such as blood tests, physical examinations, medical histories and other tests. Testosterone replacement therapy (TRT) is used to treat androgen deficiency. Topical creams, oral medications, transdermal patches and intramuscular injections are examples of TRT procedures. It is a popular treatment for men who have symptomatic hypogonadism. This book unravels the recent studies on testosterone replacement. It is compiled in such a manner, that it will provide in-depth knowledge about the assessment and management of androgen deficiency through testosterone replacement. Researchers and students in this field will be assisted by this book.

All of the data presented henceforth, was collaborated in the wake of recent advancements in the field. The aim of this book is to present the diversified developments from across the globe in a comprehensible manner. The opinions expressed in each chapter belong solely to the contributing authors. Their interpretations of the topics are the integral part of this book, which I have carefully compiled for a better understanding of the readers.

At the end, I would like to thank all those who dedicated their time and efforts for the successful completion of this book. I also wish to convey my gratitude towards my friends and family who supported me at every step.

Editor

Androgen Effects on Neural Plasticity

Nariko Kuwahara, Kate Nicholson, Lauren Isaacs, and Neil J. MacLusky*,i

Abstract
Androgens are synthesized in the brain, gonads, and adrenal glands, in both sexes, exerting physiologically important effects on the structure and function of the central nervous system. These effects may contribute to the incidence and progression of neurological disorders such as autism spectrum disorder, schizophrenia, and Alzheimer's disease, which occur at different rates in males and females. This review briefly summarizes the current state of knowledge with respect to the neuroplastic effects of androgens, with particular emphasis on the hippocampus, which has been the focus of much of the research in this field.

Keywords: testosterone; neurosteroidogenesis; hippocampus; synaptogenesis; glia

Introduction

The incidence and progression of several neurological and psychiatric disorders, including Alzheimer's disease (AD),[1] schizophrenia,[2] and depression,[3] are sexually differentiated. For example, in comparison to their male counterparts, women are more likely to develop AD and experience a more rapid decline in memory.[4] The severity of cognitive symptoms associated with many of these disorders also appears to differ between the sexes.[2] That these sex differences might be attributable, at least in part, to the actions of sex steroid hormones has prompted increased interest in the mechanisms mediating hormonal effects on the brain.

Much of the work in this field has focused on the effects of the principal ovarian steroid, estradiol, because of data indicating that circulating and locally synthesized estradiol may play a fundamental homeostatic role in the brain.[5–7] In addition to wide-ranging effects on neurotransmitter and neuropeptide systems[8,9] and cerebral energy metabolism,[5] estradiol has also been demonstrated to induce dramatic, reversible changes in cellular morphology in many regions of the brain. Estrogen-induced changes in neuroplasticity include alterations in dendritic morphology, spine synapse density, and neuron number.[10,11]

Relatively less is known about the effects of androgens on the brain, although there are similarities between their effects and those of estrogens, particularly in females, at least in part because testosterone is a substrate for estradiol biosynthesis in the brain.[12] Androgen-induced changes in cognitive functions and behavior have been reported in humans[13–15] as well as experimental animals.[16,17] In men, the gradual decline in testosterone with age has been correlated

Department of Biomedical Sciences, University of Guelph, Guelph, Ontario N1G 2W1, Canada.
iORCID ID (https://orcid.org/0000-0002-9202-0564).

*Address correspondence to: Neil J. MacLusky, PhD, Department of Biomedical Sciences, Ontario Veterinary College, University of Guelph, Guelph, Ontario N1G 2W1, Canada, Email: nmaclusk@uoguelph.ca

with cognitive performance, with lower levels of free testosterone in older men being associated with reduced performance on verbal and spatial memory tasks.[18–20]

In male rodents, gonadectomy and testosterone supplementation has been found to influence spatial and working memory, although the responses appear to be mixed, possibly due to methodological differences across studies, including the type of cognitive test used and age of the animals.[16] Associated with these effects, morphological analysis has demonstrated that androgens induce marked changes in hippocampal and cerebral cortical dendritic morphology, spine and spine synapse density, and hippocampal neurogenesis.[21–26]

Although the catalogue of reported neuroplastic effects of androgens on the brain continues to expand, how these effects are mediated remains only partially understood. In this review, we provide a brief summary of the current research on androgens and their influence on various aspects of neuroplasticity, with a particular focus on the effects of these hormones in the hippocampus and the possible mechanisms mediating these effects. We also highlight areas of uncertainty and suggest possible directions for future research.

Androgens in the Brain: An Overview

Androgens, similar to other steroid hormones, are derived from the metabolism of cholesterol (Fig. 1). The initial, rate-determining step in steroidogenesis is cleavage of the cholesterol side chain by the P450scc enzyme, associated with the inner mitochondrial membrane, to form pregnenolone. Pregnenolone acts as a substrate for the synthesis of other steroid hormones via conversion to either 17α-hydroxypregnenolone or progesterone.

These steroids are precursors for the synthesis of dehydroepiandrosterone (DHEA), androstenediol, and androstenedione, weak androgens that are themselves substrates for conversion to testosterone, the predominant androgen circulating in the bloodstream. In androgen target tissues, testosterone is further metabolized to a range of biologically active metabolites, including 5α dihydrotestosterone (DHT), via the actions of 5α-reductase, as well as estradiol via cytochrome P450-aromatase.

In addition to being a more potent androgen than testosterone, DHT is also the precursor for two other biologically active metabolites: 5α-androstane-3α,17β-diol (3α-diol) and 5α-androstane-3β,17β-diol (3β-diol). 3α-diol is an allosteric modulator of

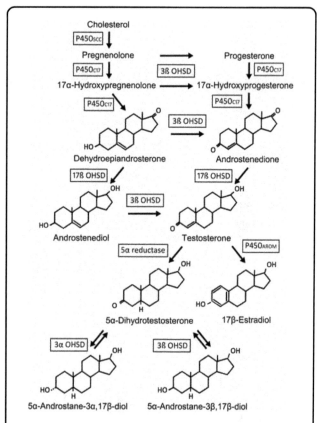

FIG. 1. Schematic illustration of the metabolic pathways involved in the biosynthesis and metabolism of the principal physiological androgens. Androgens and their major biologically active metabolites are shown with their structures; steroidal precursors for androgens are shown only by name. The enzymes mediating each metabolic conversion step are indicated by abbreviations in rectangular boxes. 17ß OHSD, 17ß hydroxysteroid dehydrogenase; 3ß OHSD, 3ß hydroxysteroid dehydrogenase; 3α OHSD, 3α-hydroxysteroid dehydrogenase; 5α reductase (3-oxo-5α-steroid 4-dehydrogenases, a family of isozymes with different tissue distributions[158]); P450$_{AROM}$, aromatase, or CYP19; P450$_{C17}$, 17α-hydroxylase/17,20 lyase or CYP17; P450$_{SCC}$, cholesterol side chain cleavage enzyme, or CYP11A1.

the GABA$_A$ receptor.[27] Both 3β-diol and, to a lesser extent 3α-diol, are ligands for estrogen receptor β (ERβ), possibly mediating some of the analgesic, anxiolytic, and cognitive-enhancing effects of circulating testosterone.[28]

This pattern of local tissue metabolism complicates elucidation of the mechanisms involved in mediating the effects of testosterone on the brain, since not only may multiple different neuronal and glial cell types be involved, but also there may be contributions from multiple receptor systems, responding to locally produced metabolites with a range of bioactivities. More detail regarding the enzymes and pathways involved in steroidogenesis is provided elsewhere.[29,30]

Although testosterone is often considered to be primarily a male sex hormone, it is present in females as well as males and exerts important physiological effects in both sexes.[31] The majority of circulating testosterone is synthesized by the Leydig cells of the testes in males and in the ovarian stroma in females,[32] although the amounts produced by the testes are ~7 to 8 times higher than those produced by the ovaries.[31] Biosynthesis of testosterone also occurs in the cortex of the adrenal gland in both sexes.[33,34]

Since androgens are nonpolar and are capable of easily diffusing across the blood–brain barrier, it was long assumed that androgens were synthesized in the periphery and passively distributed throughout the brain to exert their effects.[35] However, extensive evidence indicates that the brain itself is capable of local steroid synthesis.[6,12,36] This can occur by either local metabolism of circulating steroid intermediates or via de novo synthesis from cholesterol (reviewed in Schmidt et al.[37]).

The idea that androgens could be synthesized in the brain was first developed by Baulieu and colleagues in the 1980s. These authors found that androgens (principally the adrenal androgen DHEA) and their sulfoconjugate were present in higher concentrations in the nervous system than in the plasma, and these high levels remained long after gonadectomy and adrenalectomy of male rats.[38]

These findings led to the introduction of the term "neurosteroids" to refer to steroids synthesized locally in the brain.[36,38] Subsequently, the presence of the necessary steroidogenic enzymes in the brain was established in several species, including rodents and humans (reviewed in[39–42]). Along with the enzymes required for conversion of the primary sex steroids into biologically active metabolites,[36,43–45] the discovery of de novo neurosteroid synthesis has greatly expanded our appreciation of the diverse roles of gonadal steroids in the regulation of neuronal structure, function, and activity.[46]

Androgen action on the brain involves effects mediated via both steroid receptors of the nuclear receptor family, which bind to hormone response elements on DNA to regulate the expression of target genes,[47,48] and more rapid effects initiated via membrane receptors linked to kinase signaling cascades.[49] Nuclear steroid receptors (including the "classical" estrogen and androgen receptors [AR]) may in some instances subserve both roles, with a portion of the receptors in the cell being translocated to the plasma membrane.[50]

The AR have been found in both nuclear and extranuclear sites in hippocampal neurons,[51,52] as well as on oligodendrocytes and astroglia.[53] Estradiol, whether synthesized locally or delivered via the circulation, acts on both nuclear estrogen receptors (ERα and ERβ) and the G-protein coupled membrane estrogen receptor 1,[54] which are present in several subregions of the hippocampus and dentate gyrus (DG).[55,56]

Androgens and Long-Term Potentiation

Electrophysiological studies of long-term potentiation (LTP) in hippocampal slice preparations provided the first indication that androgens might induce functional plasticity in the hippocampus. LTP and long-term depression (LTD) are lasting changes in synaptic response following an initial stimulus that are believed to reflect key molecular mechanisms underlying learning and memory.[57–59] Gonadal hormones such as androgens have a profound influence on the induction of LTP and LTD in the hippocampus.[60]

After orchidectomy, male mice and rats displayed a reduction in LTP and a decrease in the amplitude of field excitatory postsynaptic potentials (fEPSP).[58,61] Orchidectomy also altered paired-pulse facilitation of fEPSP within the hippocampus,[61] suggesting that the removal of circulating androgens has a significant effect on presynaptic transmission, as well as on synaptic maturity.[61] These effects are multifaceted, including both positive and negative effects on hippocampal neural activity.

Thus, Skucas et al.[62] found that in adult male rats, orchidectomy resulted in increased synaptic transmission and LTP in the mossy fiber pathway, associated with a long-lasting upregulation of mossy fibers brain-derived neurotrophic factor (BDNF) immunoreactivity, compared with sham-operated rats.[62] Thus, the overall effects of androgen on hippocampal function may be mixed, enhancing some aspects of hippocampal neurotransmission while simultaneously limiting hyperexcitability and some forms of plasticity in the mossy fiber–CA3 pathway.[62]

In addition to orchidectomy-based studies, pharmacological and molecular targeting of the AR has also been used to investigate the effects of androgens on hippocampal LTP and LTD. Although administration of the AR antagonist flutamide has minimal effects on hippocampal LTP, it impairs the induction of LTD of CA1 pyramidal neurons, indicating a disruption in signaling processes.[60,63] The AR deletion in an AR mutant mouse model demonstrated a reduction in N-Methyl-D-aspartate (NMDA) receptor-mediated EPSP and high-frequency stimulation LTP of CA1 pyramidal neurons, indicating impairments in glutamate receptor activation.[64]

Although NMDA receptor levels did not differ between AR mutant and wild-type mice, this suggests that eliminating AR action leads to an overall decrease in the activation and function of NMDA receptor.[64]

The administration of androgens such as testosterone and its major 5α-reduced metabolites DHT and 3α-diol has also been shown to directly affect hippocampal synaptic transmission. *Ex vivo* administration of testosterone has been reported to facilitate LTP, increase overall excitability of CA1 pyramidal neurons in both gonadectomized male and female rats, and normalize CA3 mossy fiber fEPSP of orchiectomized males back to levels comparable to those observed in intact rats.[58,61,62] DHT has effects on LTP similar to those of testosterone, suggesting that local conversion to estradiol is not required for the response.

Treatment with the 5α-reductase inhibitor finasteride to block the metabolism of testosterone to DHT and 3α-diol in gonadally intact males resulted in a reduction in LTD and decreased fEPSP of CA1 pyramidal neurons.[65] This response was reversed with the application of DHT, but not testosterone.[65] DHT has been shown to reverse increases in mossy fiber transmission of orchiectomized rats back to the levels observed in sham-operated animals.[62] However, 3α-diol had no effect on CA3 fEPSP,[62] consistent with the view that the effects were mediated via AR-dependent mechanisms.

Androgens and Neurogenesis
The electrophysiological evidence for functional alterations in hippocampal neuroplasticity after androgen exposure led to studies aimed at defining the effects of these hormones on the hippocampal circuitry. Studies over the past 40 years have demonstrated that neurogenesis continues in regions of the adult vertebrate brain that are involved in learning and memory, notably in the vocal control centers of songbirds[66] and the

DG of the hippocampus.[67] Newly proliferated neurons in the DG subgranular zone migrate to the inner granule cell layer, where they extend long axons along the mossy fiber pathway to the CA3 subregion.[68–70]

Neurogenesis is a complex multistep process that involves the proliferation, differentiation, migration, and survival of new neurons.[71,72] A growing body of research indicates that, in the hippocampus of adult rodents, gonadal steroids affect multiple steps in this pathway. This subject is covered in detail in the article by Blankers and Galea in this special issue,[21] so we will only provide a brief summary here.

The effects of gonadal steroids on neurogenesis appear to be both sex- and hormone-specific. Thus, estradiol modulates new neuron survival and cell proliferation in the DG of adult female, but not male, rats,[73] whereas the reverse is true for the non-aromatizable androgen, DHT.[74] By contrast, in adult male voles, testosterone appears to enhance the survival of newly generated neurons in the DG, with no significant difference in cell proliferation.[75]

Similarly, castration of adult male rats led to a decrease in cell survival of new neurons within the DG, with no effect on cell proliferation.[24] However, in castrate adult male rats, 30 days of hormone replacement via injections or implants of testosterone propionate have been shown to increase neurogenesis in the DG via cell survival, relative to controls.[24,76] The dose and duration of testosterone administration appears to be an important determinant of the effects of testosterone on neurogenesis.[24,77]

Studies using metabolites of testosterone, as well as receptor-specific antagonists, suggest that the effects of testosterone on neurogenesis in the male hippocampus are probably mediated via AR, as opposed to local estrogen biosynthesis.[24,76] Consistent with this hypothesis, Okamoto et al. found that in male rats, mild exercise increased local intrahippocampal DHT synthesis, resulting in significantly increased neurogenesis, a response blocked by systemic administration of the AR antagonist, flutamide.[78]

The molecular mechanisms underlying these effects are not yet fully understood. Some studies in male rodents have detected AR protein and mRNA expression in the DG,[51,79] suggesting that androgens may influence cell survival directly via AR in newly generated neurons. However, whether the effects are actually mediated directly within the DG remains uncertain because of evidence indicating that AR are expressed in the CA1 and CA3 subregions of the hippocampus, but not the DG.[80–83]

Because AR are not expressed by immature neurons within the DG of young male mice and rats, it is possible that their effects may be mediated indirectly via target cells located elsewhere in the brain.[76,84] In particular, androgens may bind to AR on CA3 pyramidal cells, initiating the release and retrograde transport of a survival factor that may act on newborn neurons in the DG.[74,76,85] This hypothesis is consistent with observations indicating that newly formed neurons in the DG send projections to CA3, whereas damage to the CA3 has significant effects on neurogenesis in the DG.[86,87]

It also provides a striking parallel to work in the developing spinal cord, in which motoneurons in the spinal nucleus of the bulbocavernosus (SNB) are dependent for survival on androgen-dependent trophic support mechanisms via the target muscles that they innervate, even though the SNB neurons themselves do not express AR.[88]

Androgens and Hippocampal Synaptic Plasticity

A large body of evidence has demonstrated the effects of androgens on hippocampal plasticity, which may play important roles in normal physiological responses to changes in the environment. For example, in response to a stressful stimulus, males exhibit higher hip-

pocampal CA1 dendritic spine density in comparison to their female counterparts.[89] These rapid synaptic modulations may be mediated by sex steroids such as androgens because of their local and rapid synthesis within the brain.[90,91] Local synthesis results in elevated DHT, testosterone, and estradiol levels within the hippocampus, when compared with plasma levels.[90,92]

The majority of studies, however, have not been based on examination of the effects of physiological variations in steroid levels, but rather on experiments in which gonadal hormone levels are controlled by surgical gonadectomy and hormone replacement. Morphological studies often correlate changes in dendritic spine density with spine structure and the numbers and structure of spine synaptic contacts.[93] After orchidectomy, studies in both rats and non-human primate St. Kitts vervet monkeys demonstrated a significant reduction in dendritic spine synapse density in the CA1 region of the hippocampus.[22,23]

In the St. Kitts vervet monkeys, as much as 40% of spine synapse volumetric density was lost after orchidectomy.[23] Subsequently, it was demonstrated that androgen replacement restores the loss of spine synapse density in the male hippocampus that occurs after surgical gonadectomy[22,94] (Fig. 2). A similar effect has been reported in the CA1 subfield of the ovariectomized female rat hippocampus treated with testosterone.[23] However, despite

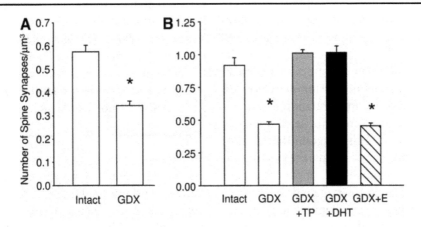

FIG. 2. **(A)** Bar graph shows the significant reduction in the number of spine synapses in the CA1 subfield of the hippocampus in GDX monkeys compared with intact monkeys. **(B)** Bar graph shows spine synapse densities in the stratum radiatum of the CA1 region in intact, GDX, GDX and testosterone propionate-treated (GDX+T), GDX and DHT-treated (GDX+DHT), or GDX and estradiol-treated (GDX+E) male rats. Spine synapse density was significantly lower in both GDX and GDX+E animals compared with controls, whereas there was no significant difference between intact animals and GDX animals treated with testosterone-propionate or DHT. Taken from MacLusky et al.[94]. DHT, dihydrotestosterone; GDX, gonadectomized.

the qualitatively similar nature of the CA1 synaptic response to testosterone in males and females, the underlying mechanisms are probably different.

When orchidectomized rats were replaced with testosterone, DHT or estradiol, only testosterone and DHT reversed the orchidectomy-induced loss of synapse density, whereas estradiol had no significant effect.[22] By contrast, in females DHT induced responses similar to those of estradiol, whereas the effects of both testosterone and DHEA on hippocampal synapse density were reversed by concomitant treatment with the aromatase inhibitor, letrozole.[23] This suggests that in males, both testosterone and DHT can stimulate spine synapse formation independently of aromatization, whereas in females the synaptic response to circulating testosterone is largely mediated via local estrogen biosynthesis.[22,94]

These findings cannot, however, be interpreted as indicating that the effects of testosterone on hippocampal synaptogenesis are mediated entirely via the cell nuclear AR system. Studies using the AR antagonist flutamide and animals expressing mutated forms of the AR have raised the possibility that other mechanisms may be involved. Thus, the administration of flutamide to orchidectomized male rats significantly increased CA1 spine synapse density compared with vehicle-treated controls, even though no significant trophic effect was observed in the ventral prostate gland, a widely used marker of androgenic biological activity (Fig. 3).

Flutamide did not block the synaptoplastic effects of either DHT or DHEA: Indeed, the responses to flutamide and the two androgens appeared to be additive, rather than inhibitory.[94,95] Further emphasizing the complex nature of this response, in testicular feminization mutant (Tfm) male rats expressing defective AR, results with both androgen and antiandrogen treatment were indistinguishable from those observed in wild-type male controls.[96] This suggests that at least in the CA1 region of the hippocampus, the synaptic effects of testosterone are retained even under conditions in which nuclear AR function is impaired.

This cannot be ascribed to local conversion of the androgen to estradiol, since estradiol does not affect hippocampal synapse density in males[22] whereas flutamide also exerts additive effects on CA1 synaptogenesis in combination with the non-aromatizable androgen, DHT.[95]

A definitive explanation for these observations remains lacking. One possibility is that the effects of flutamide may involve mechanisms other than those activated by the cell nuclear AR. As previously noted,[95] flutamide is not a completely specific antago-

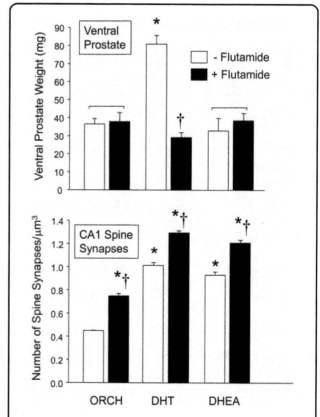

FIG. 3. Effects of DHT, DHEA, and flutamide on ventral prostate weight (top panel) and CA1 hippocampal spine synapse density (lower panel) in GDX male rats. *Significantly different from orchidectomized males given the same dose of androgen or oil vehicle; †Significantly different from orchidectomized males treated with the same doses of flutamide or vehicle, without androgen (Scheffe's test; $p < 0.05$ level). Compiled from data in MacLusky et al.[94,95]. DHEA, dehydroepiandrosterone.

nist of AR-mediated responses and may itself exert some agonist effects. Under *in vitro* cell culture conditions, the main bioactive metabolite of flutamide, hydroxyflutamide, has been reported to activate the mitogen activated protein kinase (MAPK)/extracellular regulated protein kinase (ERK) pathway, even in AR-negative cell lines.[97]

It also exerts weak benzodiazepine-like effects in the mouse brain.[98] Membrane-associated AR may be involved. Sato et al.[99] have reported that the self-reinforcing behavioral effects of androgen appear to involve membrane AR. These effects are preserved in

Tfm rats, suggesting that membrane receptor-mediated effects of androgens are retained in these animals despite the deficit in nuclear AR-activated responses.[99] Similar considerations may apply to androgen-induced synaptogenesis, which could explain the continued expression of normal androgen-induced increases in hippocampal synaptogenesis in Tfm males.

Cellular Mechanisms: How are the Neurotrophic Effects of Androgen Mediated?

The downstream signaling pathways mediating the neuroplastic effects of testosterone and its metabolites also remain only partially resolved. There are two main possibilities: first, that androgens may act directly on neurons to regulate intracellular neuronal signaling pathways contributing to growth and differentiation; and second, that androgen action on other cells, including both neurons and glia, may affect neuronal structure and function indirectly, via neurotrophic and metabolic response mechanisms. These two possibilities are, of course, not mutually exclusive and both may well contribute to testosterone action *in vivo*.

That androgens can act directly on neurons to modulate neuroplasticity has been established by a number of *in vitro* studies, using neurons in tissue culture or hippocampal tissue slices. Androgen treatment increases spine formation in hippocampal neurons in culture.[93,100,101] Using hippocampal slices from male adult rats, 2-hour treatment with DHT resulted in a significant increase in the densities of middle and large-head spine whereas 2-hour treatment with testosterone resulted in a significant increase in the density of small head spines.[93]

Incubation with letrozole did not affect testosterone's induction of spine density, suggesting that these effects may be attributed to its androgenic effects, as opposed to local conversion to estradiol.[93] Using primary cultures of rat hippocampal neurons, Guo et al. demonstrated that *in vitro* testosterone and bovine serum albumin-conjugated testosterone treatment similarly resulted in a rapid increase in spine density, consistent with the hypothesis that these effects may be mediated via membrane-associated AR.[101]

In the CA1 subregion of the hippocampus, a number of serine/threonine kinase signaling pathways have been implicated in mediating rapid structural responses to gonadal steroids. Intracellular signaling cascades that have been shown to be differentially activated by sex steroids include the MAPK/ERK, the cyclic AMP/protein kinase A (cAMP/PKA) pathways and the phosphoinositide 3-kinase/PI3K/Akt/mammalian target of rapamycin (PI3/Akt/mTOR) pathway.[54,102–105] By modulating intracellular signaling cascades, sex steroids may continuously regulate neuronal structure, dendritic spine density, and the functional plasticity of the hippocampal circuitry[62,93,106] (Fig. 4).

MAPK cascades are well known for their roles in synaptic modulation, and activation of PKC has been shown to be necessary for LTP in hippocampal slices.[107–110] Androgen-mediated increases in spine density have been correlated with increased expression of structural proteins such as synaptophysin and activation of ERK and cAMP-response element binding protein (CREB).[101]

For many years, it has been known that androgens stimulate rapid activation of PKC and ERK MAPK phosphorylation in the hippocampus and other tissues.[111–114] In cultured hippocampal neurons, PKC activation has been shown to rapidly upregulate NMDA receptor-mediated signaling[115] whereas multiple PKC isoforms are expressed within dendritic spines themselves.[116] Activation of PKC has been shown to induce activation of extracellular receptor kinase and rapid formation of new dendritic spines in cultured hippocampal neurons.[109]

ERK-1 and ERK-2 have been shown to be transiently phosphorylated after AR activation, and this has been implicated in mediating the neuroprotective effects of androgens such as testosterone and DHT.[111] New spine formation has been associated with increased functional synaptic connectivity and network activity in cultured neurons.[109] Within CA1 specifically, it has been shown that ERK MAPK mediates synaptic modulation of LTP through activation of both PKA and PKC mechanisms.[110] Although AR-dependent PKC and ERK activation has been well established in a variety of tissues,[112–114] findings from Hatanaka et al.[93] suggest that AR activation by DHT and testosterone results in activation of both PKA- and PKC-mediated ERK signaling.

Within dendritic spines, concurrent expression of these kinase cascades and ARs suggests that they may associate post-synaptically.[51] Androgen-mediated activation of ERK signaling is further supported by the data of Guo et al.,[101] who showed that in the presence of U0126 (a selective inhibitor of MAPK/ERK kinases 1 and 2), rapid testosterone-mediated increases in spine density were reversed and subsequent CREB phosphorylation was inhibited, suggesting that this rapid effect is mediated through AR-dependent ERK signaling.[101] Similarly, testosterone and DHT-induced dendritic spine formation is reduced by inhibition of ERK

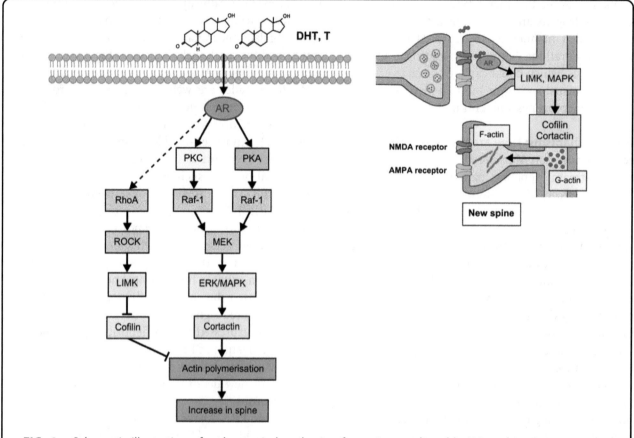

FIG. 4.   Schematic illustration of androgen-induced spine formation mediated by AR and its downstream kinase networks (adapted from Fig. 5 in Hatanaka et al.[93]). AR, androgen receptors.

MAPK, PKA, PKC, or LIMK, whereas inhibition of CAMKII or PI3K has been shown to have no effect on total spine density.[93]

The CREB is an important downstream transcriptional effector of MAPK/ERK activation.[117,118] CREB activity has been shown to be regulated by many other cell signaling mechanisms, including PI3K/Akt,[119] PKA,[120,121] CaMKIV,[122,123] and PKC.[110] Coupling of the PKA and PKC to CREB phosphorylation is mediated by the MAPK cascade within hippocampal CA1.[110]

Although CREB has been shown to be rapidly activated by DHT in hippocampal neurons, Nguyen et al. investigated the upstream signaling mechanisms responsible for this and determined that DHT mediates CREB phosphorylation through AR-dependent activation of PKC.[124] Intriguingly, subsequent studies demonstrated that androgen-induced formation of dendritic thorns within the CA3 stratum lucidum occurs via MAPK and PKC but independently of PKA signaling.[100]

Indirect mechanisms

Under *in vitro* conditions, tissue culture studies suggest that AR-mediated neuroplastic responses can be initiated directly in neurons; however, under *in vivo* conditions, lesion studies have demonstrated that androgen effects on neurogenesis and synaptic plasticity are at least partially dependent on afferent input from other areas of the brain.[86,87,125,126] Indirect androgen mediated modulation of cellular responses could theoretically involve synaptic/neurotransmitter input, and/or trophic factors released into the extracellular milieu.

A likely mediator of at least some androgen effects is the neurotrophin BDNF. BDNF and its downstream targets such as post-synaptic density protein 95 (PSD-95) play important roles in regulating spine formation. BDNF modulates functional synaptic properties in the mature and developing nervous system,[127,128] as well as hippocampal LTP.[129] Several studies have investigated androgen regulation of BDNF in the context of AR activation and synaptogenesis. For example, Jia et al.

determined that testosterone treatment significant increased CA1 spine density, BDNF, PSD-95, and CREB levels, whereas these endpoints were reduced in animals treated with flutamide.[130]

Conversely, orchidectomy has been reported to reduce protein levels of PSD-95 and BDNF in the CA1 region of the hippocampus in male mice, an effect reversed by testosterone replacement.[131] In other regions of the hippocampus, interactions between androgens and BDNF may have different consequences. Thus, after orchidectomy in rats, Skucas et al. reported increased synaptic transmission and LTP of the mossy fiber pathway along with increased BDNF levels, suggesting that androgens may play an inhibitory role in CA3 to prevent hyperexcitability and aberrant mossy fiber synaptic transmission.[62,132]

Within the cell, BDNF appears to be involved in regulating the distribution of key synaptic proteins that mediate actin cytoskeletal development.[133] For example, cortactin redistribution has been shown to be the result of a balance between BDNF and NMDA receptor activation during the development of the postsynaptic actin cytoskeleton.[133] Cortactin is an important structural protein that is known to be a target of ERK activation.

Once phosphorylated, cortactin may play an important role in spine reorganization and remodeling by grouping actin cytoskeletal matrices.[133] Cortactin contains multiple phosphorylation sites that may be phosphorylated by kinases such as PKA or PKC, which have been shown to be activated after DHT or testosterone treatment.[134] However, multiple cortactin phosphorylation sites may need to be activated to mediate androgen-induced spine formation.[93]

Potential contributions from glial-neuronal interactions

Astroglia are critical regulators of synaptic plasticity and neurotransmission.[135] The potential importance of these interactions is illustrated by data indicating that defective neuronal–glial interactions may play a key role in the etiology of common neurological disorders such as depression,[136] schizophrenia,[137] and AD.[138]

Not only are astroglia capable of androgen and estrogen biosynthesis,[139] but they may also contribute to androgen-mediated regulation of neural plasticity.[140] Androgen and estrogen receptors are expressed in astrocytes,[141–143] whereas oligodendrocytes express ERβ, which is involved in estrogen-mediated

enhancement of myelination.[144] In rats, at least after intrahippocampal injury, microglia also express immunoreactive AR.[142]

Although the study of androgen modulation of glial–neuronal interactions remains relatively limited, a few studies have reported the effects of testosterone on astroglial morphology. In male rats, Leranth et al.[23] demonstrated a significantly increased density of immunoreactive astrocytes in the cerebral cortex after orchidectomy (Fig. 5). Androgens also profoundly affect astrogliosis after neural injury. Barreto et al.[145] used an orchidectomized rat model to investigate and compare the effects of testosterone, estradiol, and non-aromatizable DHT treatment on reactive astroglia and microglial staining after a stab wound injury to the brain.

Early and delayed subcutaneous treatment with either testosterone or estradiol significantly reduced immunoreactive astrocyte and microglial staining within the hippocampus. Intriguingly, DHT had no effect on astrocyte staining but significantly reduced the volume fraction of immunoreactive microglial staining after early subcutaneous treatment. This suggests that early and late androgenic regulation of astroglia and microglia reactivity to neural injury is, at least in part, mediated through aromatization to estradiol whereas the early effects of androgens on microglia reactivity may also involve AR-specific mechanisms.

Conclusions and Future Directions

Androgen-regulated neural plasticity may play a role in both the normal development and function of the brain and in pathological states, leading to the development of sexually differentiated neurological disease states. Although progress in understanding the mechanisms involved in these effects is less well developed than is the case for estrogen-induced neuroplasticity, in part because of the range of bioactive metabolites involved in testosterone's actions, there are hints that the effects of androgens may involve unique elements that are distinct from the effects of androgens on non-neural target tissues.

Understanding these mechanisms may help to clarify the effects of androgens on neurological disorders that are expressed more commonly in males than females, potentially helping to provide improved therapeutic modalities for these disorders. In concluding this review, we will briefly consider two elements of the neurotrophic actions of androgens in which significant gaps in our understanding remain, hopefully to stimulate additional research in these remaining areas of uncertainty.

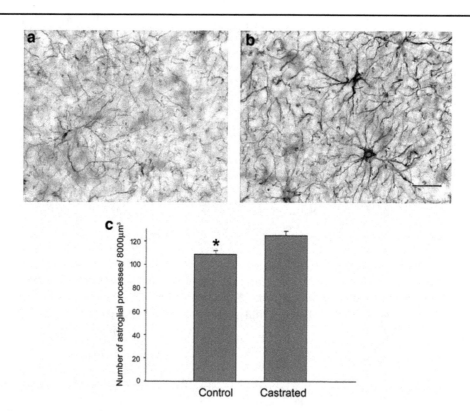

FIG. 5. Light micrographs show GFAP-immunoreactive glia and processes in vibratome sections taken from the stratum radiatum of the CA1 hippocampal subfield of a control **(a)** and a 1 month orchidectomized monkey **(b)**. Note the higher density of immunoreactive glia profiles in the hippocampus of the GDX animal **(b)**. Scale bar = 50 μm. **(C)** Bar graphs show the result of a semiquantitative calculation on the density of glia processes in the stratum radiatum of the CA1 hippocampal subfield. The surface density of glia processes is significantly higher (15%) in the orchidectomized (1 month) than control monkeys (mean ± SEM, $*p < 0.031$, $t = -3.270$, d.f. = 4). GFAP, glial fibrillary acidic protein.

A major unresolved question is: how the effects of testosterone on hippocampal synaptogenesis *in vivo* are mediated. These effects are clearly not mediated simply via conversion to estradiol.[94,22] As discussed earlier, although testosterone induction of hippocampal spine formation is mimicked by DHT, suggesting AR involvement, it is also reproduced by the much weaker androgen DHEA—at doses that do not induce a significant peripheral androgenic effect.[95]

Administration of flutamide, at a dose sufficient to block the trophic effects of DHT on the prostate, does not antagonize, but rather potentiates the effects of this androgen on hippocampal spine synapse density (Fig. 3). In male rats with the Tfm mutation, which impairs AR function, the effects of both DHT and hydroxyflutamide are indistinguishable from those in normal wild-type males.[96] Taken together, these observations suggest that the neurotrophic effects of androgens on hippocampal spine synapse density may be mediated via mechanisms distinct from those mediated through the "classical" intranuclear AR—despite the extensive evidence indicating the involvement of AR-linked kinase networks in the actions of DHT on spine plasticity in hippocampal neurons in culture.[93,100,101]

Exactly how androgens exert their effects *in vivo* remains unclear. We have previously speculated that the effects of testosterone *in vivo* may involve contributions from other mechanisms, such as potentiation of GABA-ergic transmission via the actions of 3α-diol.[94] Contributions from afferent input originating from other parts of the brain may also be involved.[125,126] Membrane AR-mediated responses may be involved,[101] since this response pathway appears to be preserved in Tfm rats.[99]

A second area of uncertainty concerns the question of how the effects of gonadal steroids on neural plasticity are integrated within the preexisting neural circuitry. For steroid induction of neurogenesis and new synaptic connections to be beneficial, it needs to be integrated with the existing neural circuitry. Otherwise, it may have detrimental consequences—disrupting rather than enhancing function.[146] How are new neurons integrated within existing neural networks? What processes ensure that androgen-induced increases in synapse density enhance function, rather than simply increasing "noise" in preexisting circuits?

An obvious possibility is that interactions between new neurons and potential synaptic targets, as has so elegantly been described for the SNB in the spinal cord,[147,148] may direct functional connectivity in androgen-sensitive circuitry in the brain. In addition to growth factor-dependent regulation, however, it seems likely that mechanisms exist to regulate connectivity at the local level. What processes determine how newly formed synapses connect? Or are the mechanisms similar to those operating normally in development, with initial synaptic over-production being subsequently refined and focused by selective pruning of under-utilized connections?[149]

These questions cannot be answered definitively at the present time. One possibility that may merit further investigation, however, is that androgens may regulate cell–cell communication via the Wnt-β-catenin-cadherin signaling pathways. Wnts are critically involved in the organization of different cell types during development, regulating interactions between neighboring cells. A key component of the Wnt signaling pathway, β-catenin, also functions as a component of the cadherin complex, which controls cell–cell adhesion and influences cell migration.

Cell adhesion molecules, including the cadherins and protocadherins,[150] are also of critical importance during embryonic development for morphogenesis of the central nervous system. This pathway is of particular interest, in the context of androgen action on the brain, for two reasons. First, the Wnt-β-catenin pathway is androgen-sensitive in the male reproductive tract,[151] as well as in prostate cancer in which androgen regulation of the Wnt signaling contributes to the progress of the disease.[152]

Second, several recent studies have demonstrated that developmental neurological disorders such as autism spectrum disorder and schizophrenia, which occur more often in males than in females, are frequently associated with mutations in the cadherin signaling pathway.[153–155] This raises the possibility that the relatively greater sensitivity of the male to these disorders might involve a genetic-hormonal interaction, with the effects of the mutations being enhanced by testosterone-induced responses.

Consistent with this hypothesis, Monks et al. have reported in rats that testosterone treatment increases expression of N-cadherin in both spinal motoneurons[156] and the hippocampus.[157] In the hippocampus, this effect was also induced by estradiol, but not by DHT,[157] suggesting possible estrogen receptor involvement. Further studies of androgen regulation of the Wnt-β-catenin-cadherin signaling pathway may shed additional light on the mechanisms involved in androgen-induced neuroplasticity.

In summary, extensive evidence supports a role for androgens, locally synthesized in the brain as well as derived from adrenal and gonadal androgens delivered via the circulation, in the regulation of cellular plasticity in the central nervous system. This plasticity involves both androgen-induced enhancement of synapse formation and increases in the formation and survival of new neurons.

These effects may play a role in the normal development and function of the brain as well as in pathological states leading to the development of sexually differentiated neurological disorders. The underlying cellular mechanisms responsible for these processes, however, still remain incompletely defined. A better understanding of these mechanisms may allow the development of improved therapeutic interventions to correct the problems associated with androgen-sensitive neurological disease.

Authors' Contributions

Concept and design of the article: N.K. and N.J.M; writing: N.K., K.N., L.I., and N.J.M; review and editing: N.K. and N.J.M; visualization: N.K. and N.J.M.

References

1. Barnes LL, Wilson RS, Bienias JL, Schneider JA, Evans DA, Bennett DA. Sex differences in the clinical manifestations of Alzheimer disease pathology. Arch Gen Psychiatry. 2005;62(6):685–691.

2. Mendrek A, Mancini-Marie A. Sex/gender differences in the brain and cognition in schizophrenia. Neurosci Biobehav Rev. 2016;67:57–78.

3. Angst J, Gamma A, Gastpar M, Lépine JP, Mendlewicz J, Tylee A. Gender differences in depression: Epidemiological findings from the European DEPRES I and II studies. Eur Arch Psychiatry Clin Neurosci. 2002;252(5): 201–209.

4. Irvine K, Laws KR, Gale TM, Kondel TK. Greater cognitive deterioration in women than men with Alzheimer's disease: A meta analysis. J Clin Exp Neuropsychol. 2012;34(9):989–998.

5. Brinton RD. Estrogen regulation of glucose metabolism and mitochondrial function: Therapeutic implications for prevention of Alzheimer's disease. Adv Drug Deliv Rev. 2008;60(13–14):1504–1511.

6. Cornil CA. On the role of brain aromatase in females: Why are estrogens produced locally when they are available systemically? J Comp Physiol A Neuroethol Sens Neural Behav Physiol. 2018;204(1):31–49.

7. Brocca ME, Garcia-Segura LM. Non-reproductive functions of aromatase in the central nervous system under physiological and pathological conditions. Cell Mol Neurobiol. 2019;39(4):473–481.

8. McEwen B. Estrogen actions throughout the brain. Recent Prog Horm Res. 2002;57:357–384.

9. Fink G, Sumner BE, Rosie R, Grace O, Quinn JP. Estrogen control of central neurotransmission: Effect on mood, mental state, and memory. Cell Mol Neurobiol. 1996;16(3):325–344.

10. Gould E, Woolley CS, Frankfurt M, McEwen BS. Gonadal steroids regulate dendritic spine density in hippocampal pyramidal cells in adulthood. J Neurosci. 1990;10(4):1286–1291.

11. Mahmoud R, Wainwright SR, Galea LAM. Sex hormones and adult hippocampal neurogenesis: Regulation, implications, and potential mechanisms. Front Neuroendocrinol. 2016;41:129–152.

12. Naftolin F, Ryan KJ, Davies IJ, et al. The formation of estrogens by central neuroendocrine tissue. Recent Prog Horm Res. 1975;31:295–319.

13. Nguyen TV, Lew J, Albaugh MD, et al. Sex-specific associations of testosterone with prefrontal-hippocampal development and executive function. Psychoneuroendocrinology. 2017;76:206–217.

14. Foland-Ross LC, Ross JL, Reiss AL. Androgen treatment effects on hippocampus structure in boys with Klinefelter syndrome. Psychoneuroendocrinology. 2019;100:223–228.

15. Panizzon MS, Hauger RL, Xian H, et al. Interactive effects of testosterone and cortisol on hippocampal volume and episodic memory in middle-aged men. Psychoneuroendocrinology. 2018;91:115–122.

16. Leonard ST, Winsauer PJ. The effects of gonadal hormones on learning and memory in male mammals: A review. Curr Zool. 2011;57:543–558.

17. Koss WA, Frick KM. Activation of androgen receptors protects intact male mice from memory impairments caused by aromatase inhibition. Horm Behav. 2019;111:96–104.

18. Holland J, Bandelow S, Hogervorst E. Testosterone levels and cognition in elderly men: A review. Maturitas. 2011;69:322–337.

19. Janowsky JS. The role of androgens in cognition and brain aging in men. Neuroscience. 2006;138(3):1015–1020.

20. Janowsky JS. Thinking with your gonads: Testosterone and cognition. Trends Cogn Sci. 2006;10:77–82.

21. Blankers SA, Galea LAM. Androgens and Adult Neurogenesis in the Hippocampus. Androgens: Clin Res Thera. 2021;2, DOI: 10.1089/andro.2021.0016.

22. Leranth C, Petnehazy O, MacLusky NJ. Gonadal hormones affect spine synaptic density in the CA1 hippocampal subfield of male rats. J Neurosci. 2003;23(5):1588–1592.

23. Leranth C, Prange-Kiel J, Frick KM, Horvath TL. Low CA1 spine synapse density is further reduced by castration in male non-human primates. Cereb Cortex. 2004;14(5):503–510.

24. Spritzer MD, Galea LAM. Testosterone and dihydrotestosterone, but not estradiol, enhance survival of new hippocampal neurons in adult male rats. Develop Neurobiol. 2007;67(10):1321–1333.

25. Hajszan T, MacLusky NJ, Leranth C. Role of androgens and the androgen receptor in remodeling of spine synapses in limbic brain areas. Horm Behav. 2008;53(5):638–646.

26. Leranth C, Szigeti-Buck K, Maclusky NJ, Hajszan T. Bisphenol A prevents the synaptogenic response to testosterone in the brain of adult male rats. Endocrinology. 2008;149(3):988–994.

27. Reddy DS, Jian K. The testosterone-derived neurosteroid androstanediol is a positive allosteric modulator of GABAA receptors. J Pharmacol Exp Ther. 2010;334(3):1031–1041.

28. Edinger KL, Frye CA. Androgens' effects to enhance learning may be mediated in part through actions at estrogen receptor-? in the hippocampus. Neurobiol Learn Mem. 2007;87(1):78–85.

29. Compagnone NA, Mellon SH. Neurosteroids: Biosynthesis and function of these novel neuromodulators. Front Neuroendocrinol. 2000;21(1):1–56.

30. Diotel N, Charlier TD, Lefebvre d'Hellencourt C, et al. Steroid transport, local synthesis, and signaling within the brain: Roles in neurogenesis, neuroprotection, and sexual behaviors. Front Neurosci. 2018;12:84–84.

31. Hammes SR, Levin ER. Impact of estrogens in males and androgens in females. J Clin Invest. 2019;129:1818–1826.

32. Celec P, Ostatníková D, Hodosy J. On the effects of testosterone on brain behavioral functions. Front Neurosci. 2015;9(12):1–17.

33. Burger HG. Androgen production in women. Fertil Steril. 2002;77:3–5.

34. Dohle GR, Smit M, Weber RFA. Androgens and male fertility. World J Urol. 2003;21(5):341–345.

35. Pardridge WM, Mietus LJ. Transport of steroid hormones through the rat blood-brain barrier. Primary role of albumin-bound hormone. J Clin Invest. 1979;64(1):145–154.

36. Mellon SH, Griffin LD. Neurosteroids: Biochemistry and clinical significance. Trends Endocrinol Metab. 2002;13:35–43.

37. Schmidt KL, Pradhan DS, Shah AH, Charlier TD, Chin EH, Soma KK. Neurosteroids, immunosteroids, and the Balkanization of endocrinology. Gen Comp Endocrinol. 2008;157:266–274.

38. Corpechot C, Robel P, Axelson M, Sjovall J, Baulieu EE. Characterization and measurement of dehydroepiandrosterone sulfate in rat brain. Proc Natl Acad Sci U S A. 1981;78(8):4704–4707.

39. Stoffel-Wagner B. Neurosteroid metabolism in the human brain. Eur J Endocrinol. 2001;145:669–679.

40. Stoffel-Wagner B. Neurosteroid Biosynthesis in the Human Brain and Its Clinical Implications. Ann N Y Acad Sci. 2003;1007:64–78.

41. Tobiansky DJ, Wallin-Miller KG, Floresco SB, Wood RI, Soma KK. Androgen regulation of the mesocorticolimbic system and executive function. Front Endocrinol. 2018;9(279):1–18.

42. Hojo Y, Kawato S. Neurosteroids in adult hippocampus of male and female rodents: Biosynthesis and actions of sex steroids. Front Endocrinol. 2018;9(183):1–8.

43. Baulieu EE, Robel P. Neurosteroids: A new brain function? J Steroid Biochem Mol Biol. 1990;37(3):395–403.

44. Melcangi RC, Froelichsthal P, Martini L, Vescovi AL. Steroid metabolizing enzymes in pluripotential progenitor central nervous system cells: Effect of differentiation and maturation. Neuroscience. 1996;72(2):467–475.

45. Taves MD, Gomez-Sanchez CE, Soma KK. Extra-adrenal glucocorticoids and mineralocorticoids: Evidence for local synthesis, regulation, and function. Am J Physiol Endocrinol Metab. 2011;301(1):E11–E24.

46. Baulieu EE, Robel P, Schumacher M. Neurosteroids: Beginning of the story. Int Rev Neurobiol. 2001;46:1–32.

47. Tsai M, O'Malley BW. Molecular Mechanisms of Action of Steroid/Thyroid Receptor Superfamily Members. Ann Rev Biochem. 1994;63(1):451–486.

48. Quigley CA. The androgen receptor: Physiology and pathophysiology. In: Testosterone (Nieschlag E, Behre HM, eds). Berlin: Springer. 1998, pp. 33–106.

49. Michels G, Hoppe UC. Rapid actions of androgens. Front Neuroendocrinol. 2008;29:182–198.

50. Hammes SR, Levin ER. Extranuclear steroid receptors: Nature and actions. Endocr Rev. 2007;28(7):726–741.

51. Tabori NE, Stewart LS, Znamensky V, et al. Ultrastructural evidence that androgen receptors are located at extranuclear sites in the rat hippocampal formation. Neuroscience. 2005;130(1):151–163.

52. Sarkey S, Azcoitia Ii, Garcia-Segura LM, Garcia-Ovejero D, DonCarlos LL. Classical androgen receptors in non-classical sites in the brain. Horm Behav. 2008;53(5):753–764.

53. Finley SK, Kritzer MF. Immunoreactivity for intracellular androgen receptors in identified subpopulations of neurons, astrocytes and oligodendrocytes in primate prefrontal cortex. J Neurobiol. 1999;40(4):446–457.

54. Frick KM, Kim J, Tuscher JJ, Fortress AM. Sex steroid hormones matter for learning and memory: Estrogenic regulation of hippocampal function in male and female rodents. Learn Mem. 2015;22:472–493.

55. Mitra SW, Hoskin E, Yudkovitz J, et al. Immunolocalization of estrogen receptor beta in the mouse brain: Comparison with estrogen receptor alpha. Endocrinology. 2003;144(5):2055–2067.

56. Hazell GGJ, Yao ST, Roper JA, Prossnitz ER, O'Carroll AM, Lolait SJ. Localisation of GPR30, a novel G protein-coupled oestrogen receptor, suggests multiple functions in rodent brain and peripheral tissues. J Endocrinol. 2009;202(2):223–236.

57. Bliss TVP, Collingridge GL. A synaptic model of memory: Long-term potentiation in the hippocampus. Nature. 1993;361:31–39.

58. Smith MD, Jones LS, Wilson MA. Sex differences in hippocampal slice excitability: Role of testosterone. Neuroscience. 2002;109(3):517–530.

59. Collingridge GL, Peineau S, Howland JG, Wang YT. Long-term depression in the CNS. Nat Rev Neurosci. 2010;11(7):459–473.

60. Pettorossi VE, Di Mauro M, Scarduzio M, et al. Modulatory role of androgenic and estrogenic neurosteroids in determining the direction of synaptic plasticity in the CA1 hippocampal region of male rats. Physiological Rep. 2013;1(7):1–12.

61. Sakata K, Tokue A, Kawai N. Altered synaptic transmission in the hippocampus of the castrated male mouse is reversed by testosterone replacement. J Urol. 2000;163(4):1333–1338.

62. Skucas VA, Duffy AM, Harte-Hargrove LC, et al. Testosterone depletion in adult male rats increases mossy fiber transmission, LTP, and sprouting in area CA3 of hippocampus. J Neurosci. 2013;33(6):2338–2355.

63. Tozzi A, Durante V, Manca P, et al. Bidirectional Synaptic Plasticity Is Driven by Sex Neurosteroids Targeting Estrogen and Androgen Receptors in Hippocampal CA1 Pyramidal Neurons. Front Cell Neurosci. 2019; 13 (534):1–13.

64. Picot M, Billard JM, Dombret C, et al. Neural androgen receptor deletion impairs the temporal processing of objects and hippocampal CA1-dependent mechanisms. PLoS One. 2016;11(2):1–16.

65. Di Mauro M, Tozzi A, Calabresi P, Pettorossi VE, Grassi S. Neo-synthesis of estrogenic or androgenic neurosteroids determine whether long-term potentiation or depression is induced in hippocampus of male rat. Front Cell Neurosci. 2015;9(376):1–13.

66. Goldman SA, Nottebohm F. Neuronal production, migration, and differentiation in a vocal control nucleus of the adult female canary brain. Proc Natl Acad Sci U S A 1983;80(8):2390–2394.

67. Pytte CL. Adult Neurogenesis in the Songbird: Region-Specific Contributions of New Neurons to Behavioral Plasticity and Stability. Brain Behav Evol 2016;87(3):191–204.

68. Ming GL, Song H. Adult neurogenesis in the mammalian central nervous system. Ann Rev Neurosci. 2005;28:223–250.

69. Van Praag H, Schinder AF, Christle BR, Toni N, Palmer TD, Gage FH. Functional neurogenesis in the adult hippocampus. Nature. 2002; 415(6875):1030–1034.

70. Zhao C, Teng EM, Summers RG, Ming G-L, Gage FH. Development/-Plasticity/Repair Distinct Morphological Stages of Dentate Granule Neuron Maturation in the Adult Mouse Hippocampus. J Neurosci. 2006; 26(1):3–11.

71. Abrous DN, Koehl M, Le Moal M. Adult neurogenesis: From precursors to network and physiology. Physiological Rev 2005;85:523–569.

72. Kempermann G, Song H, Gage FH. Neurogenesis in the adult hippocampus. Cold Spring Harbor Perspect Biol. 2015;7(9):a018812.

73. Barker JM, Galea LAM. Repeated estradiol administration alters different aspects of neurogenesis and cell death in the hippocampus of female, but not male, rats. Neuroscience. 2008;152(4):888–902.

74. Duarte-Guterman P, Lieblich SE, Wainwright SR, et al. Androgens enhance adult hippocampal neurogenesis in males but not females in an age-dependent manner. Endocrinology. 2019;160(9):2128–2136.

75. Ormerod BK, Galea LAM. Reproductive status influences the survival of new cells in the dentate gyrus of adult male meadow voles. Neurosci Lett. 2003;346(1–2):25–28.

76. Hamson DK, Wainwright SR, Taylor JR, Jones BA, Watson NV, Galea LAM. Androgens increase survival of adult-born neurons in the dentate gyrus by an androgen receptor-dependent mechanism in male rats. Endocrinology. 2013;154(9):3294–3304.

77. Zhang Z, Yang R, Zhou R, Li L, Sokabe M, Chen L. Progesterone promotes the survival of newborn neurons in the dentate gyrus of adult male mice. Hippocampus. 2010;20(3):402–412.

78. Okamoto M, Hojo Y, Inoue K, et al. Mild exercise increases dihydrotestosterone in hippocampus providing evidence for androgenic mediation of neurogenesis. Proc Natl Acad Sci U S A. 2012;109(32):13100–13105.

79. Brännvall K, Bogdanovic N, Korhonen L, Lindholm D. 19-Nortestosterone influences neural stem cell proliferation and neurogenesis in the rat brain. Eur J Neurosci. 2005;21(4):871–878.

80. Clancy AN, Bonsall RW, Michael RP. Immunohistochemical labeling of androgen receptors in the brain of rat and monkey. Life Sci. 1992;50(6): 409–417.

81. Kerr JE, Allore RJ, Beck SG, Handa RJ. Distribution and hormonal regulation of androgen receptor (AR) and AR messenger ribonucleic acid in the rat hippocampus. Endocrinology. 1995;136(8): 3213–3221.

82. Simerly RB, Swanson LW, Chang C, Muramatsu M. Distribution of androgen and estrogen receptor mRNA-containing cells in the rat brain: An in situ hybridization study. J Comp Neurol. 1990;294(1):76–95.

83. Xiao L, Jordan CL. Sex differences, laterality, and hormonal regulation of androgen receptor immunoreactivity in rat hippocampus. Horm Behav. 2002;42(3):327–336.

84. Swift-Gallant A, Duarte-Guterman P, Hamson DK, Ibrahim M, Monks DA, Galea LAM. Neural androgen receptors affect the number of surviving new neurones in the adult dentate gyrus of male mice. J Neuroendocrinol. 2018;30(4):e12578.

85. Galea LAM, Wainwright SR, Roes MM, Duarte-Guterman P, Chow C, Hamson DK. Sex, hormones and neurogenesis in the hippocampus: Hormonal modulation of neurogenesis and potential functional implications. J Neuroendocrinol. 2013;25:1039–1061.

86. Hastings NB, Gould E. Rapid extension of axons into the CA3 region by adult-generated granule cells. J Comp Neurol. 1999;413(1):146–154.

87. Liu JX, Pinnock SB, Herbert J. Novel control by the CA3 region of the hippocampus on neurogenesis in the dentate gyrus of the adult rat. PLoS One. 2011;6(3):e17562.

88. Breedlove SM. Cellular analyses of hormone influence on motoneuronal development and function. J Neurobiol. 1986;17:157–176.

89. Shors TJ, Chua C, Falduto J. Sex differences and opposite effects of stress on dendritic spine density in the male versus female hippocampus. J Neurosci. 2001;21(16):6292–6297.

90. Hojo Y, Higo S, Ishii H, et al. Comparison between hippocampus-synthesized and circulation-derived sex steroids in the hippocampus. Endocrinology. 2009;150(11):5106–5112.

91. Hojo Y, Higo S, Kawato S, et al. Hippocampal synthesis of sex steroids and corticosteroids: Essential for modulation of synaptic plasticity. Front Endocrinol. 2011;2(43):1–17.

92. Kato A, Hojo Y, Higo S, et al. Female hippocampal estrogens have a significant correlation with cyclic fluctuation of hippocampal spines. Front Neural Circuits. 2013;7(139):1–13.

93. Hatanaka Y, Hojo Y, Mukai H, et al. Rapid increase of spines by dihydrotestosterone and testosterone in hippocampal neurons: Dependence on synaptic androgen receptor and kinase networks. Brain Res. 2015;1621:121–132.

94. MacLusky NJ, Hajszan T, Prange-Kiel J, Leranth C. Androgen modulation of hippocampal synaptic plasticity. Neuroscience. 2006;138(3): 957–965.

95. MacLusky NJ, Hajszan T, Leranth C. Effects of dehydroepiandrosterone and flutamide on hippocampal CA1 spine synapse density in male and female rats: Implications for the role of androgens in maintenance of hippocampal structure. Endocrinology. 2004;145(9):4154–4161.

96. Maclusky NJ, Hajszan T, Johansen JA, Jordan CL, Leranth C. Androgen effects on hippocampal CA1 spine synapse numbers are retained in Tfm male rats with defective androgen receptors. Endocrinology. 2006; 147(5):2392–2398.

97. Lee YF, Lin WJ, Huang J, et al. Activation of mitogen-activated protein kinase pathway by the antiandrogen hydroxyflutamide in androgen receptor-negative prostate cancer cells. Cancer Res. 2002;62(21):6039–6044.

98. Ahmadiani A, Mandgary A, Sayyah M. Anticonvulsant effect of flutamide on seizures induced by pentylenetetrazole: Involvement of benzodiazepine receptors. Epilepsia. 2003;44(5):629–635.

99. Sato SM, Johansen JA, Jordan CL, Wood RI. Membrane androgen receptors may mediate androgen reinforcement. Psychoneuroendocrinology. 2010;35(7):1063–1073.

100. Hatanaka Y, Mukai H, Mitsuhashi K, et al. Androgen rapidly increases dendritic thorns of CA3 neurons in male rat hippocampus. Biochem Biophy Res Commun. 2009;381(4):728–732.

101. Guo G, Kang L, Geng D, et al. Testosterone modulates structural synaptic plasticity of primary cultured hippocampal neurons through ERK - CREB signalling pathways. Mol Cell Endocrinol. 2020;503:110671.

102. Foradori CD, Weiser MJ, Handa RJ. Non-genomic actions of androgens. Front Neuroendocrinol. 2008;29:169–181.

103. Galea LAM, Frick KM, Hampson E, Sohrabji F, Choleris E. Why estrogens matter for behavior and brain health. Neurosci Biobehav Rev. 2017;76:363–379.

104. Pike CJ, Nguyen TVV, Ramsden M, Yao M, Murphy MP, Rosario ER. Androgen cell signaling pathways involved in neuroprotective actions. Horm Behav. 2008;53:693–705.

105. Srivastava DP, Waters EM, Mermelstein PG, Kramár EA, Shors TJ, Liu F. Rapid estrogen signaling in the brain: Implications for the fine-tuning of neuronal circuitry. J Neurosci. 2011;31(45):16056–16063.

106. Harley CW, Malsbury CW, Squires A, Brown RAM. Testosterone decrease CA1 plasticity in vivo in gonadectomized male rats. Hippocampus. 2000; 10(6):693–697.

107. Angenstein F, Staak S. Receptor-mediated activation of protein kinase C in hippocampal long-term potentiation: Facts, problems and implications. Prog Neuro-Psychopharmacol Biol Psychiatry. 1997;21(3):427–454.

108. Van Der Zee EA, Luiten PGM, Disterhoft JF. Learning-induced alterations in hippocampal PKC-immunoreactivity: A review and hypothesis of its functional significance. Prog Neuro-Psychopharmacol Biologi Psychiatry. 1997;21(3):531–572.

109. Goldin M, Segal M. Protein kinase C and ERK involvement in dendritic spine plasticity in cultured rodent hippocampal neurons. European J Neurosci. 2003;17(12):2529–2539.

110. Roberson ED, English JD, Adams JP, Selcher JC, Kondratick C, Sweatt JD. The mitogen-activated protein kinase cascade couples PKA and PKC to cAMP response element binding protein phosphorylation in area CA1 of hippocampus. J Neurosci. 1999;19(11):4337–4348.

111. Nguyen TVV, Yao M, Pike CJ. Androgens activate mitogen-activated protein kinase signaling: Role in neuroprotection. J Neurochem. 2005; 94(6):1639–1651.

112. Sato K, Iemitsu M, Aizawa K, Ajisaka R. Testosterone and DHEA activate the glucose metabolism-related signaling pathway in skeletal muscle. American J Physiol Endocrinol Metab. 2008;294(5):961–968.

113. Fix C, Jordan C, Cano P, Walker WH. Testosterone activates mitogen-activated protein kinase and the cAMP response element binding protein transcription factor in Sertoli cells. Proc Natl Acad Sci U S A. 2004; 101(30):10919–10924.

114. Gatson JW, Kaur P, Singh M. Dihydrotestosterone differentially modulates the mitogen-activated protein kinase and the phosphoinositide 3-kinase/Akt pathways through the nuclear and novel membrane androgen receptor in C6 cells. Endocrinology. 2006;147(4):2028–2034.

115. Lu WY, Xiong ZG, Lei S, et al. G-protein-coupled receptors act via protein kinase C and Src to regulate NMDA receptors. Nat Neurosci. 1999;2(4): 331–338.

116. Kose A, Ito A, Saito N, Tanaka C. Electron microscopic localization of gamma- and beta II-subspecies of protein kinase C in rat hippocampus. Brain Res. 1990;518(1–2):209–217.

117. Dolmetsch RE, Pajvani U, Fife K, Spotts JM, Greenberg ME. Signaling to the nucleus by an L-type calcium channel-calmodulin complex through the MAP kinase pathway. Science. 2001;294(5541):333–339.

118. Vanhoutte P, Barnier J-V, Guibert B, et al. Glutamate induces phosphorylation of Elk-1 and CREB, along with c-fos activation, via an extracellular signal-regulated kinase-dependent pathway in brain slices. Mol Cell Biol. 1999;19(1):136–146.

119. Perkinton MS, Sihra TS, Williams RJ. Ca2+-permeable AMPA receptors induce phosphorylation of cAMP response element-binding protein through a phosphatidylinositol 3-kinase-dependent stimulation of the mitogen-activated protein kinase signaling cascade in neurons. J Neurosci. 1999;19(14):5861–5874.

120. Impey S, Obrietan K, Wong ST, et al. Cross talk between ERK and PKA is required for Ca2+ stimulation of CREB-dependent transcription and ERK nuclear translocation. Neuron. 1998;21(4):869–883.

121. Vitolo OV, Sant'Angelo A, Costanzo V, Battaglia F, Arancio O, Shelanski M. Amyloid β-peptide inhibition of the PKA/CREB pathway and long-term potentiation: Reversibility by drugs that enhance cAMP signaling. Proc Natl Acad Sci U S A. 2002;99(20):13217–13221.

122. Deisseroth K, Heist EK, Tsien RW. Translocation of calmodulin to the nucleus supports CREB phosphorylation in hippocampal neurons. Nature. 1998;392(6672):198–202.

123. Redmond L, Kashani AH, Ghosh A. Calcium regulation of dendritic growth via CaM kinase IV and CREB-mediated transcription. Neuron. 2002;34(6):999–1010.

124. Nguyen TVV, Yao M, Pike CJ. Dihydrotestosterone activates CREB signaling in cultured hippocampal neurons. Brain Res. 2009;1298:1–12.

125. Kovacs EG, MacLusky NJ, Leranth C. Effects of testosterone on hippocampal CA1 spine synaptic density in the male rat are inhibited by fimbria/fornix transection. Neuroscience. 2003;122(3):807–810.

126. Mendell AL, MacLusky NJ, Leranth C. Unilateral Fimbria/Fornix Transection Prevents the Synaptoplastic Effect of Dehydroepiandrosterone in the Hippocampus of Female, but not Male, Rats. Neurosci Med. 2013;4(3):134.

127. Gottmann K, Mittmann T, Lessmann V. BDNF signaling in the formation, maturation and plasticity of glutamatergic and GABAergic synapses. Exp Brain Res. 2009;199:203–234.

128. Zagrebelsky M, Korte M. Form follows function: BDNF and its involvement in sculpting the function and structure of synapses. Neuropharmacology. 2014;76:628–638.

129. Chen G, Kolbeck R, Barde YA, Bonhoeffer T, Kossel A. Relative contribution of endogenous neurotrophins in hippocampal long-term potentiation. J Neurosci. 1999;19(18):7983–7990.

130. Jia J-X, Cui C-L, Yan X-S, et al. Effects of testosterone on synaptic plasticity mediated by androgen receptors in male SAMP8 mice. J Toxicol Environ Health A. 2016;79(19):849–855.

131. Li M, Masugi-Tokita M, Takanami K, Yamada S, Kawata M. Testosterone has sublayer-specific effects on dendritic spine maturation mediated by BDNF and PSD-95 in pyramidal neurons in the hippocampus CA1 area. Brain Res. 2012;1484:76–84.

132. Scharfman HE, Maclusky NJ. Differential regulation of BDNF, synaptic plasticity and sprouting in the hippocampal mossy fiber pathway of male and female rats. Neuropharmacology. 2014;76:696–708.

133. Iki J, Inoue A, Bito H, Okabe S. Bi-directional regulation of postsynaptic cortactin distribution by BDNF and NMDA receptor activity. Eur J Neurosci. 2005;22(12):2985–2994.

134. Campbell DH, Sutherland RL, Daly RJ. Signaling Pathways and Structural Domains Required for Phosphorylation of EMS1/Cortactin 1. Can Res. 1999;59:5376–5385.

135. Ullian EM, Sapperstein SK, Christopherson KS, Barres BA. Control of synapse number by glia. Science. 2001;291(5504):657–661.

136. Oliveira JF, Gomes CA, Vaz SH, Sousa N, Pinto L. Editorial: Glial plasticity in depression. Front Cell Neurosci. 2016;10:163.

137. Dietz AG, Goldman SA, Nedergaard M. Glial cells in schizophrenia: A unified hypothesis. Lancet Psychiatry. 2019;7(3):272–281.

138. Dzamba D, Harantova L, Butenko O, Anderova M. Glial cells - the key elements of Alzheimer's disease. Curr Alzheimer Res. 2016;13(8):894–911.

139. Zwain IH, Yen SS. Neurosteroidogenesis in astrocytes, oligodendrocytes, and neurons of cerebral cortex of rat brain. Endocrinology. 1999;140: 3843–3852.

140. Johnson RT, Breedlove SM, Jordan CL. Sex differences and laterality in astrocyte number and complexity in the adult rat medial amygdala. J Comp Neurol. 2008;511(5):599–609.

141. Rurak GM, Woodside B, Aguilar-Valles A, Salmaso N. Astroglial cells as neuroendocrine targets in forebrain development: Implications for sex differences in psychiatric disease. Front Neuroendocrinol. 2021;60: 100897.

142. Garcia-Ovejero D, Veiga S, Garcia-Segura LM, Doncarlos LL. Glial expression of estrogen and androgen receptors after rat brain injury. J Comp Neurol. 2002;450(3):256–271.

143. Gatson JW, Singh M. Activation of a membrane-associated androgen receptor promotes cell death in primary cortical astrocytes. Endocrinology. 2007;148(5):2458–2464.

144. Khalaj AJ, Yoon J, Nakai J, et al. Estrogen receptor (ER) beta expression in oligodendrocytes is required for attenuation of clinical disease by an ERbeta ligand. Proc Natl Acad Sci U S A. 2013;110(47):19125–19130.

145. Barreto G, Veiga S, Azcoitia Ii, Garcia-Segura LM, Garcia-Ovejero D. Testosterone decreases reactive astroglia and reactive microglia after brain injury in male rats: Role of its metabolites, oestradiol and dihydrotestosterone. Eur J Neurosci. 2007;25(10):3039–3046.

146. Scharfman HE, Hen R. Neuroscience. Is more neurogenesis always better? Science. 2007;315(5810):336–338.

147. Rand MN, Breedlove SM. Androgen alters the dendritic arbors of SNB motoneurons by acting upon their target muscles. J Neurosci. 1995;15: 4408–4416.

148. Ottem EN, Beck LA, Jordan CL, Breedlove SM. Androgen-dependent regulation of brain-derived neurotrophic factor and tyrosine kinase B in the sexually dimorphic spinal nucleus of the bulbocavernosus. Endocrinology. 2007;148(8):3655–3665.

149. Sakai J. Core Concept: How synaptic pruning shapes neural wiring during development and, possibly, in disease. Proc Natl Acad Sci U S A. 2020;117(28):16096–16099.

150. Peek SL, Mah KM, Weiner JA. Regulation of neural circuit formation by protocadherins. Cell Mol Life Sci. 2017;74(22):4133–4157.

151. Lombardi AP, Royer C, Pisolato R, et al. Physiopathological aspects of the Wnt/beta-catenin signaling pathway in the male reproductive system. Spermatogenesis. 2013;3(1):e23181.

152. Murillo-Garzon V, Kypta R. WNT signalling in prostate cancer. Nat Rev Urol. 2017;14(11):683–696.

153. Hawi Z, Tong J, Dark C, Yates H, Johnson B, Bellgrove MA. The role of cadherin genes in five major psychiatric disorders: A literature update. Am J Med Genet B Neuropsychiatr Genet. 2017;177(2):168–180.

154. Evgrafov OV, Armoskus C, Wrobel BB, et al. Gene Expression in Patient-Derived Neural Progenitors Implicates WNT5A Signaling in the Etiology of Schizophrenia. Biol Psychiatry. 2020;88(3):236–247.

155. Yan P, Qiao X, Wu H, et al. An Association Study Between Genetic Polymorphisms in Functional Regions of Five Genes and the Risk of Schizophrenia. J Mol Neurosci. 2016;59(3):366–375.

156. Monks DA, Getsios S, MacCalman CD, Watson NV. N-cadherin is regulated by gonadal steroids in adult sexually dimorphic spinal motoneurons. J Neurobiol. 2001;47(4):255–264.

157. Monks DA, Getsios S, MacCalman CD, Watson NV. N-cadherin is regulated by gonadal steroids in the adult hippocampus. Proc Natl Acad Sci U S A. 2001;98(3):1312–1316.

158. Traish AM. 5α-reductases in human physiology: An unfolding story. Endocr Pract. 2012;18(6):965–975.

2

Androgens and Parkinson's Disease: A Review of Human Studies and Animal Models

Mélanie Bourque,[1] Denis Soulet,[1,2] and Thérèse Di Paolo[1,2,i,*]

Abstract

Parkinson's disease (PD) is the second most common neurodegenerative disorder after Alzheimer's disease. A greater prevalence and incidence of PD are reported in men than in women, suggesting a potential contribution of sex, genetic difference and/or sex hormones. This review presents an overview of epidemiological and clinical studies investigating sex differences in the incidence and symptoms of PD. This sex difference is replicated in animal models of PD showing an important neuroprotective role of sex steroids. Therefore, although gender and genetic factors likely contribute to the sex difference in PD, focus here will be on sex hormones because of their neuroprotective role. Androgens receive less attention than estrogen. It is well known that endogenous androgens are more abundant in healthy men than in women and decrease with aging; lower levels are reported in PD men than in healthy male subjects. Drug treatments with androgens, androgen precursors, antiandrogens, and drugs modifying androgen metabolism are available to treat various endocrine conditions, thus having translational value for PD but none have yet given sufficient positive effects for PD. Variability in the androgen receptor is reported in humans and is an additional factor in the response to androgens. In animal models of PD used to study neuroprotective activity, the androgens testosterone and dihydrotestosterone have given inconsistent results. 5α-Reductase inhibitors have shown neuroprotective activity in animal models of PD and antidyskinetic activity. Hence, androgens have not consistently shown beneficial or deleterious effects in PD but numerous androgen-related drugs are available that could be repurposed for PD.

Keywords: Parkinson's disease; androgen; testosterone; dihydrotestosterone; sex differences

Introduction

Parkinson's disease (PD) is a chronic progressive neurodegenerative disease, with clinical manifestations resulting from gradual but extensive loss of dopamine (DA) neurons in the brain substantia nigra pars compacta.[1] Except for familial cases, PD is rarely observed before age 50 years but its prevalence is about 1% in people over 60 years of age.[2] The appearance of rigidity, bradykinesia, postural instability, and resting tremor are the clinical hallmarks of PD.[1] Nonmotor symptoms are also present including a variety of cognitive, neuropsychiatric, sleep, autonomic, and sensory disturbances.[3]

PD can be linked to gene mutations in familial forms but the etiology of the majority of PD cases is currently unknown and most likely involves the interaction of genetic, epigenetic, and environmental risk factors.[4]

Sex differences in PD have been reported in epidemiological and clinical studies as well as in response to treatments.[5] Epidemiological studies have documented that both the incidence and prevalence of PD are higher in men than in women, men are at least 1.5 times more likely to develop PD than women.[6-13] The age of onset of PD appears about 2 years earlier in men.[14,15] A longer reproductive lifespan is associated

[1]Centre de Recherche du CHU de Québec-Université Laval, Axe Neurosciences, Québec, Canada.
[2]Faculté de pharmacie, Pavillon Ferdinand-Vandry, Université Laval, Québec, Canada.
[i]ORCID ID (https://orcid.org/0000-0003-1020-6566).

*Address correspondence to: Thérèse Di Paolo, PhD, Centre de recherche du CHU de Québec-Université Laval, Axe Neurosciences, T2-40, 2705, Boulevard Laurier, Québec, QC G1V 4G2, Canada, Email: therese.dipaolo@crchul.ulaval.ca

with a delay in age of onset,[14,16,17] suggesting that longer exposure to circulating endogenous estrogen levels throughout a woman's life has a positive effect and that estrogens can act as a protective agent. The epidemiological evidence of sex differences in PD suggests a possible beneficial activity of female gonadal hormones, and this aspect has been extensively reviewed.[5,18,19] Androgens have received less attention with respect to their potential effects in PD, and their implication will be reviewed here.

Endogenous Androgens and PD

Testosterone is one of the main androgenic steroids synthesized by the testis. Testosterone is biotransformed to dihydrotestosterone by 5α-reductase enzymes, or into estradiol by an aromatization process.[20] Androgens' ac-

tion is mediated by binding to classical androgen receptor or membrane androgen receptor.[21,22] The variability in the androgen receptor reported in human confers differences in receptor function and then distinct response to androgens.[23,24]

During normal aging, levels of testosterone in men slowly decrease in a progressive rate from the fourth or fifth decade.[25] Incidence of testosterone deficiency increased to 12%, 19%, 28%, and 49% for men over ages 50, 60, 70, and 80 years, respectively.[26] Since the incidence of PD is higher in men than in women and ovarian hormones could be a protective factor in women, an important question is to determine whether there is an association between androgen levels and PD in men (Table 1). Two studies,[27,28] each with a small number of PD patients, suggested a higher prevalence

Table 1. Testosterone and Clinical Studies in Parkinson's Disease

Endogenous androgen and PD		
Sample description	**Main results**	**Refs.**
PD and testosterone levels		
68 patients with PD	The prevalence of low testosterone levels in PD patient was 35%.	27
50 of the 91 patients with PD were screened with free testosterone levels.	Half the PD patients who were screened were defined as having low testosterone levels.	28
Reduction of testosterone levels and incidence of PD		
1335 patients with prostate cancer compared with 4005 age-matched patients.	Androgen deprivation therapy in patients with prostate cancer was not associated with a higher risk of PD.	31
38,931 patients with prostate cancer on continuous androgen deprivation therapy and 34,272 matched patients.	Androgen deprivation therapy in patients with prostate cancer was associated with a lower risk of PD.	32

Androgen treatment on PD symptoms			
Treatment	**Study description**	**Main results**	**Refs.**
Testosterone			
A single daily dose of testosterone topical gel (5 g/day of Androgel [equivalent of 5 mg/day of testosterone]) for 1 month. Six of the 10 patients were also followed up for 3 months.	A prospective open-labeled pilot study in 10 testosterone-deficient men with PD.	No effect on the UPDRS parts II and III, the Obeso dyskinesias rating scale. The UPDRS part IV improved at 1 month but not at 3 months. The UPDRS part I improved at the 3-month follow-up visit.	46
Intramuscular testosterone esters 100 mg monthly for 3 months and increasing to 250 mg monthly.	A case report of an 80-year-old man with PD with testosterone deficiency.	Improvement in resting tremor and fine motor control after testosterone administration correlated with serum testosterone levels.	47
200 mg/mL of testosterone enanthate every 2 weeks for 8 weeks.	A double-blind, placebo-controlled trial (15 PD patients in the placebo group, 15 PD patients in the testosterone group).	No effect on the UPDRS scale.	45
A single daily dose of testosterone topical gel (5 g/day of androgel (equivalent of 5 mg/day of testosterone)).	A retrospective analysis of five patients with combined PD and symptom of testosterone deficiency.	Several PD patients described an improvement in their PD symptoms, but this was not always associated by a change in the UPDRS motor score.	27
5α-Reductase inhibitor			
Finasteride 5 mg/day	Case reports of two PD patients with pathological gambling.	Finasteride attenuated pathological gambling symptoms of PD patients.	70
Androgen receptor inhibitor			
Spironolactone 100 mg/day	A case report of a 72-year-old man with PD and congestive heart failure.	Worsening of the ON state UPDRS part III. After withdrawal of spironolactone, motor function returns to baseline values.	59

PD, Parkinson's disease; UPDRS, Unified Parkinson Disease Rating Scale; Part I, nonmotor experiences of daily living; Part II, motor experiences of daily living; Part III, motor examination; Part IV, motor complications.

of low testosterone in these patients than during normal aging,[26] but this has to be confirmed in larger studies. In addition to androgen contents, androgen receptor levels could play a role in the effect of androgens in PD. However, the mRNA levels of the androgen receptor in substantia nigra were reported not different between male and female PD patients and matched those of controls.[29] As testosterone can be synthesized in the brain, plasma testosterone levels do not necessarily reflect the levels found in the brain. To our knowledge, measures of testosterone levels in the brain of PD patients have not been reported.

Another aspect to consider that could potentially influence testosterone levels is dopaminergic treatments. Levodopa, the precursor of DA (gold standard treatment for PD), or the DA receptor agonist pramipexole treatments in early PD, do not reduce testosterone levels but rather have been reported to slightly increase them, thus the decrease in testosterone levels does not appear to be related to dopaminergic medication.[30]

Furthermore, the use of androgen deprivation therapy in patients with prostate cancer was not associated with a greater risk of PD[31,32] (Table 1), suggesting that having low levels of androgen is not a risk factor to develop PD. The risk of developing parkinsonism at the end of the study follow-up was lower in androgen deprivation therapy users, suggesting that androgen deprivation therapy might have a slight neuroprotective effect.[32] Thus, this suggests that androgens do not play a protective role but may actually intensify toxicity of the nigrostriatal dopaminergic pathway.

Endogenous Androgens and Animal Models of PD

The effect of castration to reduce gonadal endogenous androgen levels was investigated on brain DA markers. Whereas castration in very young male mice increased glial activation, decreased striatal DA levels and tyrosine hydroxylase positive cells in striatum and substantia nigra, and impaired locomotor activities, this effect was age dependent, and castration in adult male mice did not induce any of these effects.[33] Furthermore, in the 6-hydroxydopamine (6-OHDA)-lesioned rat model of PD, castration is reported to reduce 6-OHDA-induced toxicity (Table 2): castrated male rats having less DA content or neuronal loss and a decrease in motor asymmetry and oxidative stress generation following a 6-OHDA lesion.[34–36]

Striatal DA and its metabolite dihydroxyphenylacetic acid contents in male mice were reported to be the same in intact and castrated retired breeder male mice (about 6 months old) and similarly decreased when lesioned with the neurotoxin 1-methyl-4-phenyl-1,2,3,6-tetrahydropyridine (MPTP; 4×10 mg/kg), a mouse model of PD.[37] Younger 10–12 weeks old male mice showed no difference in striatal tyrosine hydroxylase staining between intact and castrated animals and a similar loss with MPTP (4×20 mg/kg) lesioning.[38] The above studies had differences in species and age of animals as well toxins to model PD. Furthermore, for 6-OHDA-lesioned male rats and MPTP-treated male mice, testosterone or dihydrotestosterone treatment, the two more abundant, or more biologically active androgens, had no effect on toxin-induced lesion in castrated animals.[34,38]

Thus, in animal models, castration (reducing testosterone and dihydrotestosterone) did not increase susceptibility to toxin damaging the nigrostriatal system nor was testosterone or dihydrotestosterone treatment beneficial.

MPTP-lesioned male mice were reported to have reduced levels of plasma and brain testosterone and dihydrotestosterone compared with those of control mice.[39,40] Leydig cells are the major site for producing endogenous testosterone under physiological conditions and a decrease in Leydig cell counts was reported in MPTP mice.[41] This could explain the reduced plasma and brain testosterone and dihydrotestosterone levels in MPTP male mice. Activity of the steroidogenesis enzymes could also be altered by exposure to reactive oxygen species,[42,43] which are produced after MPTP administration. In the 6-OHDA-unilaterally lesioned male rat model of PD, no difference of testosterone and dihydrotestosterone striatal and cerebral cortex was measured between the ipsilateral and contralateral sides and compared with that in intact controls; by contrast, differences in progesterone metabolism were observed.[44]

Treatment with Androgens in PD

Although the effect of testosterone replacement therapy on motor symptoms of PD in patients with testosterone deficiency has been investigated, the studies are scarce, the number of patients included is small or the studies are case reports, and the results are not consistent (Table 1).

A double-blind placebo-controlled trial evaluated the effect of testosterone enanthate for 8 weeks on motor symptom in PD patients with low, but in the normal range, testosterone levels.[45] Evaluation of motor

Table 2. Effect of Endogenous and Exogenous Androgen Compounds in Animal Models of Parkinson's Disease

Animal models: effect of castration	Decreased toxicity to toxin	No change in response to toxin
6-OHDA-lesioned castrated male rats	Castrated male rats having less DA content or neuronal loss after a 6-OHDA lesion[34,35]	
MPTP castrated male mice		No difference in susceptibility to MPTP is reported[37,38]

Animal models: effect of androgen and related compound treatments	Active compounds	Inactive compounds
Neuroprotection studies		
MPTP male mice	Dutasteride[39,40]	Testosterone[50]
	DHEA[80]	Dihydrotestosterone[50]
		Finasteride[39]
MPTP castrated male mice		Testosterone[38]
6-OHDA-lesioned gonadectomized female and male rats		Dihydrotestosterone[34,51]
Dyskinesia studies		
6-OHDA-lesioned female and male rats	Finasteride[71]	
6-OHDA-lesioned male rats	Finasteride,[72] but impaired L-Dopa motor activation	
6-OHDA-lesioned male rats	Dutasteride[72]	

DA, dopamine; DHEA, dehydroepiandrosterone; MPTP, 1-methyl-4-phenyl-1,2,3,6-tetrahydropyridine; 6-OHDA, 6-hydroxydopamine.

function using the Unified Parkinson's Disease Rating Scale (UPDRS) has not shown any beneficial effect of testosterone treatment in PD patients.[45] In a prospective open-labeled pilot study in 10 testosterone-deficient men with PD, the UPDRS IV scores (Fluctuations) improved at 1 month but did not show sustainable improvement at 3 months.[46] In this study, testosterone treatment had no effect on the UPDRS (II, Activities of Daily Living; III, Motor) and the Obeso dyskinesias rating scale.[46] A case report of an 80-year-old man with PD with testosterone deficiency described a significant improvement in resting tremor and fine motor control after testosterone administration.[47]

In a retrospective analysis of five PD patients treated with testosterone for testosterone deficiency, several PD patients described an improvement in their PD symptoms, but this was not always associated by a change in the UPDRS motor score.[27] As noted by the authors, this improvement could be the result of a testosterone effect on mood and energy, rather than a direct effect on PD symptoms.

It should be taken into consideration that three of the four studies reported here have included PD patients with testosterone levels below the normal range. Among the nonspecific symptoms and signs associated with testosterone deficiency are decreased energy, impaired physical performance, and mobility limitation.[48,49] Testosterone treatment in aging men with testosterone deficiency improved energy and had a modest effect on physical function.[48,49] Thus, as testosterone therapy can act directly on symptoms and

signs associated with testosterone deficiency, it is unclear whether the improvements come from restoring testosterone levels to normal levels, thus by a direct effect on symptoms of testosterone deficiency, or rather by direct effect on motor symptoms of PD. It could also be an indirect effect through the transformation of testosterone into 17β-estradiol by aromatase.

Treatment with Androgens in Animal Models of PD

In male mice, testosterone treatment failed to induce any protective effect against MPTP toxicity[38,50] (Table 2). However, the lack of effect of testosterone may be the result of insufficient conversion to estradiol, or the lack of beneficial effect of androgen receptor stimulation. To specifically investigate the role of androgen receptor stimulation in neuroprotection, dihydrotestosterone, which is the most potent androgen, is a more appropriate compound than testosterone since it is not aromatized to estradiol. Studies performed in MPTP-treated male mice and 6-OHDA-lesioned gonadectomized female and male rats reported no beneficial effect of dihydrotestosterone treatment,[34,50,51] suggesting that stimulation of the androgen receptor was not effective in inducing a protective effect. Given the absence of protection with both testosterone and dihydrotestosterone, these results suggest that testosterone is not converted in the brain into estradiol in sufficient concentration to achieve neuroprotective levels.

When testosterone is administered to aged rats, there is an improvement in motor deficits, as well as an increase in DA transporters and tyrosine hydroxy-lase in striatum and substantia nigra of aged male rats.[52,53] Nevertheless, these results are observed in normal aging, not in pathological conditions such as occurring in PD. In conditions where oxidative stress is present, like in reserpine-treated aged male rats, testosterone worsened the deficits in behaviors and in nigrostriatal dopaminergic system.[52]

Dihydrotestosterone can be metabolized into 3β-diol and the latter is an agonist on estrogen receptors.[54] We previously reported reduced plasma testosterone, dihydrotestosterone, and 3β-diol in male MPTP mice.[40,55] In men with PD, reduced 17β-estradiol and testosterone levels were reported.[56] The reduction of gonadal androgens in PD males and MPTP mice is related to impaired Leydig cells activity. Hence, a role of 3β-diol is difficult to decipher in PD since it is a weaker estrogen receptor agonist (binding affinity of 6 nM for ERα [vs. 0.13 for 17β-estradiol] and 2 nM [vs. 0.12 for 17β-estradiol] for ERβ)[54] than 17β-estradiol, and its levels are reduced due to decreased levels of its metabolic precursor dihydrotestosterone.

Thus, animal and clinical studies do not support that androgens may modify the risk to develop PD. The potential beneficial effect of testosterone when combined with antiparkinsonian medication to improve PD symptoms requires larger studies to draw a clear conclusion.

Antiandrogenic Therapies in PD

Antiandrogenic therapies include drugs inhibiting the hypothalamic–pituitary–gonadal axis, including modulators of the gonadotrophic inhibitory hormone and Kisspeptin–Kiss1 receptor axis and gonadotrophic releasing hormone agonists (leuprolide, goserelin, and triptorelin) and antagonists (degarelix), androgen receptor inhibitors (cyproterone, spironolactone, eplerenone, and flutamide), and 5α-reductase inhibitors (finasteride and dutasteride). Androgen receptor inhibitors and 5α-reductase inhibitors provide prompter antiandrogenic actions and some were tested in PD patients. The major representatives of androgen receptor inhibitors are spironolactone and eplerenone, also acting on the mineralocorticoid receptor.[57,58]

In a case report, spironolactone was observed to worsen PD symptoms[59] and no data is available for eplerenone in PD. Flutamide was investigated in rats where it was reported that low doses of flutamide reduced haloperidol-induced catalepsy and higher doses worsen catalepsy.[60] In a dopaminergic cell line (N27 cells), flutamide inhibited testosterone-induced apo-

ptosis,[61] and apoptosis effect of testosterone was recently reported to be mediated by a membrane androgen receptor in N27 cells.[62] A case report showed that low-dose cyproterone acetate treatment reduced sexual acting out in a man with PD and dementia without relevant side effects.[63] As reviewed above, there are limited studies with the androgen receptor inhibitors in PD, whereas the 5α-reductase inhibitors have led to recent interesting findings.

5α-reductase

5α-reductase enzymes are enzymes that catalyze the conversion of progesterone into dihydroprogesterone and also metabolize testosterone into dihydrotestosterone. Both 5α-reductase types 1 and 2 are expressed in the brain.[64] In the rat brain, 5α-reductase isoform 2 is localized in neurons, but not in glial cells, whereas isoform 1 is expressed in glial cells,[65,66] suggesting different functions of these isoforms in the regulation of neuroendocrine processes. 5α-Reductase inhibitors, such as finasteride and dutasteride, are used in the clinic to treat endocrine condition such as benign prostatic hyperplasia and androgenic alopecia.[67] Finasteride inhibits selectively 5α-reductase type 2, whereas dutasteride has higher potency than finasteride in inhibiting both types 1 and 2.[68]

5α-Reductase inhibitors: PD and animal models

Studies have shown a role of 5α-reductase inhibitors in dopaminergic transmission, with potential therapeutic effects in several disorders associated with dopaminergic hyperactivity.[69] Regarding PD, a case study with two male patients with PD reports that finasteride treatment reduced pathological gambling, a side effect induced by dopaminergic medication[70] (Table 1).

In both female and male rats lesioned with 6-OHDA, finasteride reduces the development and expression of L-Dopa-induced dyskinesias[71]; this effect is also observed with dutasteride in 6-OHDA-lesioned male rats.[72] Lower dose of dutasteride compared to finasteride are required to produce this effect.[72] Moreover, dutasteride does not affect L-Dopa-induced motor activation, unlike finasteride.[72] Finasteride has been reported to attenuate behaviors induced by DA D1 and D3 receptors agonists, thus suggesting the implication of these receptors in its activity to decrease dyskinesias.[73,74] Furthermore, both dutasteride and finasteride prevent the L-Dopa-induced upregulation of striatal DA D1-receptor-related signaling pathways and D1–D3 receptor interaction.[72] These studies suggest that 5α-reductase inhibitors could be beneficial to reduce side effect related to dopaminergic medication such as L-Dopa-induced dyskinesias and compulsive behavior.

Antiandrogen Therapies in Animal Models of PD

5α-Reductase inhibitors: neuroprotective effect

Since 5α-reductase inhibitors block the conversion of progesterone into dihydroprogesterone and also testosterone into dihydrotestosterone, and thus hypothetically increasing 17β-estradiol levels through aromatization of testosterone, these are interesting molecules as they may have a neuroprotective effect by increasing the levels of the neuroprotective steroids (Table 2).

We previously showed that administration of dutasteride to male mice starting before and pursued after MPTP lesion prevented MPTP-induced loss of DA markers, but this effect was not seen when dutasteride administration was started only after MPTP, where similar change in striatal DA content between MPTP mice and MPTP mice treated with dutasteride was observed.[39,40] Thus, dutasteride did not increase MPTP toxicity when administration was initiated after injury. This is important information since this drug could be repurposed to reduce L-Dopa-induced dyskinesias in PD based on its decrease of abnormal involuntary movements in 6-OHDA-lesioned rats.[72] Finasteride was ineffective in protecting dopaminergic neurons of MPTP toxicity in male mice,[39] perhaps due to its shorter serum half-life (2 h) than dutasteride (31 h).[68]

Measures of steroid levels have shown that MPTP treatment decreased plasma and brain levels of testosterone, and dutasteride administration in MPTP mice maintains the levels of this steroid at control value, whereas the levels of dihydrotestosterone were found to be decreased in intact mice, MPTP and dutasteride-treated MPTP mice.[40] Since testosterone or dihydrotestosterone treatments in MPTP male mice did not induce any protective effect,[50] it seems unlikely that maintaining the physiological levels of testosterone could be one of the mechanisms by which dutasteride prevented the MPTP-induced toxicity, but rather support the protective effect of dutasteride.

Although 17β-estradiol levels were not assayed specifically in the striatum and the substantia nigra, levels of 17β-estradiol were under detection limits in the plasma and one brain hemisphere of control male mice and remained undetectable with the MPTP lesion and dutasteride treatment, suggesting that dutasteride

protective effect is unlikely mediated by increasing 17β-estradiol levels.[39,40]

Although plasma and brain concentrations of progesterone are at control levels with the administration of dutasteride in intact mice, MPTP and dutasteride-treated MPTP mice have elevated progesterone levels.[40] Thus, the protective effect of dutasteride does not seem to be only related to change in progesterone and testosterone contents and their metabolites.

Dutasteride increases dopamine transporter (DAT) specific binding and glycosylation in intact male mice, therefore, increasing DAT function at the membrane.[40] Whereas previous study reported that mice overexpressing the DAT are more susceptible to MPTP toxicity,[75] thus that increased DAT activity induces a detrimental effect, this is not supported by our previous study showing that the increased maturation of DAT and its activity with dutasteride treatment did not intensify MPTP toxicity, suggesting that these effects on DAT would contribute to the protection of DA neurons.[40] Neuroprotection by dutasteride in MPTP-treated mice is also associated with reduced neuroinflammation as assessed with striatal glial fibrillary acidic protein levels, thus supporting its anti-inflammatory activity in its mechanism of action.[40]

Androgen Precursors, Dehydroepiandrosterone and Pregnenolone for PD

Dehydroepiandrosterone (DHEA) and pregnenolone are steroids precursors in the synthetic pathways of androgens. Pregnenolone is an FDA-approved drug under investigation in clinical trials on psychiatric disorders with dysfunctions of DA signaling, including bipolar disorders, schizophrenia, and marijuana intoxication.[76] In the 6-OHDA unilaterally lesioned male rat model of PD, DHEA levels in the striatum and cerebral cortex were unchanged by the lesion, whereas pregnenolone levels were reduced in the lesioned and unlesioned striatum but not in the cerebral cortex.[44] Mouse brain and plasma levels of DHEA were unchanged by the MPTP lesion, whereas pregnenolone levels were reduced in the plasma and elevated in the brain by the MPTP lesion.[40]

There are limited data available on pregnenolone and DHEA in PD patients' cerebrospinal fluid, plasma, and/or brain. DHEA and its sulfate derivative were unchanged in PD patients.[77] In animal models of PD, beneficial effects of DHEA on motor behavior were reported in MPTP parkinsonian monkeys[78,79] and neuroprotection of dopaminergic markers against MPTP toxicity.[80] There is potential of pregnenolone for treatment of PD and L-Dopa-induced dyskinesias. It can rescue synaptic defects and normalize hyperdopaminergic activity and abnormal DA-dependent behavior in rats offspring exposed to cannabis during pregnancy.[81] Pregnenolone rectifies DA neuron excitability and prevents Δ9-tetrahydrocannabinol (THC)-induced enhancement of striatal DA levels. These effects were still evident when pregnenolone is cleared from the brain, indicating its long-lasting properties in counteracting pathological hyperdopaminergic states.[81]

Discussion

Aging is the primary risk factor for PD and is associated with reduced gonadal function in both men and women. In women, the loss of ovarian function at menopause around 50 years of age is abrupt, whereas in men there is a more progressive and slower reduction of gonadal function and decrease of androgens called andropause.

Considering the sex difference in PD pointing to a protective role of ovarian steroids that is lost at menopause and the abundant literature of neuroprotective activity of estrogens and progesterone in animal models of PD, hormonal replacement (estrogen and progesterone) seems a plausible approach (reviewed in Ref.[18]). However, the risk associated with estrogens has led to search for alternatives such as selective estrogen receptor modulators, raloxifene, specific agonists for estrogen receptor subtypes (estrogen receptor α, estrogen receptor β, and membrane estrogen receptor GPER1).[18] As reviewed above, androgen loss (due to aging or castration) and androgen treatment have not given solid beneficial or deleterious evidence in PD.

Although this review has mainly focused on androgens in men and PD, androgen variations throughout life are also reported in women. Serum androgen levels in women decline in the early reproductive years but levels do not decline further with the menopause transition.[82] The decline of testosterone levels in women is of 55%.[82] The higher androgens relative to estrogen in women in the postmenopausal state and its role in the increase in PD incidence after menopause remain to be investigated. Nevertheless, in gonadectomized female rats, dihydrotestosterone treatment has no effect on 6-OHDA toxicity, whereas estradiol showed protective effect,[34] suggesting that increasing androgen levels in females have no damaging effect in the dopaminergic system.

Many cellular mechanisms contributing to impaired neuronal function during aging are also present in PD,

including mitochondrial dysfunction, inflammation, oxidative stress, and impaired DA metabolism.[83–85] More specifically for brain DA in aging, there is a decrease in the synthesis of DA, DA receptors and transporters, as well as tyrosine hydroxylase positive neurons.[83,85–87] The age-related decrease in brain DA activity is associated with a decline in cognitive and motor functions for both men and women.[88–90] Changes during aging could render DA neurons more vulnerable to insults. Indeed, the toxin MPTP produces greater degeneration of DA neurons in aged monkeys and mice than in younger animals.[91,92]

Most people will age without developing PD. What causes the degeneration of DA neurons in PD is still unknown and is likely a multifactorial etiology including genetic and environmental factors.[84] The vulnerability of DA neurons observed with aging could reduce the ability of those neurons to respond to stressful events, and a therapeutic strategy that targets the multiple mechanisms contributing to DA neuron dysfunction should be useful.

Although the loss of DA nigrostriatal neurons is the major neuropathological cause of PD, other neuronal groups also degenerate to a lesser extent such as serotoninergic neurons of the raphe nucleus, noradrenergic neurons of the locus coeruleus, or cholinergic neurons of the nucleus basalis of Meynert.[93] By contrast, brain glutamate neurotransmission is reported to be increased in PD.[94] PD also involves accumulation of intracellular α-synuclein protein deposits called Lewy bodies.[95] Endocrine drugs with multiple activities could have translational value for PD. Among these activities are the anti-inflammatory action of various steroids that could be useful for PD. Indeed, neurodegenerative diseases including PD are associated with inflammation.[96]

Viral infections were proposed as potential risk factors for PD, and there is supporting although not entirely consistent epidemiological and basic science supporting evidence (review Ref.[97]). In a multihit hypothesis of PD, Sadasivan et al. demonstrated that prior exposure of mice to non-neurotropic pandemic influenza A/California/04/2009 H1N1 virus, which triggers brain inflammation, exacerbates their vulnerability to a parkinsonian toxin, MPTP, 1 month later, resulting in heightened loss of DA neurons.[98] This finding raises a concern for survivors of viral infections, who could be more susceptible to other potential environmental PD triggers, which independently are not considered sufficient to elicit PD phenotypes.

Since men have been shown to be over-represented among those severely affected by coronavirus disease (COVID-19), repurposing drugs for COVID-19 with an endocrine perspective has been recently reviewed.[99] Interestingly, 5-α reductase inhibitors (finasteride and dutasteride) were recently shown to have beneficial effects in males with COVID-19.[99–102] Therefore, with the possible increase of parkinsonism post-COVID-19 infection and the higher incidence of men in both these diseases, possible converging endocrine treatments open interesting opportunities for drug repurposing.

Conclusion

Although it is now well documented that PD is more prevalent in men than in women, androgens have not consistently shown beneficial or a deleterious effect on PD symptoms or disease progression. Numerous antiandrogen drugs are available to treat endocrine conditions, thus offering opportunities to repurpose them for PD. The 5α-reductase inhibitors have shown neuroprotective and antidyskinetic activities and need to be further investigated. Although the effect of dutasteride was observed only when started before injury, the lack of increased damage to dopaminergic neurons when used after the lesion makes it an attractive drug for repurposing in PD patients for its antidyskinetic properties.[72]

Moreover, although testosterone derivatives and related compounds (such as anabolic-androgenic steroids) are frequently misused by athletes, they offer possibilities that could be helpful in PD neurodegeneration condition (reviewed Ref.[103]). Selective androgen receptor modulators (SARMs) are compounds developed to be tissue-selective androgen receptor ligands.[103,104] SARMs give an alternative for androgens therapy (osteoporosis, prostate cancer, and muscle wasting), but are presently recognized as forbidden substances by the World Anti-Doping Agency.[104] Flutamide, initially classified as an androgen receptor inhibitor, is now considered as an SARM. The activity of SARMs in the normal brain and in PD brain is yet to be investigated.

Authors' Contributions

All three authors contributed to the conception or design of the study, drafted the study or revising it critically, gave final approval of the version to be published, and agreed to be accountable for the study.

References

1. Armstrong MJ, Okun MS. Diagnosis and treatment of parkinson disease: A review. JAMA. 2020;323(6):548–560.
2. de Lau LM, Breteler MM. Epidemiology of Parkinson's disease. Lancet Neurol. 2006;5(6):525–535.
3. Park A, Stacy M. Non-motor symptoms in Parkinson's disease. J Neurol. 2009;256 Suppl 3:293–298.
4. Lesage S, Brice A. Parkinson's disease: From monogenic forms to genetic susceptibility factors. Hum Mol Genet. 2009;18(R1):R48–R59.
5. Meoni S, Macerollo A, Moro E. Sex differences in movement disorders. Nat Rev Neurol. 2020;16(2):84–96.
6. Pringsheim T, Jette N, Frolkis A, Steeves TD. The prevalence of Parkinson's disease: A systematic review and meta-analysis. Mov Disord. 2014; 29(13):1583–1590.
7. Baldereschi M, Di Carlo A, Rocca WA, et al. Parkinson's disease and parkinsonism in a longitudinal study: Two-fold higher incidence in men. ILSA Working Group. Italian Longitudinal Study on Aging. Neurology. 2000;55(9):1358–1363.
8. Hirsch L, Jette N, Frolkis A, Steeves T, Pringsheim T. The incidence of Parkinson's disease: A systematic review and meta-analysis. Neuroepidemiology. 2016;46(4):292–300.
9. Shulman LM, Bhat V. Gender disparities in Parkinson's disease. Expert Rev Neurother. 2006;6(3):407–416.
10. Swerdlow RH, Parker WD, Currie LJ, et al. Gender ratio differences between Parkinson's disease patients and their affected relatives. Parkinsonism Relat Disord. 2001;7(2):129–133.
11. Taylor KS, Cook JA, Counsell CE. Heterogeneity in male to female risk for Parkinson's disease. J Neurol Neurosurg Psychiatry. 2007;78(8):905–906.
12. Van Den Eeden SK, Tanner CM, Bernstein AL, et al. Incidence of Parkinson's disease: Variation by age, gender, and race/ethnicity. Am J Epidemiol. 2003;157(11):1015–1022.
13. Wooten GF, Currie LJ, Bovbjerg VE, Lee JK, Patrie J. Are men at greater risk for Parkinson's disease than women? J Neurol Neurosurg Psychiatry. 2004;75(4):637–639.
14. Haaxma CA, Bloem BR, Borm GF, et al. Gender differences in Parkinson's disease. J Neurol Neurosurg Psychiatry. 2007;78(8):819–824.
15. Twelves D, Perkins KS, Counsell C. Systematic review of incidence studies of Parkinson's disease. Mov Disord. 2003;18(1):19–31.
16. Frentzel D, Judanin G, Borozdina O, et al. Increase of reproductive life span delays age of onset of Parkinson's disease. Front Neurol. 2017;8:397.
17. Ragonese P, D'Amelio M, Callari G, et al. Age at menopause predicts age at onset of Parkinson's disease. Mov Disord. 2006;21(12):2211–2214.
18. Bourque M, Morissette M, Di Paolo T. Repurposing sex steroids and related drugs as potential treatment for Parkinson's disease. Neuropharmacology. 2019;147:37–54.
19. Jurado-Coronel JC, Cabezas R, Avila Rodriguez MF, et al. Sex differences in Parkinson's disease: Features on clinical symptoms, treatment outcome, sexual hormones and genetics. Front Neuroendocrinol. 2018;50: 18–30.
20. Do Rego JL, Seong JY, Burel D, et al. Neurosteroid biosynthesis: Enzymatic pathways and neuroendocrine regulation by neurotransmitters and neuropeptides. Front Neuroendocrinol. 2009;30(3):259–301.
21. McEwan IJ, Brinkmann AO. Androgen physiology: Receptor and metabolic disorders. In: Endotext. (Feingold KR, et al., ed). South Dartmouth, MA. MDText.com, Inc. 2000.
22. Thomas P. Membrane androgen receptors unrelated to nuclear steroid receptors. Endocrinology. 2019;160(4):772–781.
23. Callewaert L, Christiaens V, Haelens A. et al. Implications of a polyglutamine tract in the function of the human androgen receptor. Biochem Biophys Res Commun. 2003;306(1):46–52.

24. Tirabassi G, Cignarelli A, Perrini S. et al. Influence of CAG repeat poly-morphism on the targets of testosterone action. Int J Endocrinol. 2015; 2015:298107.

25. Kaufman JM, Lapauw B, Mahmoud A, T'Sjoen G, Huhtaniemi IT. Aging and the male reproductive system. Endocr Rev. 2019;40(4):906–972.

26. Harman SM, Metter EJ, Tobin JD, et al. Longitudinal effects of aging on serum total and free testosterone levels in healthy men. Baltimore Longitudinal Study of Aging. J Clin Endocrinol Metab. 2001;86(2):724–731.

27. Okun MS, McDonald WM, DeLong MR. Refractory nonmotor symptoms in male patients with Parkinson disease due to testosterone deficiency: A common unrecognized comorbidity. Arch Neurol. 2002;59(5):807–811.

28. Okun MS, Crucian GP, Fischer L, et al. Testosterone deficiency in a Par-kinson's disease clinic: Results of a survey. J Neurol Neurosurg Psychia-try. 2004;75(1):165–166.

29. Luchetti S, Bossers K, Frajese GV, Swaab DF. Neurosteroid biosynthetic pathway changes in substantia nigra and caudate nucleus in Parkinson's disease. Brain Pathol. 2010;20(5):945–951.

30. Okun MS, Wu SS, Jennings D, et al. Testosterone level and the effect of levodopa and agonists in early Parkinson disease: Results from the INSPECT cohort. J Clin Mov Disord. 2014;1:8.

31. Chung SD, Lin HC, Tsai MC, et al. Androgen deprivation therapy did not increase the risk of Alzheimer's and Parkinson's disease in patients with prostate cancer. Andrology. 2016;4(3):481–485.

32. Young JW,S., Sutradhar R, Rangrej J, et al. Androgen deprivation therapy and the risk of parkinsonism in men with prostate cancer. World J Urol. 2017;35(9):1417–1423.

33. Khasnavis S, Ghosh A, Roy A, Pahan K. Castration induces Parkinson disease pathologies in young male mice via inducible nitric-oxide syn-thase. J Biol Chem. 2013;288(29):20843–20855.

34. Murray HE, Pillai AV, McArthur SR, et al. Dose- and sex-dependent effects of the neurotoxin 6-hydroxydopamine on the nigrostriatal dopaminer-gic pathway of adult rats: Differential actions of estrogen in males and females. Neuroscience. 2003;116(1):213–222.

35. Tamas A, Lubics A, Lengvari I, Reglodi D. Effects of age, gender, and gonadectomy on neurochemistry and behavior in animal models of Parkinson's disease. Endocrine. 2006;29(2):275–287.

36. Cunningham RL, Macheda T, Watts LT, et al. Androgens exacerbate motor asymmetry in male rats with unilateral 6-hydroxydopamine le-sion. Horm Behav. 2011;60(5):617–624.

37. Antzoulatos E, Jakowec MW, Petzinger GM, Wood RI. MPTP neurotoxicity and testosterone induce dendritic remodeling of striatal medium spiny neurons in the C57Bl/6 mouse. Parkinsons Dis. 2011;2011:138471.

38. Dluzen DE. Effects of testosterone upon MPTP-induced neurotoxicity of the nigrostriatal dopaminergic system of C57/B1 mice. Brain Res. 1996; 715(1–2):113–118.

39. Litim N, Bourque M, Al Sweidi S, Morissette M, Di Paolo T. The 5alpha-reductase inhibitor Dutasteride but not Finasteride protects dopamine neurons in the MPTP mouse model of Parkinson's disease. Neurophar-macology. 2015;97:86–94.

40. Litim N, Morissette M, Caruso D, Melcangi RC, Di Paolo T. Effect of the 5alpha-reductase enzyme inhibitor dutasteride in the brain of intact and parkinsonian mice. J Steroid Biochem Mol Biol. 2017;174:242–256.

41. Ruffoli R, Giambelluca MA, Scavuzzo MC, et al. MPTP-induced Parkin-sonism is associated with damage to Leydig cells and testosterone loss. Brain Res. 2008;1229:218–223.

42. Allen JA, Diemer T, Janus P, Hales KH, Hales DB. Bacterial endotoxin li-popolysaccharide and reactive oxygen species inhibit Leydig cell ste-roidogenesis via perturbation of mitochondria. Endocrine. 2004;25(3): 265–275.

43. Lee SY, Gong EY, Hong CY, et al. ROS inhibit the expression of testicular steroidogenic enzyme genes via the suppression of Nur77 transactiva-tion. Free Radic Biol Med. 2009;47(11):1591–1600.

44. Melcangi RC, Caruso D, Levandis G. et al. Modifications of neuroactive steroid levels in an experimental model of nigrostriatal degeneration: Potential relevance to the pathophysiology of Parkinson's disease. J Mol Neurosci. 2012;46(1):177–183.

45. Okun MS, Fernandez HH, Rodriguez RL, et al. Testosterone therapy in men with Parkinson disease: Results of the TEST-PD Study. Arch Neurol. 2006;63(5):729–735.

46. Okun MS, Walter BL, McDonald WM, et al. Beneficial effects of testos-terone replacement for the nonmotor symptoms of Parkinson disease. Arch Neurol. 2002;59(11):1750–1753.

47. Mitchell E, Thomas D, Burnet R. Testosterone improves motor function in Parkinson's disease. J Clin Neurosci. 2006;13(1):133–136.

48. Bhasin S, Brito JP, Cunningham GR, et al. Testosterone therapy in men with hypogonadism: An Endocrine Society Clinical Practice Guideline. J Clin Endocrinol Metab. 2018;103(5):1715–1744.

49. Rodrigues Dos Santos M, Bhasin S. Benefits and risks of testosterone treatment in men with age-related decline in testosterone. Annu Rev Med. 2021;72:75–91.

50. Ekue A, Boulanger JF, Morissette M, Di Paolo T. Lack of effect of tes-tosterone and dihydrotestosterone compared to 17beta-oestradiol in 1-methyl-4-phenyl-1,2,3,6, tetrahydropyridine-mice. J Neuroendocrinol. 2002;14(9):731–736.

51. Gillies GE, Murray HE, Dexter D, McArthur S. Sex dimorphisms in the neuroprotective effects of estrogen in an animal model of Parkinson's disease. Pharmacol Biochem Behav. 2004;78(3):513–522.

52. Cui R, Kang Y, Wang L, et al. Testosterone propionate exacerbates the deficits of nigrostriatal dopaminergic system and downregulates Nrf2 expression in reserpine-treated aged male rats. Front Aging Neurosci. 2017;9:172.

53. Cui R, Zhang G, Kang Y, et al. Amelioratory effects of testosterone pro-pionate supplement on behavioral, biochemical and morphological parameters in aged rats. Exp Gerontol. 2012;47(1):67–76.

54. Kuiper GG, Carlsson B, Grandien K, et al. Comparison of the ligand binding specificity and transcript tissue distribution of estrogen recep-tors alpha and beta. Endocrinology. 1997;138(3):863–870.

55. Bourque M, Morissette M, Di Paolo T. Raloxifene activates G protein-coupled estrogen receptor 1/Akt signaling to protect dopamine neu-rons in 1-methyl-4-phenyl-1,2,3,6-tetrahydropyridine mice. Neurobiol Aging. 2014;35(10):2347–2356.

56. Nitkowska M, Tomasiuk R, Czyzyk M, Friedman A. Prolactin and sex hormones levels in males with Parkinson's disease. Acta Neurol Scand. 2015;131(6):411–416.

57. Georgianos PI, Vaios V, Eleftheriadis T, Zebekakis P, Liakopoulos V. Mineralocorticoid antagonists in ESRD: An overview of clinical trial evi-dence. Curr Vasc Pharmacol. 2017;15(6):599–606.

58. Hermidorff MM, Faria Gde O, Amancio Gde C, de Assis LV, Isoldi MC. Non-genomic effects of spironolactone and eplerenone in cardiomyo-cytes of neonatal Wistar rats: Do they evoke cardioprotective pathways? Biochem Cell Biol. 2015;93(1):83–93.

59. Teive HA, Munhoz RP, Werneck LC. Worsening of motor symptoms and gynecomastia during spironolactone treatment in a patient with Par-kinson's disease and congestive heart failure. Mov Disord. 2007;22(11): 1678–1679.

60. Majidi Zolbanin N, Zolali E, Mohajjel Nayebi A. Testosterone replace-ment attenuates haloperidol-induced catalepsy in male rats. Adv Pharm Bull. 2014;4(3):237–241.

61. Cunningham RL, Giuffrida A, Roberts JL. Androgens induce dopami-nergic neurotoxicity via caspase-3-dependent activation of protein ki-nase Cdelta. Endocrinology. 2009;150(12):5539–5548.

62. Duong P, Tenkorang MAA, Trieu J, et al. Neuroprotective and neurotoxic outcomes of androgens and estrogens in an oxidative stress environ-ment. Biol Sex Differ. 2020;11(1):12.

63. Haussermann P, Goecker D, Beier K, Schroeder S. Low-dose cyproterone acetate treatment of sexual acting out in men with dementia. Int Psy-chogeriatr. 2003;15(2):181–186.

64. Giatti S, Diviccaro S, Falvo E, Garcia-Segura LM, Melcangi RC. Physiopa-thological role of the enzymatic complex 5alpha-reductase and 3alpha/beta-hydroxysteroid oxidoreductase in the generation of pro-gesterone and testosterone neuroactive metabolites. Front Neuroen-docrinol. 2020;57:100836.

65. Melcangi RC, Garcia-Segura LM, Mensah-Nyagan AG. Neuroactive ste-roids: State of the art and new perspectives. Cell Mol Life Sci. 2008;65(5): 777–797.

66. Castelli MP, Casti A, Casu A. et al. Regional distribution of 5alpha-reductase type 2 in the adult rat brain: An immunohistochemical anal-ysis. Psychoneuroendocrinology. 2013;38(2):281–293.

67. Finn DA, Beadles-Bohling AS, Beckley EH, et al. A new look at the 5alpha-reductase inhibitor finasteride. CNS Drug Rev. 2006;12(1):53–76.

68. Xu Y, Dalrymple SL, Becker RE, Denmeade SR, Isaacs JT. Pharmacologic basis for the enhanced efficacy of dutasteride against prostatic cancers. Clin Cancer Res. 2006;12(13):4072–4079.
69. Paba S, Frau R, Godar SC, et al. Steroid 5alpha-reductase as a novel therapeutic target for schizophrenia and other neuropsychiatric disorders. Curr Pharm Des. 2011;17(2):151–167.
70. Bortolato M, Cannas A, Solla, et al. Finasteride attenuates pathological gambling in patients with Parkinson disease. J Clin Psychopharmacol. 2012;32(3):424–425.
71. Frau R, Savoia P, Fanni S. et al. The 5-alpha reductase inhibitor finasteride reduces dyskinesia in a rat model of Parkinson's disease. Exp Neurol. 2017;291:1–7.
72. Fanni S, Scheggi S, Rossi F, et al. 5alpha-reductase inhibitors dampen L-DOPA-induced dyskinesia via normalization of dopamine D1-receptor signaling pathway and D1-D3 receptor interaction. Neurobiol Dis. 2019;121:120–130.
73. Frau R, Mosher LJ, Bini V, et al. The neurosteroidogenic enzyme 5alpha-reductase modulates the role of D1 dopamine receptors in rat sensorimotor gating. Psychoneuroendocrinology. 2016;63:59–67.
74. Frau R, Pillolla G, Bini V. et al. Inhibition of 5alpha-reductase attenuates behavioral effects of D1-, but not D2-like receptor agonists in C57BL/6 mice. Psychoneuroendocrinology. 2013;38(4):542–551.
75. Masoud ST, Vecchio LM, Bergeron Y. et al. Increased expression of the dopamine transporter leads to loss of dopamine neurons, oxidative stress and l-DOPA reversible motor deficits. Neurobiol Dis. 2015;74:66–75.
76. Vallee M. Neurosteroids and potential therapeutics: Focus on pregnenolone. J Steroid Biochem Mol Biol. 2016;160:78–87.
77. Azuma T, Matsubara T, Shima Y, et al. Neurosteroids in cerebrospinal fluid in neurologic disorders. J Neurol Sci. 1993;120(1):87–92.
78. Belanger N, Gregoire L, Bedard P, Di Paolo T. Estradiol and dehydroepiandrosterone potentiate levodopa-induced locomotor activity in 1-methyl-4-phenyl-1,2,3,6-tetrahydropyridine monkeys. Endocrine. 2003;21(1):97–101.
79. Belanger N, Gregoire L, Bedard PJ, Di Paolo T. DHEA improves symptomatic treatment of moderately and severely impaired MPTP monkeys. Neurobiol Aging 2006;27(11):1684–1693.
80. D'Astous M, Morissette M, Tanguay B, Callier S, Di Paolo T. Dehydroepiandrosterone (DHEA) such as 17beta-estradiol prevents MPTP-induced dopamine depletion in mice. Synapse. 2003;47(1):10–14.
81. Frau R, Miczan V, Traccis F, et al. Prenatal THC exposure produces a hyperdopaminergic phenotype rescued by pregnenolone. Nat Neurosci. 2019;22(12):1975–1985.
82. Davison SL, Bell R, Donath S, Montalto JG, Davis SR. Androgen levels in adult females: Changes with age, menopause, and oophorectomy. J Clin Endocrinol Metab. 2005;90(7):3847–3853.
83. Collier TJ, Kanaan NM, Kordower JH. Ageing as a primary risk factor for Parkinson's disease: Evidence from studies of non-human primates. Nat Rev Neurosci. 2011;12(6):359–366.
84. Collier TJ, Kanaan NM, Kordower JH. Aging and Parkinson's disease: Different sides of the same coin? Mov Disord. 2017;32(7):983–990.
85. Reeve A, Simcox E, Turnbull D. Ageing and Parkinson's disease: Why is advancing age the biggest risk factor? Ageing Res Rev. 2014;14:19–30.
86. Darbin O. The aging striatal dopamine function. Parkinsonism Relat Disord. 2012;18(5):426–432.
87. Rollo CD. Dopamine and aging: Intersecting facets. Neurochem Res. 2009;34(4):601–629.
88. Erixon-Lindroth N, Farde L, Wahlin TB, et al. The role of the striatal dopamine transporter in cognitive aging. Psychiatry Res. 2005;138(1):1–12.
89. Volkow ND, Gur RC, Wang GJ, et al. Association between decline in brain dopamine activity with age and cognitive and motor impairment in healthy individuals. Am J Psychiatry. 1998;155(3):344–349.
90. Volkow ND, Logan J, Fowler JS, et al. Association between age-related decline in brain dopamine activity and impairment in frontal and cingulate metabolism. Am J Psychiatry. 2000;157(1):75–80.
91. Jiang N, Bo H, Song C, et al. Increased vulnerability with aging to MPTP: The mechanisms underlying mitochondrial dynamics. Neurol Res. 2014;36(8):722–732.
92. McCormack AL, Di Monte DA, Delfani K, et al. Aging of the nigrostriatal system in the squirrel monkey. J Comp Neurol. 2004;471(4):387–395.
93. Lang AE. The progression of Parkinson disease: A hypothesis. Neurology. 2007;68(12):948–952.
94. Jenner P. Molecular mechanisms of L-DOPA-induced dyskinesia. Nat Rev Neurosci. 2008;9(9):665–677.
95. Siderowf A, Stern M. Update on Parkinson disease. Ann Intern Med. 2003;138(8):651–658.
96. Gundersen V. Parkinson's disease: Can targeting inflammation be an effective neuroprotective strategy? Front Neurosci. 2020;14:580311.
97. Smeyne RJ, Noyce AJ, Byrne M, Savica R, Marras C. Infection and risk of Parkinson's disease. J Parkinsons Dis. 2021;11(1):31–43.
98. Sadasivan S, Sharp B, Schultz-Cherry S, Smeyne RJ. Synergistic effects of influenza and 1-methyl-4-phenyl-1,2,3,6-tetrahydropyridine (MPTP) can be eliminated by the use of influenza therapeutics: Experimental evidence for the multi-hit hypothesis. NPJ Parkinsons Dis. 2017;3:18.
99. Cadegiani FA. Repurposing existing drugs for COVID-19: An endocrinology perspective. BMC Endocr Disord. 2020;20(1):149.
100. Cadegiani FA, McCoy J, Gustavo Wambier C, Goren A. Early antiandrogen therapy with dutasteride reduces viral shedding, inflammatory responses, and time-to-remission in males with COVID-19: A Randomized, Double-Blind, Placebo-Controlled Interventional Trial (EAT-DUTA AndroCoV Trial—Biochemical). Cureus. 2021;13(2):e13047.
101. McCoy J, Cadegiani FA, Wambier CG, et al. 5-alpha-reductase inhibitors are associated with reduced frequency of COVID-19 symptoms in males with androgenetic alopecia. J Eur Acad Dermatol Venereol. 2021;35(4):e243–e246.
102. Lazzeri M, Duga S, Azzolini E, et al. Impact of chronic exposure to 5-alpha reductase inhibitors on the risk of hospitalization for COVID-19: A case-control study in male population from two COVID-19 regional centers of Lombardy (Italy). Minerva Urol Nefrol. 2021;33439572.
103. Tauchen J, Jurasek M, Huml L, Rimpelova S. Medicinal use of testosterone and related steroids revisited. Molecules. 2021;26(4):33672087.
104. Gorczyca D, Kwiatkowska D. Duality nature of selective androgen receptor modulators and specific steroids substance. Disaster Emerg Med J. 2019;4(2):60–62.

3

Androgens and Their Role in Regulating Sex Differences in the Hypothalamic/Pituitary/Adrenal Axis Stress Response and Stress-Related Behaviors

Julietta A. Sheng,[1,i] Sarah M.L. Tan,[1] Taben M. Hale,[2,*] and Robert J. Handa[1,†]

Abstract

Androgens play a pivotal role during development. These gonadal hormones and their receptors exert organizational actions that shape brain morphology in regions controlling the stress regulatory systems in a male-specific manner. Specifically, androgens drive sex differences in the hypothalamic/pituitary/adrenal (HPA) axis and corresponding hypothalamic neuropeptides. While studies have examined the role of estradiol and its receptors in sex differences in the HPA axis and associated behaviors, the role of androgens remains far less studied. Androgens are generally thought to modulate the HPA axis through the activation of androgen receptors (ARs). They can also impact the HPA axis through reduction to estrogenic metabolites that can bind estrogen receptors in the brain and periphery. Such regulation of the HPA axis stress response by androgens can often result in sex-biased risk factors for stress-related disorders, such as anxiety and depression. This review focuses on the biosynthesis pathways and molecular actions of androgens and their nuclear receptors. The impact of androgens on hypothalamic neuropeptide systems (corticotropin-releasing hormone, arginine vasopressin, oxytocin, dopamine, and serotonin) that control the stress response and stress-related disorders is discussed. Finally, this review discusses potential therapeutics involving androgens (androgen replacement therapies, selective AR modulator therapies) and ongoing clinical trials.

Keywords: androgen; estrogen; glucocorticoids; HPA axis; SARMs; androgen therapy

Introduction

Androgens exert many neurobiological effects, one of which is to regulate the hypothalamic function.[1,2] In part, these actions occur through androgenic regulation of the hypothalamic/pituitary/adrenal (HPA) and the hypothalamic/pituitary gonadal axes, thereby influencing important neurobiological functions such as autonomic and neuroendocrine function, feeding and metabolism, and stress-related and reproductive behaviors.[3] Acute exposure to glucocorticoids (GCs),

[1]Department of Biomedical Sciences, Colorado State University, Fort Collins, Colorado, USA.
[2]Department of Basic Medical Science, University of Arizona College of Medicine - Phoenix, Arizona, USA.
[i]ORCID ID (https://orcid.org/0000-0002-6192-1060).
[†]Deceased, August 27, 2021.

*Address correspondence to: Taben M. Hale, PhD, Department of Basic Medical Science, University of Arizona College of Medicine, 425 North 5th Street, Phoenix, AZ 85004, USA, Email: tabenh@arizona.edu

the product of the activation of the HPA axis, can be beneficial and enhance cognition and increase metabolism, whereas chronic exposure can lead to cardiovascular disease, metabolic and feeding disorders, neurological disorders, and behavioral disruption.[4,5]

Both neuroendocrine axes are intertwined with changes in the levels of circulating GCs, in part, regulated by gonadal steroid hormone action on hypothalamic function. Gonadal hormones are further implicated as the underlying cause for sex differences in neurological disorders.[6] Whereas many studies have examined the role of estrogens and estrogen receptors (ERs) in regulating the HPA axis and related behaviors,[7] the role for androgens and androgen receptors (ARs) is not as widely explored.

The focus of this review is to examine the HPA axis function and related regulatory neuropeptide (arginine vasopressin [AVP], oxytocin [OT], corticotropin-releasing factor [CRH], serotonin [5-HT], and dopamine [DA]) expression and action as they relate to androgens.[7] The role of androgens and ARs in stress-related disorders and potential therapeutic methods are discussed.[8]

Molecular Actions of Androgens in the Brain

The sexual differentiation of the male phenotype is heavily driven by androgens. Androgens exert organizational actions during development to program lasting sex differences in the brain. There is a prenatal surge of testosterone (T) during late gestation (gestation day 18 in the rat) and a second surge that occurs immediately following parturition, both of which masculinizes and defeminizes the brain in males.[9-11] Similarly, humans are exposed to a surge of T during gestation that also allows for sexual differentiation of the brain and development of sex differences in behavior and hormone release during development.[12] T is produced primarily in the testis.

Dehydroepiandrosterone (DHEA) is first converted to 4-androstenedione by the enzyme 3β-hydroxysteroid dehydrogenase (3β-HSD), followed by the conversion to T by enzyme 17β-hydroxysteroid dehydrogenase (17β-HSD). T is then converted into estradiol (E2) by aromatase or into dihydrotestosterone (DHT) by 5α-reductase (5αR) in tissues in which these enzymes are expressed (Fig. 1). Dysregulations of such enzymes are implicated in various androgen-related disorders. Individuals with decreased expressions of 17β-HSD or 5αR lead to male pseudohermaphroditism present with ambiguous female virilization and external genitalia around puberty.[6]

The actions of androgens are largely mediated by the AR. AR is expressed in a wide range of tissues, with levels that vary during development and throughout the life span.[13] AR is a member of a family of steroid nuclear receptors that share similar structural and functional identity.[14,15] Nuclear receptors share a crystal structure composed of a β-sheet (S1/S2) and 12 α-helices (H1–H12). H4–H6 and H9 are found between H1–H3 on one end and H7 and H10–H11 on the other end.[16] The first step in AR activation is the binding of a ligand (e.g., T) in the binding pocket of cytoplasmic AR. This activates AR by inducing release of several heat shock proteins. AR can then interact with the DNA at its specific androgen response element (ARE).

Interestingly, the consensus sequence of the ARE, GG(A/T)ACAnnnTGTTCT, is very similar to the consensus sequence of GC response elements (GREs). Therefore, when ARE is activated, the nearby GRE is also detected, implicating the interaction of GC receptor (GR), AR, and mineralocorticoid receptor (MR) with similar sequences.[17] Once AR is bound to ARE on the DNA, components important for transcription are recruited. The recruitment of these components is mediated by the interaction between AR N-terminus, TATA box-binding protein, and TFIIF compound.[18] Mechanisms of inhibition of AR actions are less understood. When AR is bound to an antagonist ligand, inhibitory proteins are recruited.

Such inhibitory proteins compete with coactivators of transcription, prevent the entry of AR into the nucleus to interact with the DNA, or induce binding of AR to the DNA.[19] Specifically, coinhibitor, short heterodimer partner (SHIP), prevents AR from entering the nucleus by tethering it to the cytoplasm.[20] Gobinet et al.[21] hypothesize that SHIP also competes with coactivators and attracts additional inhibitory proteins to AR to inhibit it. Further research on inhibitory mechanisms of AR could allow better understanding of dysregulations between androgens and their receptor-mediated effects.

Androgens Regulate the HPA Axis Stress Response in a Sex-Dependent Manner

Sex-dependent regulation of HPA axis activation

The HPA axis is an intricate stressor-responsive system that allows central communication between hypothalamic neurons, the pituitary gland, and the adrenal glands in the periphery. Activation of the HPA axis occurs by afferent inputs to the paraventricular nucleus of the hypothalamus (PVN). While some inputs to the PVN arise from upstream extrahypothalamic and

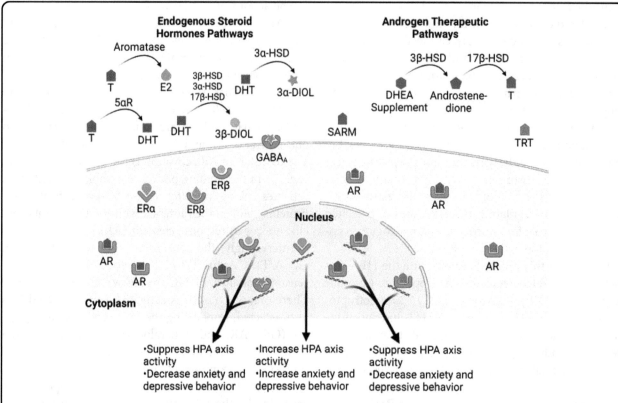

FIG. 1. Endogenous steroid hormone pathways and androgen replacement therapies. T is converted to DHT and E2 by 5αR and aromatase, respectively. DHT is further metabolized to 3β-diol by 3β-HSD, 3α-HSD, or 17β-HSD, and 3α-diol by 3α-HSD. Both T and DHT bind AR in the cytoplasm and enter the nucleus to bind the DNA. E2 binds either ERα or ERβ. 3β-diol also binds ERβ while 3α-diol binds GABA$_A$. ERα, ERβ, and GABA$_A$ are translocated to the nucleus to bind DNA and drive changes to the HPA axis and related behavior. SARMs, TRT, and T derived from DHEA additionally bind cytoplasmic AR. These therapies also bind nuclear DNA to suppress HPA axis activity and decrease anxiety and depressive behaviors. Figure created with BioRender.com. 3α-diol, 3α-androstanediol glucuronide; 3β-diol, 5α-androstane-3β, 17β diol; 3α-HSD, 3α-hydroxysteroid; 3β-HSD, 3β-hydroxysteroid dehydrogenase; 5αR, 5α-reductase; 17β-HSD, 17β-hydroxysteroid dehydrogenase; ERα, estrogen receptor α; ERβ, estrogen receptor β; AR, androgen receptor; DHEA, dehydroepiandrosterone; DHT, dihydrotestosterone; E2, estradiol; GABA, gamma-aminobutyric acid; HPA, hypothalamic/pituitary/adrenal; SARM, selective androgen receptor modulator; T, testosterone; TRT, testosterone replacement therapy.

limbic regions through direct serotonergic or catecholaminergic pathways, others activate the PVN directly.[9]

Upon activation of the HPA axis, parvocellular neurons in the PVN synthesize several neuropeptides (CRH, AVP, and OT) that are released into the hypophyseal portal vasculature to drive secretion of adrenocorticotropic hormone (ACTH) from the anterior pituitary. Release of ACTH into the general circulation drives further secretion of GC synthesis and release from the adrenal cortex[22-25] (cortisol in humans, and corticosterone [CORT] in rats and mice). Circulating

GCs act upon peripheral tissue to elicit a myriad of effects. Acute stress-induced GC exposure is beneficial in that it improves cognition and augments physiological responses and energy required in the fight-or-flight response while simultaneously suppressing digestive and reproductive functions.

While short-term elevations of GCs are beneficial for physiological function and survival, chronic exposure to elevated GCs has the opposite effect. Long-term exposure to GCs suppresses immune and neural functions through inhibiting neuronal and glial resilience, glucose uptake, and energy balance, leading to neurotoxicity.[22,23] Moreover, chronic elevations of GC can also alter social, anxiety-, depressive-like, and reproductive behaviors,[24,26] increasing the risk for metabolic and neuropsychiatric disorders.[25,27]

Sex differences in HPA axis activity have been reported in numerous publications over the past 50 years. In rodents, females show a more robust and prolonged CORT and ACTH response to acute stressors than males.[28,29] Levels of *Crh* mRNA in the PVN and the ACTH precursor protein, proopiomelanocortin, in the anterior pituitary are also greater in females. Together, such data indicate an enhanced HPA axis stress response and decreased GC negative feedback.[30] At rest, females display higher baseline levels of CORT than males, suggesting increased basal HPA axis function.

Importantly, gonadectomy (GDX) of male and female rodents has been shown to decrease basal levels of CORT in females and raise levels in males. GDX with hormone replacement (E2 in females, T in males) reinstates the sex difference in CORT to that of intact animals, indicating a significant role of gonadal hormones in CORT secretion.[7]

Corticosteroid binding globulin (CBG) is another important player to consider when examining sex differences in HPA axis function. CBG is a circulating glycoprotein of liver origin, which binds circulating corticosteroids following their release by the adrenal gland. It is thought that the primary role of CBG is to prevent degradation of corticosteroid during transport to target tissues. At the target tissues, corticosteroids are released from CBG and can bind their intracellular receptors.[31,32]

Hence, CBGs directly regulate the availability of plasma free-CORT and its ability to act upon target tissues. Baseline CBG levels in females are shown to be twofold higher than in males, whereas bioavailable free CORT is not different between the two sexes.[33] Therefore, increased levels of CBG could be acting as a buffer against the increased basal and stress-induced CORT found in females. It is also likely that the higher CBG levels in females may partly contribute to the blunted HPA axis negative feedback mechanism seen after an acute stressor since corticosteroids can only bind target tissues when not bound to CBG.[31,34]

Sex-dependent regulation of negative feedback inhibition of the HPA axis

GC feedback inhibition on the HPA axis returns levels of adrenal hormones to baseline following stress-induced increases and prevents baseline CORT levels from getting too high or too low under nonstress conditions.

Two types of corticosteroid receptors are important in the negative feedback mechanism: the type I or MR and the type II or GR. MR and GR are both found in varying densities within hypothalamic and hippocampal regions, with highest levels of GR in the hypothalamic PVN and the CA1 region of the hippocampus, whereas MR is found at high levels in all hippocampal CA regions (greatest in CA2) with lower but significant amount in the PVN.[35] MRs have a high binding affinity (Kd) for GCs reportedly in the range of 0.1 nM and receptors are predominantly occupied by the lower levels of GCs found during basal secretion.

Meanwhile GR possesses a binding affinity that is 10-fold less (Kd = 1–2 nM) than MR and becomes mainly bound during significant elevations of GCs (e.g., following acute stressor).[36] This is an important mechanism to extend the range of sensitivity to circulating CORT levels, which can undergo wide excursions in amplitude depending on the time of day and the environment in which the animals are facing. Many studies report sex differences in MR and GR as potentially contributing to more blunted negative feedback in females. Reduced density of GR and MR in the hypothalamus and hippocampus corresponds with the weaker negative feedback on the HPA axis in females and higher basal CORT secretions.[37]

Stress studies in rodents also show females with reduced GC binding and attenuated upregulation of GR in the hypothalamus[38,39] following acute stressors, potentially resulting in a less robust negative feedback.

Androgens and their steroid hormone receptors

The potent actions of T and DHT to suppress the HPA axis stress response[40–42] work through binding to ARs (Fig. 1). Moreover, metabolites of T and DHT can additionally bind ERs, gamma-aminobutyric acid, and other receptors to induce changes in the HPA axis[43–46] (Fig. 1). Hence, it is important to consider studies involving AR-deficient rodents to confirm the role of AR in altering stress reactivity.[47] In rodent studies examining testicular feminization mutation (Tfm), AR is rendered mostly nonfunctional. Tfm rat males exhibit higher levels of T than wild types, but still have elevated CORT following acute stress.

Experiments in Cre-lox AR knockout mice with induced testicular feminization mutation (iTfm) further demonstrate increased basal and stress-induced CORT in iTfm mice treated with T than wild-type mice treated with T.[47–49] iTfm mice also display increased anxiety-like behavior in light/dark box, open field, and elevated plus maze assays,[47–50] implicating a role for AR in mediation of stress-related behavior. Williams et al.[51] recently demonstrated a T-dependent reduction in anhedonia-like behavior with subchronic variable stress. Anhedonia-like behavior is also increased in AR-deficient rodents following chronic stress.[52]

Taken together, these data further emphasize the important role played by AR for androgenic suppression of the HPA axis. In humans, androgens are similarly thought to enhance mood through actions at the AR. Studies in prostate cancer patients demonstrate that treatment with flutamide increases depression symptoms.[53–55] Moreover, another study by Wang et al.[56] showed that males with complete dysfunctional AR with androgen insensitivity syndrome exhibit increased rates of depression.[57]

Androgens regulate HPA axis function through actions on estrogen receptor alpha (ERα) via metabolites of T, such as its conversion of T to E2 by aromatase (Fig. 1). This contrasts with AR-mediated inhibition of the HPA axis. Treatment with the selective ERα agonists, propylpyrazoletriol (PPT) and moxestral, increased levels of ACTH and CORT after stress in both sexes of rats.[58] Studies also report the effect of ERα on the inhibition of negative feedback to the HPA axis, a more female-typical phenotype. Central implants of PPT near the PVN increased the diurnal peak of CORT and stress responsive increases in CORT and ACTH, while the estrogen receptor beta (ERβ) agonist, diarylpropionitrile (DPN), decreased stress hormone levels.[59]

Binding of ERα is generally thought to drive anxiogenic behavior in rodents. Pharmacological stimulation with PPT increases anxiety-like behavior.[60,61] Downregulation of ERα induced by delivery of an adeno-associated viral vector into the medial preoptic area and posterodorsal amygdala of GDX rats showed decreased anxiety-like behavior in open field and light/dark box tests.[62] Global knockout of ERα does not appear to influence anxiety-like behavior in female mice,[63] but increases it in males,[64] indicating possible sex differences in the actions of ERα. Such data suggest a potential role for ERα in stimulating the neuroendocrine stress response and related anxiogenic mood disorders mediated by the HPA axis activity.

Androgens also influence the HPA axis actions by E2 on ERβ. Metabolites of DHT such as 5α-androstane-3β, 17β diol (3β-diol), have relatively high binding affinity for ERβ,[65,66] and numerous reports suggest an inhibitory role for ERβ on the HPA axis and stress-related behaviors (Fig. 1). Central administration of DPN, a selective ERβ agonist, diminishes ACTH and CORT stress responses in male and female rodents,[58,59,67,68] but has no effect in ERβ knockout mice.[69] GDX adult males further show a suppression of stress-induced ACTH and CORT by 3β-diol.[58] Tamoxifen, a nonselective ER antagonist, when coadministered with DHT, minimized the suppressing effects of DHT on stress-induced CORT and ACTH.[58]

These data suggest a blockade of 3β-diol action at ERβ, which drives the suppression of the neuroendocrine stress response. Unlike ERα, ERβ has anxiolytic behavior effects. In male and female rodents, central implants of ERβ agonists, DPN and WAY-200070, decrease anxiety-like behavior in the open field and elevated plus maze tests.[56,68] Hence, androgens may suppress anxiety-like behavior mediated through actions of 3β-diol, and binding to ERβ. Reports further demonstrate that 3β-diol does not alter anxiety-like behavior in ERβ knockout mice.[70]

Such data indicate that the effect of 3β-diol on anxiolytic behavior depends on functional ERβ. In support, ERβ knockout mice show increased anxiety-like behavior in open field and elevated plus maze in females,[63] and increased depressive-like behavior in sucrose preference following inescapable foot shock in males.[71] Data suggest that the lack of ERβ increases susceptibility for stress-related anxiogenic behaviors. In humans, the role of ERβ has been examined to a much lesser extent. Individuals with variations to the *Esr2* allele, rs1256049 and rs4986938, reported to experience increased major depression disorder and anxiety disorder, predominantly in females.[72,73]

Androgens and Neuropeptide Systems in the Stress Response

Dopamine

DA is a catecholaminergic neurotransmitter synthesized in the medulla of the adrenal gland that is responsible for modulating the HPA-axis alongside 5-HT and norepinephrine. DA also has a key role in the pathogenesis of schizophrenia and Huntington's disease, where high DA levels or DA receptor sensitivity contributes to schizophrenia and Huntington's development, and low brain levels of DA have been associated with causing Parkinson's disease.[74,75]

In addition, DA plays a role in reward and motivation responses, where a decrease in DA correlates to depressive-like symptoms including lack of motivation and loss of interest.[76] In response to stress and CRH production, DA levels and dopaminergic neuronal activity increase in the mesolimbic DA system (MDS).[77] Acute, short-term stressors in rodents (e.g., tail pinch, predator odor, immobilization) resulted in immediate significant increases in DA levels in the mesolimbic pathway.[78,79]

Comparatively, chronic stressors (e.g., food and water restriction, damp home cage bedding) in rats were associated with decreased DA levels or dampened DA neuronal activity.[80,81] This difference suggests that when acutely stressed, high DA levels strengthen the motivation to escape, but when chronically stressed, low DA levels are associated with a maladaptive stress-induced depression. DA receptors, specifically DA receptor 1 (D1) and DA receptor 2 (D2), also play a role in maintaining activation of the HPA-axis poststress, as rats who were given specific D1 and D2 antagonists showed lower and shorter lasting periods of HPA response to a postimmobilization stressor.[82]

Gonadal hormones work to modulate DA levels where E2 is a negative influencer and T is a positive influencer of DA.[83,84] Reduction of circulating E2 following ovariectomy in adult female rats resulted in greater DA transporter binding levels and D2 density in the MDS compared with their intact control rats.[83] E2 has a biphasic mechanism involving a downregulation of D2 binding in response to an acute administration, and an upregulation of binding after chronic treatment.[84]

In contrast, T contributes to stimulating DA synthesis and metabolism, where midbrain DA neurons in male rats express ERs and ARs and are responsive to gonadal steroids.[85] In a GDX study, DA-dependent spatial and learning tasks (e.g., lever pressing for a water reward) had lower breakpoints compared with control intact animals, where supplementation of T propionate attenuated the effects.[86] In addition, GDX animals showed a depletion of medial prefrontal DA innervation in relation to their intact control group,[86] implicating the role of T in DA pathways.

It has been suggested that treatment of T propionate acts as a protectant to dopaminergic neurons to age-induced oxidative damage in male rats.[87] Such data indicate that androgens support the production of DA, while decreased T and DA levels correlate with increased risk for stress-related neuropsychiatric disease.

Corticotropin-releasing hormone

Corticotropin-releasing hormone signaling via corticotropin-releasing factor receptor 1 (CRFR1) and corticotropin-releasing factor receptor 2 (CRFR2) in the pituitary is generally thought to regulate ACTH secretion.[88] CRH secretion and binding to CRFR1 and CRFR2 have been demonstrated to mediate HPA axis responses and stress-related behaviors.[89] In support of this, CRFR1 knockouts or CRFR1 antagonists suppress the HPA axis stress response and reduce anxiety- and depressive-like behaviors,[90] while CRFR1 stimulation does the opposite.[91] Unlike CRFR1 deletion, deletion of CRFR2 increases anxiogenic behavior and the HPA axis stress response.[92,93]

Sex differences have been observed in the roles of CRFR1 and CRFR2 in varying regions of the brain. There are higher levels of CRFR1 in the male PVN compared with females, with a decrease in CRFR1 in male PVN to female levels after GDX.[94-96] Androgens have also been shown to upregulate CRFR2 in various brain regions. DHT propionate (DHTP) administration increases CRFR2 expression levels within the hypothalamus, hippocampus, and lateral septum (LS).[97] Taken together, these data demonstrate that androgens decrease the HPA axis response and stress-related behaviors.[98,99]

The presence of AREs or estrogen response elements (EREs) in the promoter region of the *Crh* gene and its receptors allows androgens to directly alter the expression of CRFR1 and CRFR2.[100,101] CRH and CRFR1 expressing neurons have also been shown to coexpress ARs and ERs.[94] For instance, in rats and mice, CRH neurons in the PVN coexpress ERβ,[102] suggesting that androgens may induce effects on the HPA axis through EREs in the upstream regulatory regions of CRH. Reports further show high coexpression CRFR1 and AR in PVN cells.[96] While few neurons express both CRH and AR in the PVN, there is a large percentage of coexpression in the bed nucleus stria terminalis (BnST).[94]

Various studies in rodents additionally demonstrate that androgens can mediate CRH expression in the brain. For example, one study in males showed an increase in CRH 3 weeks after GDX. Androgen supplementation with DHT reversed this effect.[103] DHTP treatment in GDX males further reduced PVN CRH expression following restraint.[60] In contrast, CRH levels in the dorsolateral BnST have been shown to decrease following GDX of male rats and these effects were reversed with androgen treatment.[104]

Seale et al.[105] reported a reduction in CRH cell expression in the female adult BnST when they were provided with neonatal T supplementation, suggesting that adult CRH levels are also influenced by neonatal androgens. These findings supported the concept that androgens suppress CRH expression in the PVN and ultimately the HPA axis response to stressors, potentially a mechanism that leads to lower depressive- and anxiety-like behaviors.

Serotonin

5-HT is a monoamine neurotransmitter that stems from the median and dorsal raphe nuclei of the brainstem to stimulate the HPA-axis and stress response via directly activating CRH neurons in the PVN, increasing ACTH production and CORT release.[106,107] In particular, the 5-HT receptors 5-HT1A and 5-HT2A have high degrees of colocalization in the PVN CRH neurons where agonists of these receptors resulted in increased ACTH secretion.[108] Review articles have summarized the complex relationship between the 5-HT receptor subtypes, where agonist actions at specific 5-HT receptors (i.e., 1A, 1B, 2C, 4, 6) and blocking others (i.e., 2A, 2C, 3, 6, 7) produce antidepressive behaviors comparable with selective 5-HT reuptake inhibitors.[109,110]

Low levels of 5-HT have been associated with numerous illnesses, including anxiety and depression. G-protein-coupled ERs desensitize the 5-HT receptor signaling.[111] Specifically, E2 actions at ERβ lead to modulation of the expression of 5-HT neurotransmitters via enhancing the expression of tryptophan hydroxyase-2, the rate-limiting enzyme in 5-HT synthesis, and decrease HPA-axis activation with lowered despair-like responses to stressors.[112,113]

With respect to sex differences, female mice had greater CORT production after administration of a selective 5-HT reuptake inhibitor—an effect that could be attenuated by T.[114] E2 has shown a positive relationship between cortical 5-HT receptor binding in men, whereas T had no direct effect.[115] Moreover, hormone replacement therapy administered to postmenopausal women improved 5-HT receptor binding and 5-HT signaling.[116] Regarding T, there are different proposed mechanisms regarding the ability of this hormone to modulate 5-HT.

In one study, T was shown to be negatively associated with global 5-HT$_4$R levels, which led authors to suggest that higher T levels correlated with a higher cerebral 5-HT level at baseline.[117] However, 5-HT$_4$R expression has been associated with low 5-HT and antidepressant-like behavior, which is in opposition to the conclusions of Perfalk et al.[117]

A study by Kranz et al.[118] also concluded that a treatment of high-dose T in transgender men resulted in an increased 5-HT reuptake transporter binding and expression. The authors also proposed that T acts indirectly on serotonergic neurons by first converting to E2, as ERβ has been localized in serotonergic neurons, while ARs have not.[118] Therefore, while E2 produces higher levels of 5-HT and CORT, and stimulation of the HPA-axis, the specific actions of AR stimulation by T or DHT have not been fully elucidated.

Arginine vasopressin

The nonapeptide, AVP, is produced in hypothalamic neurons found in the PVN, BnST, supraoptic nucleus, and medial amygdala (MeA). When released to the general circulation via the posterior pituitary gland, the primary functions of AVP are to increase water reabsorption in the kidneys, and to constrict arterioles resulting in a higher arterial blood pressure. The release of AVP also affects behaviors related to anxiety and depression as it has been associated to work in conjunction with CRH to modulate the production of ACTH.[119,120]

In adult rodents, the number of AVP-expressing cells in the BnST and MeA is greater in males than females, while the number of AVP-expressing cells in the PVN was comparable between sexes.[121,122] Studies also show that gonadal steroid hormones can modulate PVN AVP expression resulting in a greater number of AVP neurons in the certain brain areas of males compared with females.[104,123] For example, implanting DHT into the BnST increased AVP PVN levels, whereas the introduction of hydroxyflutamide, a nonsteroidal antiandrogen, caused a decrease in PVN AVP expression.[123]

It has been hypothesized that in rats, since there is a low population of AR in PVN AVP neurons, androgens likely act indirectly to regulate expression via other brain regions such as the BnST and MeA.[124] In both these areas, AVP neurons coexpress ARs and ERs, and therefore, these can provide direct regulation by androgens.[125] Alternatively, because the PVN AVP neurons express ERβ, it could be argued that androgen metabolites such as 3β-diol can also act on the neurons directly.[126,127] Studies using in vitro reporter gene assays show that 3β-diol can directly upregulate AVP promoter activity through binding to ERβ.[128]

Androgens have also been reported to modulate depressive-like behaviors and stress responses via directly promoting AVP neurons in the LS.[129] Singewald et al.[130] demonstrated that the LS is also a key region contributing to androgen inhibition of the HPA axis. For example, when rats had increased activation of AVP neurons in the LS, they were shown to have reduced immobility compared with control animals in the forced swim test,[129] suggesting that AVP neurons in the LS can play a role in regulating and improving depressive-like behaviors and the response to androgens.

Oxytocin
OT, a nonapeptide closely related to AVP, is produced in the hypothalamic PVN and SON and influences reproductive, postpartum, and social behavior, as well as playing a role to suppress the HPA axis and associated stress responses.[131–133] Central infusion of supplemental OT diminishes PVN activation and secretion of ACTH and CORT, leading to an overall decrease in anxiety-like behaviors after stressors.[134,135] Antagonizing OT receptors does the opposite and activates the PVN and increases anxiety-like behaviors.[132] Moreover, OT receptor knockout male mice had an overactivation of the HPA axis following stress,[136] supporting the role of OT in reducing the HPA axis activity.

ARs have been colocalized with OT in the medial parvocellular region of the hypothalamic PVN.[124] OT has also been shown to be directly regulated by the androgen metabolite, 3β-diol, using in vitro reporter gene assays where 3β-diol and ERβ were transfected into human and rodent cell lines.[137] These effects were traced to a composite response element lying in the proximal OT promoter.

In vivo studies show that GDX male rats administered T propionate had significantly higher amounts of OT release from PVN neurons and subsequent binding in the ventromedial hypothalamus (VMH) and BnST.[138] It could be hypothesized that estrogenic metabolites of androgens regulate OT neuron function through an action mediated by ERβ, whereas receptor numbers are regulated through ERα.

Patisaul et al.[139] demonstrated that treatment with E2 and progesterone in GDX female mice increased OT transcripts in the PVN, suggesting an estrogen-dependent role of ERβ in OT regulation. Treatment with E2 also enhanced OT receptor binding in the MeA and VMH in mice and rats.[139] Interestingly, in the MeA and VMH, regions where ERα is predomi-

nantly expressed at higher levels than ERβ, OT receptor binding in ERβ knockout and wild-type mice was similarly increased following E2 treatment.[139] This indicates that ERα is essential for the regulation of OT receptors in these regions, while ERβ does not appear to play a role. Moreover, OT antagonists minimize effects of the ERβ antagonist DPN on anxiety-like behaviors.

Taken together, these data indicate that androgen-mediated OT production and binding potentially suppress the HPA axis through these mechanisms, which can influence anxiolytic behaviors and attenuate stress-related responses.[140]

Androgens and Their Role in Therapeutic Treatments
The physiological response to acute stress is beneficial and enhances cognition, immune function, and metabolism to increase chances of survival.[18] For instance, short-term release of GCs (cortisol in humans, and CORT in rats and mice) can induce gluconeogenesis to break down glucose stores and provide the proper nutrients and energy in response to an acute stressor.[141] In contrast, chronic activation of the stress response has deleterious effects on immune system activity and neurotoxicity. Such long-term insults to the HPA axis stress response ultimately increases risk for cardiovascular, immune, metabolic, and neuropsychiatric diseases.[142]

These stress-related disorders arise differently in males versus females, given that the sex differences have been reported in the function of the HPA axis.[143,144] For example, males are two to three times less likely to develop depression than females[145] and exhibit decreased subclinical symptoms and decreased rates of comorbid anxiety due to increased circulating levels of T.[146,147] Similarly, men with prostate cancer undergoing androgen-deprivation therapy present with increased stress-related disorders, including anxiety and depression.[148] Male rats display reduced anxiety- and depressive-like behaviors compared with females due to elevated levels of androgens, namely T.

A large body of research implicates androgens in the attenuation of the integrated central stress response. Therefore, a role for androgens in the treatment of stress-related neuropsychiatric disorders (Fig. 1), such as depression and anxiety, is emerging.[29,149]

Testosterone replacement therapy (TRT) is a common treatment for hypogonadal men. A recent meta-analysis found that men diagnosed with hypogonadism undergoing TRT presented with decreased depressive-like symptoms and improved mood.[150,151] Moreover, men with diabetes mellitus type 2 and hypogonadism in a double-blinded placebo study received intramuscular TRT or a placebo for 30 weeks.

Subjects were evaluated by the Aging Male Symptom Scale, based on the Hospital Anxiety and Depression Scale and Global Efficacy Questionnaire to evaluate overall mood. Scores were significantly increased in those who received TRT in contrast to the placebo group, implicating the role of T in attenuating depressive- and anxiety-like symptoms.[152] Such effects of T treatment are further demonstrated in animal models. In rodents, T administration increased the synthesis and release of 5-HT from the dorsal raphe nuclei and increased neuroplasticity in the hippocampus to induce antidepressive-like states and improved mood.[153] T treatment also reduced anxiety and depressive-like behavior in male rodents.[154–156]

Hence, the correlation between T and anxiolytic activity suggests high efficacy of T therapeutics in treating stress-related disorders. Although TRT has been shown to be efficacious in hypogonadal men in improving mood disorders, evaluation of long-term health risks will be important.

Administration of DHEA and its metabolite, DHEA sulfate, has also been proposed for the treatment of neuropsychiatric disease. Levels of DHEA and DHEA-sulfate decrease with age, leading to fatigue, anxiety, and depression.[157] Evidence further suggests that there is a negative correlation between plasma DHEA and DHEA sulfate levels and cortisol in stress and anxiety.[158,159] Supplementation with these compounds increases androgen levels, attenuates stress-induced cortisol output, and improves mood disorders.[160]

In human studies, DHEA or DHEA sulfate displayed improvement in anxiety and depressive symptoms.[161,162] To support these findings, DHEA and DHEA-sulfate doses decreased depressive-like symptoms and enhanced cognition in patients after 6 months of administration. Interestingly, depressive-like symptoms and cognition worsened following the withdrawal of treatment.[157] A meta-analysis of randomized-controlled trials further demonstrated that DHEA treatment had a beneficial effect on depressive symptoms in 853 females and male subjects. Side effects from DHEA treatment were uncommon and transient in trials.[162,163] Such data suggest an important role of DHEA in affective mood disorders and a promising outlook on DHEA as a therapeutic.[162–164]

The AR is an additional target for the therapeutic use of androgens. Selective AR modulators (SARMs) were first discovered near the end of the 20th century.[165] SARMs are small-molecule drugs engineered to selectively bind AR in target tissues. The tissue type allows the ligand to exert both antagonistic and agonistic effects based on the types of coregulator proteins and cofactors present.[166] In contrast, TRT is often associated with numerous off-target effects due to the lack of tissue selectivity that occurs with classical steroid treatment.[167,168] The tissue-specific effects of SARMs make them an ideal candidate for androgen-based therapeutics.[167]

Androgen modulators are being studied as a potential treatment of cognition and mood disorders, including anxiety and depression. GDX male mice treated with a SARM for 4 months displayed enhanced cognition in the Morris water maze test. Chronic SARM treatment further decreased anxiety-like behavior in the elevated plus maze and open field tests.[169] Such data implicate SARMs as a potential therapeutic for stress-related disorders. However, the development of SARMs is still in the early stages and undergoing clinical trials.[170–172] Further studies are necessary to examine their efficacy and safety, but they remain a promising strategy for androgen therapy.[173,174]

Conclusions

Androgens are an important factor to consider when examining sex differences in the HPA axis and stress-related behaviors. Several studies have been performed to assess the mechanism of action of androgens and androgen metabolites and their receptors involved in HPA axis regulation. These support their roles in driving sex-specific HPA axis phenotypes. It is important to consider that androgens and androgen metabolites exert varying hormonal and behavior effects depending on the brain region in which their associated receptor is located.

Future studies that examine the sites of these actions would be beneficial to understanding the role androgens play in the stress response. Abundant evidence additionally supports a role for androgens in neuropeptide systems that interact with the HPA axis (CRH, AVP, OT, 5-HT, and DA), but precise circuitries remain undescribed. Further research in these areas will fill these gaps in our knowledge in how steroidal gonadal hormones contribute to sex differences in important stress regulatory systems and related neuropsychiatric disorders. Moreover, therapeutic methods involving androgens and SARMs present a positive outlook.

Androgen replacement therapies such as TRT are clinically demonstrated to successfully attenuate stress disorders, such as anxiety and depression, in males and females. However, due to the potential adverse off-target effects of TRT, SARMs have become more of an interest in the present field of androgen therapies. SARMs are chemically engineered to target specific tissues expressing ARs, allowing them to be better tolerated and highly selective.

However, while SARMs have been studied in several Phase I and Phase II clinical trials,[170-172] and pre-clinical data suggest a positive outcome, they are not yet FDA approved. Nevertheless, SARMs appear to have great potential for the revolutionary treatment of numerous androgen-mediated medical challenges.

Authors' Contributions

Conception, design, and drafting of the article by J.A.S. and S.M.L.T. Critical revision by R.J.H. and T.M.H., and final approval of the article by T.M.H.

References

1. Romeo RD. The metamorphosis of adolescent hormonal stress reactivity: A focus on animal models. Front Neuroendocrinol. 2018;49:43–51.
2. Munck A, Guyre PM, Holbrook NJ. Physiological functions of glucocorticoids in stress and their relation to pharmacological actions. Endocr Rev. 1984;5(1):25–44.
3. Green MR, McCormick CM. Sex and stress steroids in adolescence: Gonadal regulation of the hypothalamic-pituitary-adrenal axis in the rat. Gen Comp Endocrinol. 2016;234:110–116.
4. Goldstein JM, Holsen L, Huang G, et al. Prenatal stress-immune programming of sex differences in comorbidity of depression and obesity/metabolic syndrome. Dialogues Clin Neurosci. 2016;18(4): 425–436.
5. Castro-Vale I, Carvalho D. The pathways between cortisol-related regulation genes and PTSD psychotherapy. Healthcare (Basel). 2020; 8(4):376.
6. Mendell AL, MacLusky NJ. Neurosteroid metabolites of gonadal steroid hormones in neuroprotection: Implications for sex differences in neurodegenerative disease. Front Mol Neurosci. 2018;11:359.
7. Heck AL, Handa RJ. Sex differences in the hypothalamic-pituitary-adrenal axis' response to stress: An important role for gonadal hormones. Neuropsychopharmacology. 2019;44(1):45–58.
8. Lombardo MV, Auyeung B, Pramparo T, et al. Sex-specific impact of prenatal androgens on social brain default mode subsystems. Mol Psychiatry. 2020;25(9):2175–2188.
9. Weisz J, Ward IL. Plasma testosterone and progesterone titers of pregnant rats, their male and female fetuses, and neonatal offspring. Endocrinology. 1980;106(1):306–316.
10. Corbier P, Edwards DA, Roffi J. The neonatal testosterone surge: A comparative study. Arch Int Physiol Biochim Biophys. 1992;100(2):127–131.
11. Sheng JA, Bales NJ, Myers SA, et al. The hypothalamic-pituitary-adrenal axis: development, programming actions of hormones, and maternal-fetal interactions. Front Behav Neurosci. 2020;14(256):601939.
12. Zuloaga DG, Puts DA, Jordan CL, et al. The role of androgen receptors in the masculinization of brain and behavior: What we've learned from the testicular feminization mutation. Horm Behav. 2008;53(5):613–626.
13. Supakar PC, Song CS, Jung MH, et al. A novel regulatory element associated with age-dependent expression of the rat androgen receptor gene. J Biol Chem. 1993;268(35):26400–26408.
14. Handa RJ, Weiser MJ. Gonadal steroid hormones and the hypothalamo-pituitary-adrenal axis. Front Neuroendocrinol. 2014;35(2):197–220.
15. Thomas P. Membrane androgen receptors unrelated to nuclear steroid receptors. Endocrinology. 2019;160(4):772–781.
16. Rochel N, Wurtz JM, Mitschler A, et al. The crystal structure of the nuclear receptor for vitamin D bound to its natural ligand. Mol Cell. 2000;5(1): 173–179.
17. Downes M, Verdecia MA, Roecker AJ, et al. A chemical, genetic, and structural analysis of the nuclear bile acid receptor FXR. Mol Cell. 2003; 11(4):1079–1092.
18. McEwan IJ, Gustafsson J. Interaction of the human androgen receptor transactivation function with the general transcription factor TFIIF. Proc Natl Acad Sci U S A. 1997;94(16):8485–8490.
19. Koivisto PA, Rantala I. Amplification of the androgen receptor gene is associated with P53 mutation in hormone-refractory recurrent prostate cancer. J Pathol. 1999;187(2):237–241.
20. Trevino LS, Gorelick DA. The interface of nuclear and membrane steroid signaling. Endocrinology. 2021;162(8).
21. Gobinet J, Poujol N, Sultan C. Molecular action of androgens. Mol Cell Endocrinol. 2002;198(1-2):15–24.
22. Borrow AP, Heck AL, Miller AM, et al. Chronic variable stress alters hypothalamic-pituitary-adrenal axis function in the female mouse. Physiol Behav. 2019;209:112613.
23. Jauregui-Huerta F, Ruvalcaba-Delgadillo Y, Gonzalez-Castaneda R, et al. Responses of glial cells to stress and glucocorticoids. Curr Immunol Rev. 2010;6(3):195–204.
24. Packard AE, Egan AE, Ulrich-Lai YM. HPA axis interactions with behavioral systems. Compr Physiol. 2016;6(4):1897–1934.
25. Davis MT, Holmes SE, Pietrzak RH, et al. Neurobiology of chronic stress-related psychiatric disorders: Evidence from molecular imaging studies. Chronic Stress (Thousand Oaks). 2017;1:1–21.
26. Levy MJF, Boulle F, Steinbusch HW, et al. Neurotrophic factors and neuroplasticity pathways in the pathophysiology and treatment of depression. Psychopharmacology (Berl). 2018;235(8):2195–2220.
27. Price RB, Duman R. Neuroplasticity in cognitive and psychological mechanisms of depression: An integrative model. Mol Psychiatry. 2020; 25(2):530–543.
28. Babb JA, Masini CV, Day HE, et al. Stressor-specific effects of sex on HPA axis hormones and activation of stress-related neurocircuitry. Stress. 2013;16(6):664–677.
29. Oyola MG, Handa RJ. Hypothalamic-pituitary-adrenal and hypothalamic-pituitary-gonadal axes: Sex differences in regulation of stress responsivity. Stress. 2017;20(5):476–494.
30. Viau V, Bingham B, Davis J, et al. Gender and puberty interact on the stress-induced activation of parvocellular neurosecretory neurons and corticotropin-releasing hormone messenger ribonucleic acid expression in the rat. Endocrinology. 2005;146(1):137–146.
31. Moisan MP. Sexual dimorphism in glucocorticoid stress response. Int J Mol Sci. 2021;22(6):3139.
32. Panagiotakopoulos L, Neigh GN. Development of the HPA axis: Where and when do sex differences manifest? Front Neuroendocrinol. 2014; 35(3):285–302.
33. Gala RR, Westphal U. Corticosteroid-binding globulin in the rat: Studies on the sex difference. Endocrinology. 1965;77(5):841–851.
34. McCormick CM, Linkroum W, Sallinen BJ, et al. Peripheral and central sex steroids have differential effects on the HPA axis of male and female rats. Stress. 2002;5(4):235–247.

35. Figueiredo HF, Dolgas CM, Herman JP. Stress activation of cortex and hippocampus is modulated by sex and stage of estrus. Endocrinology. 2002;143(7):2534–2540.

36. Reul JM, de Kloet ER. Two receptor systems for corticosterone in rat brain: Microdistribution and differential occupation. Endocrinology. 1985;117(6):2505–2511.

37. Solomon MB, Loftspring M, de Kloet AD, et al. neuroendocrine function after hypothalamic depletion of glucocorticoid receptors in male and female mice. Endocrinology. 2015;156(8):2843–2853.

38. Turner BB, Weaver DA. Sexual dimorphism of glucocorticoid binding in rat brain. Brain Res. 1985;343(1):16–23.

39. Karandrea D, Kittas C, Kitraki E. Contribution of sex and cellular context in the regulation of brain corticosteroid receptors following restraint stress. Neuroendocrinology. 2000;71(6):343–353.

40. Acevedo-Rodriguez A, Kauffman AS, Cherrington BD, et al. Emerging insights into hypothalamic-pituitary-gonadal axis regulation and interaction with stress signalling. J Neuroendocrinol. 2018;30(10):e12590.

41. Handa RJ, Nunley KM, Lorens SA, et al. Androgen regulation of adrenocorticotropin and corticosterone secretion in the male rat following novelty and foot shock stressors. Physiol Behav. 1994;55(1):117–124.

42. Handa RJ, Kudwa AE, Donner NC, et al. Central 5-alpha reduction of testosterone is required for testosterone's inhibition of the hypothalamo-pituitary-adrenal axis response to restraint stress in adult male rats. Brain Res. 2013;1529:74–82.

43. Handa RJ, Weiser MJ, Zuloaga DG. A role for the androgen metabolite, 5alpha-androstane-3beta,17beta-diol, in modulating oestrogen receptor beta-mediated regulation of hormonal stress reactivity. J Neuroendocrinol. 2009;21(4):351–358.

44. Belelli D, Lambert JJ. Neurosteroids: Endogenous regulators of the GABA(A) receptor. Nat Rev Neurosci. 2005;6(7):565–575.

45. Lambert JJ, Harney SC, Belelli D, et al. Neurosteroid modulation of recombinant and synaptic GABAAA receptors. Int Rev Neurobiol. 2001;46: 177–205.

46. Mouton JC, Duckworth RA. Maternally derived hormones, neurosteroids and the development of behaviour. Proc Biol Sci. 2021;288(1943): 20202467.

47. Chen CV, Brummet JL, Lonstein JS, et al. New knockout model confirms a role for androgen receptors in regulating anxiety-like behaviors and HPA response in mice. Horm Behav. 2014;65(3):211–218.

48. Zuloaga DG, Jordan CL, Breedlove SM. The organizational role of testicular hormones and the androgen receptor in anxiety-related behaviors and sensorimotor gating in rats. Endocrinology. 2011;152(4):1572–1581.

49. Hamson DK, Jones BA, Csupity AS, et al. Androgen insensitive male rats display increased anxiety-like behavior on the elevated plus maze. Behav Brain Res. 2014;259:158–163.

50. Zuloaga DG, Morris JA, Jordan CL, et al. Mice with the testicular feminization mutation demonstrate a role for androgen receptors in the regulation of anxiety-related behaviors and the hypothalamic-pituitary-adrenal axis. Horm Behav. 2008;54(5):758–766.

51. Williams ES, Manning CE, Eagle AL, et al. Androgen-dependent excitability of mouse ventral hippocampal afferents to nucleus accumbens underlies sex-specific susceptibility to stress. Biol Psychiatry. 2020;87(6): 492–501.

52. Hung YY, Huang YL, Chang C, et al. Deficiency in androgen receptor aggravates the depressive-like behaviors in chronic mild stress model of depression. Cells. 2019;8(9):1021.

53. Lee M, Jim HS, Fishman M, et al. Depressive symptomatology in men receiving androgen deprivation therapy for prostate cancer: A controlled comparison. Psychooncology. 2015;24(4):472–477.

54. Sanchez-Martinez V, Buigues C, Navarro-Martinez R, et al. Analysis of brain functions in men with prostate cancer under androgen deprivation therapy: A one-year longitudinal study. Life (Basel). 2021;11(3):227.

55. Hoogland AI, Jim HSL, Gonzalez BD, et al. Systemic inflammation and symptomatology in patients with prostate cancer treated with androgen deprivation therapy: Preliminary findings. Cancer. 2021;127(9): 1476–1482.

56. Wang SS, Kamphuis W, Huitinga I, et al. Gene expression analysis in the human hypothalamus in depression by laser microdissection and real-time PCR: The presence of multiple receptor imbalances. Mol Psychiatry. 2008;13(8):786–799, 741.

57. Fliegner M, Krupp K, Brunner F, et al. Sexual life and sexual wellness in individuals with complete androgen insensitivity syndrome (CAIS) and Mayer-Rokitansky-Kuster-Hauser Syndrome (MRKHS). J Sex Med. 2014; 11(3):729–742.

58. Lund TD, Hinds LR, Handa RJ. The androgen 5alpha-dihydrotestosterone and its metabolite 5alpha-androstan-3beta, 17beta-diol inhibit the hypothalamo-pituitary-adrenal response to stress by acting through estrogen receptor beta-expressing neurons in the hypothalamus. J Neurosci. 2006;26(5):1448–1456.

59. Weiser MJ, Handa RJ. Estrogen impairs glucocorticoid dependent negative feedback on the hypothalamic-pituitary-adrenal axis via estrogen receptor alpha within the hypothalamus. Neuroscience. 2009;159(2): 883–895.

60. Lund TD, Munson DJ, Haldy ME, et al. Dihydrotestosterone may inhibit hypothalamo-pituitary-adrenal activity by acting through estrogen receptor in the male mouse. Neurosci Lett. 2004;365(1):43–47.

61. Borrow AP, Handa RJ. Estrogen receptors modulation of anxiety-like behavior. Vitam Horm. 2017;103:27–52.

62. Spiteri T, Musatov S, Ogawa S, et al. The role of the estrogen receptor alpha in the medial amygdala and ventromedial nucleus of the hypothalamus in social recognition, anxiety and aggression. Behav Brain Res. 2010;210(2):211–220.

63. Krezel W, Dupont S, Krust A, et al. Increased anxiety and synaptic plasticity in estrogen receptor beta-deficient mice. Proc Natl Acad Sci U S A. 2001;98(21):12278–12282.

64. Imwalle DB, Scordalakes EM, Rissman EF. Estrogen receptor alpha influences socially motivated behaviors. Horm Behav. 2002;42(4):484–491.

65. Kuiper GG, Carlsson B, Grandien K, et al. Comparison of the ligand binding specificity and transcript tissue distribution of estrogen receptors alpha and beta. Endocrinology. 1997;138(3):863–870.

66. Kovacs T, Szabo-Meleg E, Abraham IM. Estradiol-induced epigenetically mediated mechanisms and regulation of gene expression. Int J Mol Sci. 2020;21(9):3177.

67. Dombret C, Naule L, Trouillet AC, et al. Effects of neural estrogen receptor beta deletion on social and mood-related behaviors and underlying mechanisms in male mice. Sci Rep. 2020;10(1):6242.

68. Ravi M, Stevens JS, Michopoulos V. Neuroendocrine pathways underlying risk and resilience to PTSD in women. Front Neuroendocrinol. 2019; 55:100790.

69. Oyola MG, Portillo W, Reyna A, et al. Anxiolytic effects and neuroanatomical targets of estrogen receptor-beta (ERbeta) activation by a selective ERbeta agonist in female mice. Endocrinology. 2012;153(2):837–846.

70. Frye CA, Koonce CJ, Edinger KL, et al. Androgens with activity at estrogen receptor beta have anxiolytic and cognitive-enhancing effects in male rats and mice. Horm Behav. 2008;54(5):726–734.

71. Georgiou P, Zanos P, Jenne CE, et al. Sex-specific involvement of estrogen receptors in behavioral responses to stress and psychomotor activation. Front Psychiatry. 2019;10:81.

72. Ryan J, Scali J, Carriere I, et al. Oestrogen receptor polymorphisms and late-life depression. Br J Psychiatry. 2011;199(2):126–131.

73. Keyes K, Agnew-Blais J, Roberts AL, et al. The role of allelic variation in estrogen receptor genes and major depression in the Nurses Health Study. Soc Psychiatry Psychiatr Epidemiol. 2015;50(12):1893–1904.

74. Birtwistle J, Baldwin D. Role of dopamine in schizophrenia and Parkinson's disease. Br J Nurs. 1998;7(14):832–834, 836, 838–841.

75. Seeman P, Bzowej NH, Guan HC, et al. Human brain dopamine receptors in children and aging adults. Synapse. 1987;1(5):399–404.

76. Belujon P, Grace AA. Dopamine system dysregulation in Major Depressive Disorders. Int J Neuropsychopharmacol. 2017;20(12):1036–1046.

77. Payer D, Williams B, Mansouri E, et al. Corticotropin-releasing hormone and dopamine release in healthy individuals. Psychoneuroendocrinology. 2017;76:192–196.

78. Renoldi G, Invernizzi RW. Blockade of tachykinin NK1 receptors attenuates stress-induced rise of extracellular noradrenaline and dopamine in the rat and gerbil medial prefrontal cortex. J Neurosci Res. 2006;84(5): 961–968.

79. Moriya S, Yamashita A, Kawashima S, et al. Acute aversive stimuli rapidly increase the activity of ventral tegmental area dopamine neurons in awake mice. Neuroscience. 2018;386:16–23.

80. Holly EN, Miczek KA. Ventral tegmental area dopamine revisited: Effects of acute and repeated stress. Psychopharmacology (Berl). 2016;233(2): 163–186.

81. Moreines JL, Owrutsky ZL, Grace AA. Involvement of infralimbic pre-frontal cortex but not lateral habenula in dopamine attenuation after chronic mild stress. Neuropsychopharmacology. 2017;42(4):904–913.
82. Belda X, Armario A. Dopamine D1 and D2 dopamine receptors regulate immobilization stress-induced activation of the hypothalamus-pituitary-adrenal axis. Psychopharmacology (Berl). 2009;206(3):355–365.
83. Chavez C, Hollaus M, Scarr E, et al. The effect of estrogen on dopamine and serotonin receptor and transporter levels in the brain: An autora-diography study. Brain Res. 2010;1321:51–59.
84. Yoest KE, Cummings JA, Becker JB. Estradiol, dopamine and motivation. Cent Nerv Syst Agents Med Chem. 2014;14(2):83–89.
85. Sinclair D, Purves-Tyson TD, Allen KM, et al. Impacts of stress and sex hormones on dopamine neurotransmission in the adolescent brain. Psychopharmacology (Berl). 2014;231(8):1581–1599.
86. Kritzer MF, Brewer A, Montalmant F, et al. Effects of gonadectomy on performance in operant tasks measuring prefrontal cortical function in adult male rats. Horm Behav. 2007;51(2):183–194.
87. Cui R, Kang Y, Wang L, et al. Testosterone propionate exacerbates the deficits of nigrostriatal dopaminergic system and downregulates Nrf2 expression in reserpine-treated aged male rats. Front Aging Neurosci. 2017;9:172.
88. Deussing JM, Chen A. The corticotropin-releasing factor family: Physi-ology of the stress response. Physiol Rev. 2018;98(4):2225–2286.
89. Bale TL, Vale WW. CRF and CRF receptors: Role in stress responsivity and other behaviors. Annu Rev Pharmacol Toxicol. 2004;44:525–557.
90. Muller MB, Zimmermann S, Sillaber I, et al. Limbic corticotropin-releasing hormone receptor 1 mediates anxiety-related behavior and hormonal adaptation to stress. Nat Neurosci. 2003;6(10):1100–1107.
91. Britton KT, Lee G, Vale W, et al. Corticotropin releasing factor (CRF) re-ceptor antagonist blocks activating and 'anxiogenic' actions of CRF in the rat. Brain Res. 1986;369(1-2):303–306.
92. Bale TL, Contarino A, Smith GW, et al. Mice deficient for corticotropin-releasing hormone receptor-2 display anxiety-like behaviour and are hypersensitive to stress. Nat Genet. 2000;24(4):410–414.
93. Kishimoto T, Radulovic J, Radulovic M, et al. Deletion of crhr2 reveals an anxiolytic role for corticotropin-releasing hormone receptor-2. Nat Genet. 2000;24(4):415–419.
94. Heck AL, Thompson MK, Uht RM, et al. Sex-dependent mechanisms of glucocorticoid regulation of the mouse hypothalamic corticotropin-releasing hormone gene. Endocrinology. 2020;161(1):bqz012.
95. Rosinger ZJ, Jacobskind JS, Bulanchuk N, et al. Characterization and gonadal hormone regulation of a sexually dimorphic corticotropin-releasing factor receptor 1cell group. J Comp Neurol. 2019;527(6):1056–1069.
96. Rosinger ZJ, Jacobskind JS, De Guzman RM, et al. A sexually dimorphic distribution of corticotropin-releasing factor receptor 1 in the paraven-tricular hypothalamus. Neuroscience. 2019;409:195–203.
97. Weiser MJ, Goel N, Sandau US, et al. Androgen regulation of corticotropin-releasing hormone receptor 2 (CRHR2) mRNA expression and receptor binding in the rat brain. Exp Neurol. 2008;214(1):62–68.
98. Jiang Z, Rajamanickam S, Justice NJ. Local corticotropin-releasing factor signaling in the hypothalamic paraventricular nucleus. J Neurosci. 2018; 38(8):1874–1890.
99. Jiang Z, Rajamanickam S, Justice NJ. CRF signaling between neurons in the paraventricular nucleus of the hypothalamus (PVN) coordinates stress responses. Neurobiol Stress. 2019;11:100192.
100. Catalano RD, Kyriakou T, Chen J, et al. Regulation of corticotropin-releasing hormone type 2 receptors by multiple promoters and alter-native splicing: Identification of multiple splice variants. Mol Endocrinol. 2003;17(3):395–410.
101. Chen XN, Zhu H, Meng QY, et al. Estrogen receptor-alpha and -beta regulate the human corticotropin-releasing hormone gene through similar pathways. Brain Res. 2008;1223:1–10.
102. Oyola MG, Thompson MK, Handa AZ, et al. Distribution and chemical composition of estrogen receptor beta neurons in the paraventricular nucleus of the female and male mouse hypothalamus. J Comp Neurol. 2017;525(17):3666–3682.
103. Bingaman EW, Magnuson DJ, Gray TS, et al. Androgen inhibits the in-creases in hypothalamic corticotropin-releasing hormone (CRH) and CRH-immunoreactivity following gonadectomy. Neuroendocrinology. 1994;59(3):228–234.
104. Viau V, Soriano L, Dallman MF. Androgens alter corticotropin releasing hormone and arginine vasopressin mRNA within forebrain sites known to regulate activity in the hypothalamic-pituitary-adrenal axis. J Neuroendocrinol. 2001;13(5):442–452.
105. Seale JV, Wood SA, Atkinson HC, et al. Postnatal masculinization alters the HPA axis phenotype in the adult female rat. J Physiol. 2005;563(Pt 1): 265–274.
106. Holsboer F, Barden N. Antidepressants and hypothalamic-pituitary-adrenocortical regulation. Endocr Rev. 1996;17(2):187–205.
107. Heisler LK, Zhou L, Bajwa P, et al. Serotonin 5-HT(2C) receptors regulate anxiety-like behavior. Genes Brain Behav. 2007;6(5):491–496.
108. Osei-Owusu P, James A, Crane J, et al. 5-Hydroxytryptamine 1A receptors in the paraventricular nucleus of the hypothalamus mediate oxytocin and adrenocorticotropin hormone release and some behavioral com-ponents of the serotonin syndrome. J Pharmacol Exp Ther. 2005;313(3): 1324–1330.
109. Carr GV, Lucki I. The role of serotonin receptor subtypes in treating depression: A review of animal studies. Psychopharmacology (Berl). 2011;213(2-3):265–287.
110. Yohn CN, Gergues MM, Samuels BA. The role of 5-HT receptors in de-pression. Mol Brain. 2017;10(1):28.
111. McAllister CE, Creech RD, Kimball PA, et al. GPR30 is necessary for estradiol-induced desensitization of 5-HT1A receptor signaling in the paraventricular nucleus of the rat hypothalamus. Psychoneuroendocri-nology. 2012;37(8):1248–1260.
112. Donner N, Handa RJ. Estrogen receptor beta regulates the expression of tryptophan-hydroxylase 2 mRNA within serotonergic neurons of the rat dorsal raphe nuclei. Neuroscience. 2009;163(2):705–718.
113. Valdes-Sustaita B, Estrada-Camarena E, Gonzalez-Trujano ME, et al. Estrogen receptors-beta and serotonin mediate the antidepressant-like effect of an aqueous extract of pomegranate in ovariectomized rats. Neurochem Int. 2021;142:104904.
114. Goel N, Bale TL. Sex differences in the serotonergic influence on the hypothalamic-pituitary-adrenal stress axis. Endocrinology. 2010;151(4): 1784–1794.
115. Kranz GS, Kasper S, Lanzenberger R. Reward and the serotonergic sys-tem. Neuroscience. 2010;166(4):1023–1035.
116. Kugaya A, Epperson CN, Zoghbi S, et al. Increase in prefrontal cortex serotonin 2A receptors following estrogen treatment in postmeno-pausal women. Am J Psychiatry. 2003;160(8):1522–1524.
117. Perfalk E, Cunha-Bang SD, Holst KK, et al. Testosterone levels in healthy men correlate negatively with serotonin 4 receptor binding. Psycho-neuroendocrinology. 2017;81:22–28.
118. Kranz GS, Wadsak W, Kaufmann U, et al. High-dose testosterone treat-ment increases serotonin transporter binding in transgender people. Biol Psychiatry. 2015;78(4):525–533.
119. Scott LV, Dinan TG. Vasopressin and the regulation of hypothalamic-pituitary-adrenal axis function: Implications for the pathophysiology of depression. Life Sci. 1998;62(22):1985–1998.
120. Gillies GE, Linton EA, Lowry PJ. Corticotropin releasing activity of the new CRF is potentiated several times by vasopressin. Nature. 1982; 299(5881):355–357.
121. Bredewold R, Veenema AH. Sex differences in the regulation of social and anxiety-related behaviors: Insights from vasopressin and oxytocin brain systems. Curr Opin Neurobiol. 2018;49:132–140.
122. de Vries GJ. Sex differences in vasopressin and oxytocin innervation of the brain. Prog Brain Res. 2008;170:17–27.
123. Bingham B, Myung C, Innala L, et al. Androgen receptors in the posterior bed nucleus of the stria terminalis increase neuropeptide expression and the stress-induced activation of the paraventricular nucleus of the hypothalamus. Neuropsychopharmacology. 2011;36(7):1433–1443.
124. Zhou L, Blaustein JD, De Vries GJ. Distribution of androgen receptor immunoreactivity in vasopressin- and oxytocin-immunoreactive neu-rons in the male rat brain. Endocrinology. 1994;134(6):2622–2627.
125. Axelson JF, Leeuwen FW. Differential localization of estrogen receptors in various vasopressin synthesizing nuclei of the rat brain. J Neuroendocrinol. 1990;2(2):209–216.
126. Kanaya M, Higo S, Ozawa H. Neurochemical characterization of neurons expressing estrogen receptor beta in the hypothalamic nuclei of rats using in situ hybridization and immunofluorescence. Int J Mol Sci. 2019; 21(1):115–.

127. Simonian SX, Herbison AE. Differential expression of estrogen receptor alpha and beta immunoreactivity by oxytocin neurons of rat paraventricular nucleus. J Neuroendocrinol. 1997;9(11):803–806.

128. Pak TR, Chung WC, Hinds LR, et al. Estrogen receptor-beta mediates dihydrotestosterone-induced stimulation of the arginine vasopressin promoter in neuronal cells. Endocrinology. 2007;148(7):3371–3382.

129. Ebner K, Wotjak CT, Holsboer F, et al. Vasopressin released within the septal brain area during swim stress modulates the behavioural stress response in rats. Eur J Neurosci. 1999;11(3):997–1002.

130. Singewald GM, Rjabokon A, Singewald N, et al. The modulatory role of the lateral septum on neuroendocrine and behavioral stress responses. Neuropsychopharmacology. 2011;36(4):793–804.

131. Kim S, Soeken TA, Cromer SJ, et al. Oxytocin and postpartum depression: Delivering on what's known and what's not. Brain Res. 2014;1580:219–232.

132. Neumann ID, Kromer SA, Toschi N, et al. Brain oxytocin inhibits the (re)activity of the hypothalamo-pituitary-adrenal axis in male rats: Involvement of hypothalamic and limbic brain regions. Regul Pept. 2000;96(1-2):31–38.

133. Windle RJ, Kershaw YM, Shanks N, et al. Oxytocin attenuates stress-induced c-fos mRNA expression in specific forebrain regions associated with modulation of hypothalamo-pituitary-adrenal activity. J Neurosci. 2004;24(12):2974–2982.

134. Windle RJ, Gamble LE, Kershaw YM, et al. Gonadal steroid modulation of stress-induced hypothalamo-pituitary-adrenal activity and anxiety behavior: Role of central oxytocin. Endocrinology. 2006;147(5):2423–2431.

135. Ochedalski T, Subburaju S, Wynn PC, et al. Interaction between oestrogen and oxytocin on hypothalamic-pituitary-adrenal axis activity. J Neuroendocrinol. 2007;19(3):189–197.

136. Mantella RC, Vollmer RR, Amico JA. Corticosterone release is heightened in food or water deprived oxytocin deficient male mice. Brain Res. 2005;1058(1-2):56–61.

137. Hiroi R, Lacagnina AF, Hinds LR, et al. The androgen metabolite, 5alpha-androstane-3beta,17beta-diol (3beta-diol), activates the oxytocin promoter through an estrogen receptor-beta pathway. Endocrinology. 2013;154(5):1802–1812.

138. Johnson AE, Ball GF, Coirini H, et al. Time course of the estradiol-dependent induction of oxytocin receptor binding in the ventromedial hypothalamic nucleus of the rat. Endocrinology. 1989;125(3):1414–1419.

139. Patisaul HB, Scordalakes EM, Young LJ, et al. Oxytocin, but not oxytocin receptor, is regulated by oestrogen receptor beta in the female mouse hypothalamus. J Neuroendocrinol. 2003;15(8):787–793.

140. Kudwa AE, McGivern RF, Handa RJ. Estrogen receptor beta and oxytocin interact to modulate anxiety-like behavior and neuroendocrine stress reactivity in adult male and female rats. Physiol Behav. 2014;129:287–296.

141. McEwen BS. Hormones and behavior and the integration of brain-body science. Horm Behav. 2020;119:104619.

142. Heck AL, Sheng JA, Miller AM, et al. Social isolation alters hypothalamic pituitary adrenal axis activity after chronic variable stress in male C57BL/6 mice. Stress. 2020;23(4):457–465.

143. Kuhlman KR, Chiang JJ, Horn S, et al. Developmental psychoneuroendocrine and psychoneuroimmune pathways from childhood adversity to disease. Neurosci Biobehav Rev. 2017;80:166–184.

144. Kokras N, Hodes GE, Bangasser DA, et al. Sex differences in the hypothalamic-pituitary-adrenal axis: An obstacle to antidepressant drug development? Br J Pharmacol. 2019;176(21):4090–4106.

145. Kang HJ, Park Y, Yoo KH, et al. Sex differences in the genetic architecture of depression. Sci Rep. 2020;10(1):9927.

146. Labonte B, Engmann O, Purushothaman I, et al. Sex-specific transcriptional signatures in human depression. Nat Med. 2017;23(9):1102–1111.

147. Kessler RC, McGonagle KA, Nelson CB, et al. Sex and depression in the National Comorbidity Survey. II: Cohort effects. J Affect Disord. 1994;30(1):15–26.

148. Baillargeon J, Kuo YF, Fang X, et al. Long-term exposure to testosterone therapy and the risk of high grade prostate cancer. J Urol. 2015;194(6):1612–1616.

149. Jezova D, Herman JP. Stress and stress-related disease states as topics of multi-approach research. Stress. 2020;23(6):615–616.

150. Elliott J, Kelly SE, Millar AC, et al. Testosterone therapy in hypogonadal men: A systematic review and network meta-analysis. BMJ Open. 2017;7(11):e015284.

151. Walther A, Breidenstein J, Miller R. Association of testosterone treatment with alleviation of depressive symptoms in men: A systematic review and meta-analysis. JAMA Psychiatry. 2019;76(1):31–40.

152. Bhasin S, Brito JP, Cunningham GR, et al. Testosterone therapy in men with hypogonadism: An Endocrine Society Clinical Practice Guideline. J Clin Endocrinol Metab. 2018;103(5):1715–1744.

153. Paizanis E, Hamon M, Lanfumey L. Hippocampal neurogenesis, depressive disorders, and antidepressant therapy. Neural Plast. 2007;2007:73754.

154. Fernandez-Guasti A, Martinez-Mota L. Anxiolytic-like actions of testosterone in the burying behavior test: Role of androgen and GABA-benzodiazepine receptors. Psychoneuroendocrinology. 2005;30(8):762–770.

155. Aikey JL, Nyby JG, Anmuth DM, et al. Testosterone rapidly reduces anxiety in male house mice (Mus musculus). Horm Behav. 2002;42(4):448–460.

156. Hodosy J, Zelmanova D, Majzunova M, et al. The anxiolytic effect of testosterone in the rat is mediated via the androgen receptor. Pharmacol Biochem Behav. 2012;102(2):191–195.

157. Wolkowitz OM, Reus VI, Roberts E, et al. Dehydroepiandrosterone (DHEA) treatment of depression. Biol Psychiatry. 1997;41(3):311–318.

158. Jin RO, Mason S, Mellon SH, et al. Cortisol/DHEA ratio and hippocampal volume: A pilot study in major depression and healthy controls. Psychoneuroendocrinology. 2016;72:139–146.

159. Jiang X, Zhong W, An H, et al. Attenuated DHEA and DHEA-S response to acute psychosocial stress in individuals with depressive disorders. J Affect Disord. 2017;215:118–124.

160. Bentley C, Hazeldine J, Greig C, et al. Dehydroepiandrosterone: A potential therapeutic agent in the treatment and rehabilitation of the traumatically injured patient. Burns Trauma. 2019;7:26.

161. Strous RD, Maayan R, Lapidus R, et al. Dehydroepiandrosterone augmentation in the management of negative, depressive, and anxiety symptoms in schizophrenia. Arch Gen Psychiatry. 2003;60(2):133–141.

162. Peixoto C, Jose Grande A, Gomes Carrilho C, et al. Dehydroepiandrosterone for depressive symptoms: A systematic review and meta-analysis of randomized controlled trials. J Neurosci Res. 2020;98(12):2510–2528.

163. Peixoto C, Grande AJ, Mallmann MB, et al. Dehydroepiandrosterone (DHEA) for depression: A systematic review and meta-analysis. CNS Neurol Disord Drug Targets. 2018;17(9):706–711.

164. Uh D, Jeong HG, Choi KY, et al. Dehydroepiandrosterone sulfate level varies nonlinearly with symptom severity in Major Depressive Disorder. Clin Psychopharmacol Neurosci. 2017;15(2):163–169.

165. Dalton JT, Mukherjee A, Zhu Z, et al. Discovery of nonsteroidal androgens. Biochem Biophys Res Commun. 1998;244(1):1–4.

166. Hikichi Y, Yamaoka M, Kusaka M, et al. Selective androgen receptor modulator activity of a steroidal antiandrogen TSAA-291 and its cofactor recruitment profile. Eur J Pharmacol. 2015;765:322–331.

167. Solomon ZJ, Mirabal JR, Mazur DJ, et al. Selective androgen receptor modulators: Current knowledge and clinical applications. Sex Med Rev. 2019;7(1):84–94.

168. Handlon AL, Schaller LT, Leesnitzer LM, et al. Optimizing ligand efficiency of Selective Androgen Receptor Modulators (SARMs). ACS Med Chem Lett. 2016;7(1):83–88.

169. George S, Petit GH, Gouras GK, et al. Nonsteroidal selective androgen receptor modulators and selective estrogen receptor beta agonists moderate cognitive deficits and amyloid-beta levels in a mouse model of Alzheimer's disease. ACS Chem Neurosci. 2013;4(12):1537–1548.

170. Crawford J, Prado CM, Johnston MA, et al. Study design and rationale for the Phase 3 Clinical Development Program of Enobosarm, a Selective Androgen Receptor Modulator, for the Prevention and Treatment of Muscle Wasting in Cancer Patients (POWER Trials). Curr Oncol Rep. 2016;18(6):37.

171. Dobs AS, Boccia RV, Croot CC, et al. Effects of enobosarm on muscle wasting and physical function in patients with cancer: A double-blind, randomised controlled phase 2 trial. Lancet Oncol. 2013;14(4):335–345.

172. Dalton JT, Barnette KG, Bohl CE, et al. The selective androgen receptor modulator GTx-024 (enobosarm) improves lean body mass and physical function in healthy elderly men and postmenopausal women: Results of a double-blind, placebo-controlled phase II trial. J Cachexia Sarcopenia Muscle. 2011;2(3):153–161.

173. Narayanan R, Coss CC, Dalton JT. Development of selective androgen receptor modulators (SARMs). Mol Cell Endocrinol. 2018;465:134–142.

174. Krishnan V, Patel NJ, Mackrell JG, et al. Development of a selective androgen receptor modulator for transdermal use in hypogonadal patients. Andrology. 2018;6(3):455–464.

Abbreviations Used

17β-HSD = 17β-hydroxysteroid dehydrogenase
3α-diol = 3α-androstanediol glucuronide
3β-diol = 5α-androstane-3β, 17β diol
3β-HSD = 3β-hydroxysteroid dehydrogenase
5αR = 5α-reductase
5-HT = serotonin
ACTH = adrenocorticotropin hormone
AR = androgen receptor
ARE = androgen response element
AVP = arginine vasopressin
BnST = bed nucleus stria terminalis
CBG = corticosteroid binding globulin
CORT = corticosterone
CRFR1 = corticotropin-releasing factor receptor 1
CRFR2 = corticotropin-releasing factor receptor 2
CRH = corticotropin-releasing factor
DA = dopamine

D1 = DA receptor 1
D2 = DA receptor 2
DHEA = dehydroepiandrosterone
DHT = dihydrotestosterone
DHTP = DHT propionate
DPN = diarylpropionitrile
E2 = estradiol
ER = estrogen receptor
ERE = estrogen response element
ERα = estrogen receptor alpha
ERβ = estrogen receptor beta
GABA = gamma-aminobutyric acid
GC = glucocorticoids
GDX = gonadectomy
GR = GC receptor
GREs = GC response elements
HPA = hypothalamic/pituitary/adrenal
iTfm = induced testicular feminization mutation
LS = lateral septum
MDS = mesolimbic DA system
MeA = medial amygdala
MR = mineralocorticoid receptor
OT = oxytocin
PPT = propylpyrazoletriol
PVN = paraventricular nucleus of the hypothalamus
SARM = selective AR modulator
SHIP = short heterodimer partner
T = testosterone
Tfm = testicular feminization mutation
TRT = testosterone replacement therapy
VMH = ventromedial hypothalamus

4

Androgens and Adult Neurogenesis in the Hippocampus

Samantha A. Blankers[1,2] and Liisa A.M. Galea[1–3,*,i]

Abstract

Adult neurogenesis in the hippocampus is modulated by steroid hormones, including androgens, in male rodents. In this review, we summarize research showing that chronic exposure to androgens, such as testosterone and dihydrotestosterone, enhances the survival of new neurons in the dentate gyrus of male, but not female, rodents, via the androgen receptor. However, the neurogenesis promoting the effect of androgens in the dentate gyrus may be limited to younger adulthood as it is not evident in middle-aged male rodents. Although direct exposure to androgens in adult or middle age does not significantly influence neurogenesis in female rodents, the aromatase inhibitor letrozole enhances neurogenesis in the hippocampus of middle-aged female mice. Unlike other androgens, androgenic anabolic steroids reduce neurogenesis in the hippocampus of male rodents. Collectively, the research indicates that the ability of androgens to enhance hippocampal neurogenesis in adult rodents is dependent on dose, androgen type, sex, duration, and age. We discuss these findings and how androgens may be influencing neuroprotection, via neurogenesis in the hippocampus, in the context of health and disease.

Keywords: dentate gyrus; sex differences; aging; dihydrotestosterone; testosterone; cognition

Introduction

Efforts to characterize the postnatal production of new neurons have been ongoing since the concept was first introduced through experiments by Joseph Altman in the 1960s.[1] Although Altman's findings were initially dismissed by the scientific community, the notion of structural plasticity of dendritic spines in the adult brain gained acceptance with time[2–4] (reviewed in Bosch and Hayashi[5]) and studies in songbirds confirmed that new cells produced postnatally were morphologically similar to neurons.[6,7] Great progress has been made since these initial findings, through extensive research in neurogenic brain regions, including the hippocampus and olfactory bulb.[8–18] Even in the early studies by Altman, it was suspected that androgens may be involved in the regulation of neurogenesis in the hippocampus.[1] Indeed, decades later, it was noted that seasonal fluctuations in hippocampal neurogenesis coincide with changes in gonadal hormone levels in meadow voles[19] and in black-capped chickadees[20] of both sexes. Moreover, sex differences have been identified in the maturation and attrition of new neurons in the hippocampus of rats[21] and in response to certain stimuli such as stress in rats[22,23]; for review see Ref.[24] These findings warranted further investigation into the role of sex-steroid hormones in the regulation of hippocampal neurogenesis, including the sex-specific effects of estrogens and androgens. Thus, in this review, we discuss the stages and function of adult neurogenesis in the hippocampus, followed by the influence of androgens on different stages of hippocampal neurogenesis and in response to injury or disease. Within each section, we discuss sex differences in the influence of androgens, if known.

[1]Graduate Program in Neuroscience, The University of British Columbia, Vancouver, Canada.
[2]Djavad Mowafaghian Centre for Brain Health, The University of British Columbia, Vancouver, Canada.
[3]Department of Psychology, The University of British Columbia, Vancouver, Canada.
[i]ORCID ID (https://orcid.org/0000-0003-2874-9972).

*Address correspondence to: Liisa A.M. Galea, PhD, Graduate Program in Neuroscience, The University of British Columbia, 2215 Wesbrook Mall, Vancouver V6T 1Z3, British Columbia, Canada, Email: liisa.galea@ubc.ca

Androgens

Androgens are sex steroid hormones produced in Leydig cells of the testes and thecal–interstitial cells of the ovaries, as well as in the zona reticularis of the adrenal glands in both males and females.[25,26] In addition, androgens are produced in the brain itself, via either local production or *de novo* synthesis of steroids.[27–30] It is also important to recognize that the systemic levels of androgens are associated with levels in the hippocampus[31] and influence local and *de novo* production of androgens,[32] although more studies are needed. Some of the widely studied androgens include testosterone, 5α-dihydrotestosterone (DHT), androstenedione, and dehydroepiandrosterone (DHEA) among others.[33] Testosterone can be metabolized to other androgens or to estradiol, the most potent of the natural estrogens, and thus can exert its effects via androgen receptors (ARs) or estrogen receptors (ERs) depending on the availability of enzymes. Testosterone can be reduced to the potent androgen DHT via the enzyme 5α-reductase. DHT can be further metabolized to 5α-androstane-3α,17β-diol (3α-diol) and 5α-androstane-3β,17β-diol (3β-diol).[34] Both 3α-diol and 3β-diol possess weak affinity for ARs,[35] although 3β-diol displays preferential activity at ERβ.[36] Testosterone can also be aromatized to estradiol,[34] which binds to ERα, ERβ, and the G protein-coupled ER (GPER). The ARs and ERs are most often found in intracellular locations or on the nucleus, but they can also be located on the membrane.[37–39] Ligand binding, when located in the intracellular compartment, causes the AR or ER to be transported to the nucleus, where they may influence transcription of target genes to elicit genomic effects that occur on a scale of hours to days.[40] In addition, estradiol can bind to membrane-associated ERs such as GPER to induce rapid non-genomic effects through second-messenger signaling.[39]

The ERs are abundant in the hippocampus, with a high concentration of GPER in CA1, CA3, and the dentate gyrus[41] and the highest density of ERα and ERβ in CA3 region compared with the other subregions of the hippocampus in male and female rats.[42,43] On the other hand, ARs are not abundant in the dentate gyrus relative to the CA1 and CA3 regions of the hippocampus in both sexes.[44–48]. Indeed, the highest expression of ARs in the hippocampus is in the CA1 region in both sexes, which will vary by hormonal status (intact vs. gonadectomized).[44–48] Studies have found that the density of ARs in the hippocampus increases with age, as serum testosterone levels decline.[47,49] Sex differences in AR expression have been detected, as the density of AR in the CA1 region of males is greater than that of the CA1 region of females[48] but this is not seen in all studies,[47] likely due to differences in whether gonadectomized versus intact rats were used. Indeed, intact males had higher AR expression in the CA1 region compared with intact females[49] but there are no significant sex differences in AR expression when comparing gonadectomized rats.[47] In addition, the gene encoding the AR protein contains a polymorphic cytosine-adenine-guanine (CAG) microsatellite of variable lengths ranging from 6 to 39 repeats at the N-terminal transactivation domain.[50] The functionality of ARs depends on the number of CAG repeats, as transactivation of AR decreases with CAG repeat expansion.[51] Therefore, androgens act through ERs or ARs that are expressed in the hippocampus and influenced by several factors such as age, sex, and genetics.

Adult Neurogenesis

Neurogenesis is defined as the creation and functional integration of new neurons produced from neural stem/progenitor cells. There are several stages of neurogenesis that include cell proliferation, migration, differentiation, and survival of newly generated neurons (Fig. 1). Various internal and external factors have been identified as regulators of neurogenesis in each one of these stages; therefore, it is critical to be aware of the stage of neurogenesis being evaluated within an individual experiment. There are many methods available for the detection of newly formed neurons, each with their own strengths and limitations.[53,56,57] Endogenous proteins, such as Ki67, are expressed during all stages of the cell cycle except G_0 and are used to measure cell proliferation.[53] Doublecortin (DCX), another endogenous protein, is used to measure the presence of immature neurons, as it is expressed during proliferation until approximately day 21 in rats.[54] Exogenous DNA-markers, such as ³H-thymidine, or synthetic nucleosides, such as 5-bromo-2-deoxyuridine (BrdU), may be used to monitor the production and survival of new neurons depending on the time between injection and perfusion. These markers are incorporated during DNA synthesis and may be visualized postmortem to detect newly generated cells in a region of interest.[58,59] The timing between administration of DNA synthesis markers and perfusion of the animal is significant, as different time spans will measure different stages of neurogenesis. If animals are perfused 24 h or less after BrdU administration, this will be a measure of cell proliferation, whereas a span of >24 h

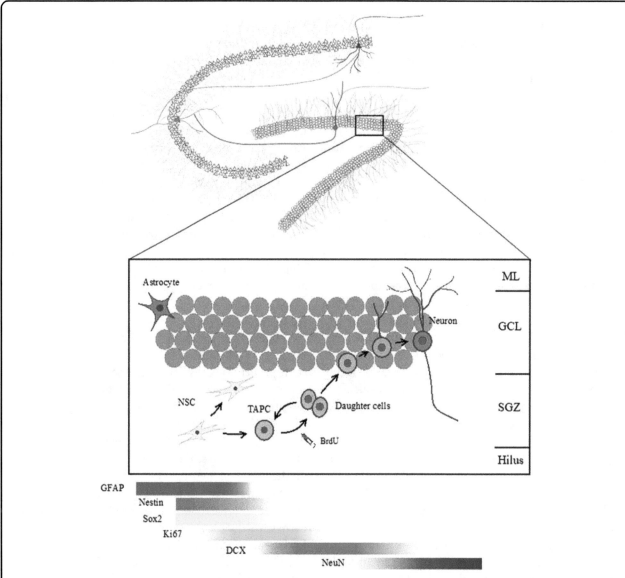

FIG. 1. Schematic image of a coronal section of the rodent hippocampus and stages of adult neurogenesis. An NSC can give rise to a TAPC, which is divided into two NPCs that migrate in the GCL of the dentate gyrus, differentiate into neurons, and send dendrites to the ML.[52] The NSCs express the glia cell marker, GFAP, and NSC markers, Nestin, and Sox2.[52] Ki67 is a nuclear protein that is expressed during all active phases of the cell cycle and thus is a marker of cell proliferation.[53] DCX is a microtubule-associated protein expressed in the cytoplasm of dividing NPC and immature neurons.[54] NeuN protein is expressed in new neurons beginning about 1 week after mitosis in rats and 2 weeks after mitosis in mice and is used as a nuclear marker for mature neurons.[55] BrdU is a DNA synthesis marker that is incorporated into cells that are actively synthesized DNA within the 2 h after injection (and in effect time stamps when the cell was produced). Depending on the length of time between injection and perfusion, BrdU-immunoreactive cells will label cell proliferation or the survival of new cells. Zif268 is an immediate early gene and will indicate whether a cell has been recently active (action potential). Reprinted with permission from Yagi et al.[21] BrdU, 5-bromo-2-deoxyuridine; DCX, doublecortin; GCL, granular cell layer; GFAP, glial fibrillary acidic protein; ML, molecular layer; NeuN, neuronal nuclei; NPC, neural progenitor cells; NSC, neural stem cell; SGZ, subgranular zone; TAPC, transient amplifying progenitor cell.

will measure survival of the daughter cells.[56,60] Further, the timing of experimental manipulation in relation to BrdU administration is important, as this will capture survival of new neurons either dependent or independent of the influence of cell proliferation; for review see Refs.[56,61] It is noteworthy that endogenous markers of mature neurons must be used in combination with thymidine analogues to determine whether newly formed cells are new neurons; therefore, the co-expression of BrdU with endogenous markers such as neuronal nuclei is often used to detect new neurons versus the use of glial fibrillary acidic protein used for the detection of new glial cells.[62]

As expected, neurogenesis occurs at a high level during development and diminishes in adulthood, and this has been observed across a wide variety of species, including primates[8,9] and rodents.[10,11] Under normal conditions, neurogenesis occurs in two distinct regions of the brain: the subventricular zone (SVZ), the lining of the lateral ventricles and the subgranular zone (SGZ) of the hippocampus. The SVZ contains mostly multipotent neural stem cells (NSCs), whereas the proliferative precursor cells of the SGZ were previously identified as mainly neural progenitor cells (NPC).[63,64] However, studies have revealed the presence of multipotent NSCs in the SGZ,[65–67] which ultimately give rise to NPC[68] that proliferate and migrate to the granular layer where most will differentiate into granule cells.[1,69] Multipotent NSCs have the capacity for self-renewal and can give rise to multiple types of mature neural cells.[70] The NPC are distinct, as they have a limited capacity for self-renewal and usually differentiate into one specific type of neural cell.[70] The NPC originating in the SGZ proliferate and migrate to the granular layer, where most will differentiate into granule cells.[1,69] Intriguingly, a few studies suggest that there is little decline in the number of new immature neurons throughout adulthood in humans.[16–18] Evidence for neurogenesis in the hippocampus of humans has been demonstrated in a multitude of studies using a variety of techniques.[12–18] Thus, these studies support the consensus that neurogenesis in the human hippocampus is evident throughout adult life, although this claim is not entirely undisputed.[71,72] This review will focus on the influence of androgens in hippocampal neurogenesis, and the reader is directed to other reviews on hormones and the SVZ.[73,74]

Function of Adult Hippocampal Neurogenesis

It is one thing to produce new neurons in the adult brain, but do these new neurons form meaningful connections to alter the function of the hippocampus? It is important to recognize that a new neuron could make aberrant connections that might interfere with the normal function of the dentate gyrus.[75,76] Ectopic new neurons can interfere with normal activity of the dentate gyrus, as seen with hippocampal neurogenesis after seizures in animal models of temporal lobe epilepsy.[75,77] Populations of these new neurons form aberrant axon projections that are characteristic of those seen in postmortem humans with temporal lobe epilepsy,[77,78] and this abnormal cytoarchitecture may result in long-term alterations of hippocampal circuitry.[75] Indeed, seizure-induced increases in neurogenesis is commensurate with reduced memory, and when neurogenesis is reduced in response to seizures, memory is improved.[75] On the other hand, voluntary wheel-running increases both hippocampal neurogenesis and performance on several new memory tasks in mice.[79–81] Jakubs et al. used whole cell-patch clamp recordings to compare the properties of new neurons generated on exposure to either running or induced seizures in rats. Both running and seizures will increase neurogenesis in the hippocampus, but new neurons generated in runners demonstrated higher excitatory synaptic drive and lower inhibitory synaptic drive compared with new neurons generated with seizures.[76] Together, these findings demonstrate that new neurons may have distinct functional properties that are dependent on the circumstances of which neurogenesis was induced; thus, increased neurogenesis is not always beneficial to the individual if atypical integration occurs; for review see Refs.[82–84]

New neurons appropriately integrated into the hippocampal circuit are believed to influence and support brain functioning in a variety of ways.[24,52,61,68,85] The hippocampus is critical in forming contextually rich memories[86] due to the neuronal characteristics of the dentate gyrus. That is, discrete representations of memory are possible because neurons of the dentate gyrus are able to discriminate between small differences in cortical input patterns.[87] Briefly, adult hippocampal neurogenesis is critical in discrimination between highly similar situations,[88–92] a phenomenon known as pattern separation.[93] Other studies have shown that hippocampal neurogenesis is critical for context encoding in spatial discrimination tasks and contextual/trace fear conditioning[89,94–97] in both male and female mice; for review see Refs.[98,99] Functional differences exist between the dorsal and ventral hippocampus due in part to their distinct connections to extra-hippocampal structures, receptor density patterns, and gene expression patterns.[100,101] The dorsal hippocampus is responsible for cognitive processing whereas the ventral hippocampus regulates emotional processing, including mood and stress.[102] It has been proposed that hippocampal neurogenesis, particularly in the ventral hippocampus, is implicated in this emotional regulation.[103] Animal models of depression in male and female rodents decrease neurogenesis in the ventral dentate gyrus[104] and chronic, but not acute, treatment with pharmacological antidepressants restores neurogenesis in the dentate gyrus of male and female rodents.[24,105,106] In primates, the anterior hippocampus is akin to the ventral hippocampus of rodents, and humans with major depressive disorder show decreased cell proliferation[107] which is increased with antidepressant exposure[107] in the anterior hippocampus, dependent on factors such as age and sex.[108] Further, Surget et al.[109] found that the antidepressant fluoxetine was not effective in restoring a dysregulated hippocampal-driven response to chronic stress unless an intact neurogenic system was present in the ventral hippocampus of male mice. Therefore, numerous lines of evidence suggest that neurogenesis in adulthood influences various aspects of brain function, including mood, stress, and cognition, dependent on the brain region in which new neurons are integrating.

Androgens and Adult Hippocampal Neurogenesis

In the following sections, we discuss the influence of androgen manipulations on hippocampal neurogenesis in males and females across the adult lifespan and in response to injury or disease.

Castration and Adult Hippocampal Neurogenesis

Reproductive status influences neurogenesis in the hippocampus of male rodents.[110,111] Reproductively active male meadow voles had increased survival of new neurons compared with reproductively inactive male meadow voles.[110] Castrated adult rats and mice show decreased survival of new neurons or fewer immature neurons in the dentate gyrus compared with intact males.[111-114] On the other hand, castration before adolescence does not have the same effect on hippocampal neurogenesis as it increased neurogenesis in the hippocampus of male rhesus macaque monkeys[115] and had no significant influence on hippocampal neurogenesis in male rats.[116] These studies collectively indicate that

the timing of castration during the lifespan matters for the influence on hippocampal neurogenesis, with adult castration decreasing but adolescent castration either increasing or not affecting neurogenesis in the hippocampus.

Androgens and Adult Hippocampal Neurogenesis in Males

Chronic exposure to androgens generally upregulates neurogenesis in the hippocampus of male, but not female, rodents via enhancement of new neuron survival in a dose-dependent manner.[47,111] Thirty days of testosterone or DHT exposure enhances neurogenesis by promoting the survival of new neurons in male rodents.[111] Interestingly, this effect is not seen with shorter testosterone replacement schedules of 15–21 days,[106,117] indicating that 30 days of testosterone replacement is necessary to observe increased survival of new neurons in the hippocampus. The influence of testosterone to promote neurogenesis in the hippocampus may be independent of any effects on cell proliferation, as 21 days of testosterone did not influence cell proliferation.[106] However, long-term but not short-term castration in adulthood decreases cell proliferation in rats,[111,112] suggesting that there may be an influence of longer-term androgen exposure on cell proliferation in the dentate gyrus.

Several lines of evidence support the notion that testosterone exerts its influence on hippocampal neurogenesis by interacting with the AR. First, treatment with estradiol has no significant effect on the survival of new neurons in adult males,[111] indicating that ER activation is not responsible for neurogenic effects of androgens in males. On the other hand, DHT, which directly stimulates the AR, increased the survival of new neurons, similar to testosterone.[44,111] The neurogenesis-promoting effect of DHT was blocked in the presence of flutamide, a competitive AR antagonist.[44] Moreover, chronic testosterone had no effect on the survival of new neurons in rats with a testicular feminization mutation, which lack a functional AR,[44] indicating that androgens influence neurogenesis through an AR-mediated mechanism. However, considering that testosterone and DHT increase neurogenesis by promoting the survival of new neurons, it is a matter of curiosity that ARs are not located on immature neurons (DCX-expressing cells) in male rats or mice in the dentate gyrus.[44,114] On the other hand, ARs are expressed in the CA3 region of the hippocampus,[45-47] which is the axonal projection site of newly formed neurons.[118,119] Androgens, via the AR, rapidly increase thorny excrescences in the CA3 region, which are the post-synaptic regions of the mossy fibers.[120] Therefore, it is possible that the small number of ARs located in the dentate gyrus and/or ARs located in the terminal region for granule cells in the CA3 region are responsible, at least in part, for the AR-dependent promotion of neurogenesis in the hippocampus.

Androgens and Adult Hippocampal Neurogenesis in Females

Although androgens promote neurogenesis in males, 30 days of testosterone or DHT treatment do not affect neurogenesis in young adult or middle-aged female rats.[47] Although these findings suggest that androgens do not support neurogenesis in females, Chaiton et al.[121] found that chronic treatment with letrozole, an aromatase inhibitor, increased neurogenesis (cell proliferation and density of immature neurons) in the hippocampus of middle-aged female mice. As letrozole inhibits the conversion of androgens into estradiol (Fig. 2), this result implies that the increase in neurogenesis may be related to the increase in androgens induced by letrozole, and/or the decrease in estradiol synthesis. Although letrozole increased the number of doublecortin cells (immature neurons) of middle-aged females, it suppresses the cell proliferation of cultured neurons from postnatal day 5 female rats,[122] indicating age differences in the influence of letrozole on neurogenesis in the hippocampus.

In adult females, the influence of estradiol on adult hippocampal neurogenesis is complex, as it is dependent

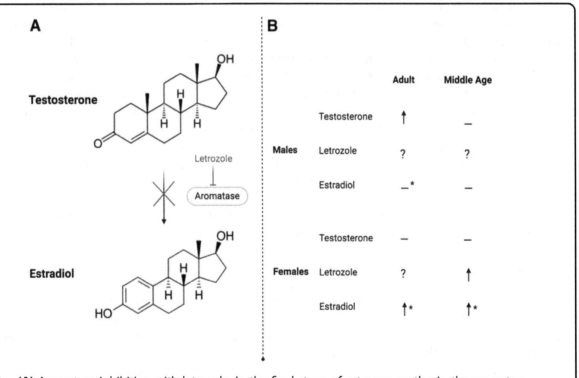

FIG. 2. **(A)** Aromatase inhibition with letrozole. In the final stage of estrogen synthesis, the aromatase inhibitor letrozole prevents the aromatization of testosterone into estradiol. **(B)** Testosterone, letrozole, and estradiol effects on survival of new neurons in the hippocampus of adult roents. In males, testosterone, but not estradiol, treatment increases the survival of new neurons in adults, although no significant effect is seen in middle age. The influence of letrozole has yet to be studied in males. In females, testosterone does not influence cell survival in either adulthood or middle age. Letrozole increases new neuron survival in middle-aged females, although studies in adults have yet to be completed. Lastly, estradiol increases the survival of new neurons in both adult and middle-aged females, although the paradigm used in the experiment influences the resulting effects on new neuron survival as indicated with an asterisk (*). Figure created using Biorender.com.

on dose, sex, age, reproductive experience, and timing of estradiol exposure[123–127]; for review see Ref.[24] As mentioned earlier, the survival of new neurons is enhanced by chronic exposure to testosterone and DHT, but not estradiol, in adult male rats.[111] However, other studies show that brief exposure to estradiol can increase neurogenesis in male meadow voles when administered during the time when new neurons are extending their axons.[125] Together, these results demonstrate that sex hormone-mediated regulation of hippocampal neurogenesis is distinct in males compared with females, with more neurogenic effects of androgens in males and more neurogenic effects of estrogens in females.

Age Effects of Androgens and Hippocampal Neurogenesis

Age is an additional factor that influences the effects of androgens on neurogenesis in males. Chronic DHT treatment increased new neuron survival in young, but not middle-aged, adult gonadectomized male rats.[47] Consistent with this, Moser et al.[128] found that 12 weeks of testosterone failed to increase neurogenesis (DCX-expressing cells) in both intact middle-aged and aged male rats. These findings are in contrast with the increased neurogenesis observed in young adult males with chronic testosterone or DHT,[111] suggesting that aging influences the ability of the dentate gyrus to respond to the pro-neurogenic effects of androgen signaling in male rats. This is a matter of curiosity, as ARs are evident in the dentate gyrus of middle-aged rodents, potentially at even higher levels than in young adults.[47,49] Although AR levels may be higher in aged males compared with young males,[47,49] it is possible that AR functionality decreases with age. Further, it is noteworthy that long-term castration resulted in loss of granule neurons in the dentate gyrus of adult male rats, which can be ameliorated by early but not late chronic DHT treatment,[129] indicating a critical window for the neuroplasticity-promoting effect of DHT. Whether or not this critical window exists with respect to DHT's ability to increase adult hippocampal neurogenesis has not yet been studied. However, it is evident that androgens are not promoting neurogenesis in intact or gonadectomized middle-aged animals, but it remains to be determined whether this has to do with dose, critical window, or the functionality of AR with aging.

Here, we concentrate our discussion on adult neurogenesis in the hippocampus, but it is important to consider that androgen exposure during gestation or the early postpartum period influences neurogenesis of the developing offspring in both sexes.[130–133] Briefly, mothers exposed to a hyperandrogenic environment during gestation produced offspring with decreased survival of new neurons in the dentate gyrus of both male and female rats.[130] On the other hand, there is evidence that androgens promote the survival of new neurons during the postpartum period in rats of both sexes.[132,133] Thus, there are likely distinct mechanisms by which androgens influence neurogenesis during gestation and early development.

Effects of DHEA and Androstenedione on Hippocampal Neurogenesis

Although the majority of studies on androgens and neurogenesis have focused on testosterone and DHT, there is some evidence for the pro-neurogenic effects of DHEA.[134–137] DHEA has distinct cellular effects from other androgens, such as DHT and testosterone, as DHEA preferentially activates ERβ while also demonstrating affinity for ERα and AR[138–140] along with other nuclear and membrane-bound receptors (reviewed in Prough et al.[141]). The NSCs derived from the human male fetal cortex demonstrated increased cell survival with DHEA treatment compared with controls.[137] In adult and middle-aged male rats, DHEA increases the survival of new neurons after repeated or chronic treatment.[134,135] Short-term treatment (12 days) with DHEA increased the number of new neurons as well as cell proliferation in the dentate gyrus of adult male rats, and pretreatment with DHEA was protective against corticosterone injections, which inhibit neurogenesis.[135] The same study found that pretreatment with androstenedione had no influence on the inhibition of neurogenesis seen with corticosterone administration[135] but did not evaluate androstenedione alone. In adult male songbirds, although DHEA increased immature neurons (DCX-expressing cells) in the HVC, a brain region involved in song production, it did not do so in the hippocampus.[136] Thus, DHEA promotes the survival of new neurons in multiple species, increasing cell proliferation and protecting against stress in adult male rats specifically.

Androgenic Anabolic Steroids and Hippocampal Neurogenesis

Other compounds of interest include androgenic anabolic steroids (AAS) such as the testosterone analogue 19-nortestosterone, also known as nandrolone. Excessive use of AAS has been linked to mood disturbances[142] such as mania and major depression in humans. On the cellular level, nandrolone elicits its effects in the brain by binding to the AR and repeated administration causes AR upregulation.[143] A study utilizing rat NSCs in culture and in the dentate gyrus revealed that the administration of nandrolone for 5 days decreased the number of new neurons detected in the dentate gyrus through an AR-mediated mechanism.[144] Another study showed that chronic (28 days) treatment with supraphysiological doses of nandrolone eliminated the strength training-induced enhancement of cell proliferation in the dentate gyrus of adult male Wistar rats.[145] These studies indicate that AAS reduce hippocampal neurogenesis in a manner distinct from that of testosterone and DHT, which may be linked to the supraphysiological doses used or the molecular differences between these androgens.

Androgens and Adult Hippocampal Neurogenesis: Implications for Health and Disease

Androgen treatments in clinical disease may afford neuroprotection via their influence on neurogenesis in the hippocampus.[146] Low levels of androgens are associated with an increased risk for stroke, cerebrovascular disease, major depressive disorders, and dementia.[147–150] Androgens have been used to treat these diseases with some success, which depends on a variety of factors.[146] In addition, androgens play a role in neuroprotective factors that boost neurogenesis, such as exercise. Exercise-induced neurogenesis is inhibited in the presence of the AR antagonist flutamide, and mild exercise stimulates DHT production in male rats, which, in turn, enhances neurogenesis in the hippocampus.[151] Thus, androgens may be involved in some of the neurogenic responses to environmental factors and demonstrate neuroprotective effects against injury and disease.

Ischemic stroke is associated with impairments in memory along with increased neurogenesis,[152] but as with seizure-induced neurogenesis in the hippocampus[76] these new neurons form aberrant connections.[152] Indeed, the reduction of post-stroke neurogenesis aids in the retention of memory formation. Intriguingly, although castration and flutamide did not alter hippocampal neurogenesis 1 week after stroke, supraphysiological doses of testosterone and DHT reduced post-stroke hippocampal neurogenesis in the same study.[153] Thus, one way that androgens may afford protection in the face of stroke is to reduce ischemia-induced neurogenesis in the

hippocampus that may be related to aberrant connections tied to poorer memory outcomes.

Androgens play an important role in reducing depression in hypogonadal males, as meta-analyses demonstrate that testosterone treatment in hypogonadal men effectively reduces the symptoms of depression.[146,154,155] Castration increased the susceptibility to depressive-like endophenotypes in the face of chronic unpredictable stress,[112] which was commensurate with reduced neurogenesis in the hippocampus. However, testosterone treatment did not rescue the decrease in cell proliferation observed under social isolation stress in castrated males.[117,156] Interestingly, testosterone and the tricyclic antidepressant imipramine increased cell proliferation in the hippocampus more than antidepressant treatment alone in response to social isolation stress, an effect observed in males but not females.[156] Further, testosterone in conjunction with imipramine increased polysialylated neuronal cell adhesion molecule (PSA-NCAM)-ir cells in the dentate gyrus, but not neurogenesis *per se*, after exposure to chronic unpredictable stress.[106] In another model of depression using olfactory bulbectomy, the androgen DHEA prevented depressive-like behavior and increased the number of 1-week-old new neurons in response to bulbectomy in adult male mice.[157] DHEA has antidepressant effects[157] and works synergistically with fluoxetine, a selective serotonin reuptake inhibitor, causing an otherwise ineffective dose of fluoxetine to increase cell proliferation in the dentate gyrus of adult male rats.[158] Thus, collectively these data demonstrate that androgens can rescue depressive-like behavior and facilitate antidepressant efficacy, perhaps via its ability to stimulate neurogenesis.

In epilepsy, androgens can influence seizure susceptibility in males.[159–163] In males with epilepsy, lower levels of free testosterone and sexual dysfunction can be observed[164] but the directionality of this effect and whether treatments for epilepsy compound this relationship are not clear.[164,165] However, in animal studies, castrated rodents are more susceptible to pentylenetetrazol, picrotoxin, and perforant pathway stimulation-induced seizures compared with intact males, and testosterone administration decreases seizure activity in castrated males.[159–161] There is also evidence to suggest that the testosterone metabolite 3α-diol is protective against gamma-aminobutyric acid (GABA)$_A$ receptor antagonist-induced seizures in male mice,[162,163] which is interesting as 3α-diol has a weak affinity for ARs.[41] However, the relationship between sex steroid hormones and epilepsy has proven difficult to discern as various factors such as experimental conditions and biological variability can greatly influence study outcomes (reviewed in Scharfman and MacLusky[166]). Although the mechanisms of androgens' influence on seizure activity are not yet clear, it should be recalled that seizures induce aberrant hippocampal neurogenesis[75,77]; thus, it is plausible that androgens may be protective via their effects on neurogenesis in the dentate gyrus to reduce the aberrant connectivity of new neurons.

Finally, androgens may play a protective role in neurodegenerative diseases such as Alzheimer's disease (AD); for review see Ref.[167] Low levels of free testosterone may be a risk factor for AD in males,[168–170] and males with AD exhibit lower levels of testosterone in the periphery and in the brain compared with age-matched controls.[149,171,172] Two copies of the *APOEe4* allele confer a greater risk to develop sporadic late-onset AD[173,174] and female *APOEe4* carriers have disproportionately increased phosphorylated Tau (p-Tau), a neuropathological feature of AD, compared with male carriers.[175] Further, low serum testosterone in both males and females corresponded to increased p-Tau,[176] suggesting that the low levels of testosterone in both sexes may confer a greater risk of neuropathology related to AD. Testosterone treatment given to males with AD or mild cognitive impairment, a prodromal state to AD, increased scores on certain forms of memory, including spatial memory.[177] Thus, androgens may improve certain types of memory in both sexes with age and given that the hippocampus undergoes early degeneration with AD, it is possible that androgens may promote cognition during aging and in AD, via its effects on hippocampal neurogenesis. Intriguingly, neurogenesis in the hippocampus is decreased in people with AD when compared with healthy aging controls.[12,13,178] In addition, low testosterone coupled with APOEe4 genotype was related to lower hippocampal volume[179] and poorer verbal episodic memory.[180] Thus, several studies suggest that the androgens are related to hippocampal structure and function and more work is needed to explore the relationship between androgens and neurogenesis in AD and aging.

Conclusion

Chronic but not acute exposure to a variety of androgens generally increases neurogenesis in the hippocampus of adult males, an effect not seen in females or in middle-aged males. Despite the progress in this field, it is currently not known how or where ARs work to promote neurogenesis in the dentate gyrus with chronic testosterone or DHT, and whether androgen-induced new neurons are contributing to the function of the dentate gyrus. The addition of new neurons in the dentate gyrus has functional implications, but improper integration of new neurons may be deleterious to the function of these circuits. In addition, environmental influences such as central nervous system injury, disease, stress, and exercise all play a role in the neurogenic response to androgens. Sex differences observed in the neurogenic response to sex steroid hormones indicate that males and females have distinct hormonal mechanisms for the control of neurogenesis, and further work should explore the benefits of androgens to influence neurogenesis in males and possibly females, particularly in relation to health and disease.

Authors' Contributions

S.A.B. and L.A.M.G. co-wrote the review.

References

1. Altman J, Das GD. Autoradiographic and histological evidence of postnatal hippocampal neurogenesis in rats. J Comp Neurol. 1965;124(3): 319–335.
2. Raisman G. Neuronal plasticity in the septal nuclei of the adult rat. Brain Res. 1969;14(1):25–48.
3. Van Harreveld A, Fifkova E. Swelling of dendritic spines in the fascia dentata after stimulation of the perforant fibers as a mechanism of post-tetanic potentiation. Exp Neurol. 1975;49(3):736–749.
4. Greenough W, West R, DeVoogd T. Subsynaptic plate perforations: Changes with age and experience in the rat. Science. 1978;202(4372): 1096–1098.
5. Bosch M, Hayashi Y. Structural plasticity of dendritic spines. Curr Opin Neurobiol. 2012;22(3):383–388.
6. Goldman SA, Nottebohm F. Neuronal production, migration, and differentiation in a vocal control nucleus of the adult female canary brain. Proc Natl Acad Sci. 1983;80(8):2390–2394.
7. Nottebohm F. Neuronal replacement in adulthood. Ann N Y Acad Sci. 1985;457(1):143–161.
8. Kornack DR, Rakic P. Continuation of neurogenesis in the hippocampus of the adult macaque monkey. Proc Natl Acad Sci. 1999;96(10):5768–5773.
9. Ngwenya LB, Peters A, Rosene DL. Maturational sequence of newly generated neurons in the dentate gyrus of the young adult rhesus monkey. J Comp Neurol. 2006;498(2):204–216.
10. Maslov AY, Barone TA, Plunkett RJ, Pruitt SC. Neural stem cell detection, characterization, and age-related changes in the subventricular zone of mice. J Neurosci. 2004;24(7):1726–1733.

11. Kempermann G, Gast D, Kronenberg G, Yamaguchi M, Gage FH. Early determination and long-term persistence of adult-generated new neurons in the hippocampus of mice. Development. 2003;130(2):391–399.

12. Moreno-Jiménez EP, Flor-García M, Terreros-Roncal J, et al. Adult hippocampal neurogenesis is abundant in neurologically healthy subjects and drops sharply in patients with Alzheimer's disease. Nat Med. 2019; 25:554–560.

13. Tobin MK, Musaraca K, Disouky A, et al. Human hippocampal neurogenesis persists in aged adults and Alzheimer's disease patients. Cell Stem Cell. 2019;24(6):974–982.

14. Eriksson PS, Perfilieva E, Björk-Eriksson T, et al. Neurogenesis in the adult human hippocampus. Nat Med. 1998;4:1313–1317.

15. Mathews KJ, Allen KM, Boerrigter D, Ball H, Shannon Weickert C, Double KL. Evidence for reduced neurogenesis in the aging human hippocampus despite stable stem cell markers. Aging Cell. 2017;16(5):1195–1199.

16. Knoth R, Singec I, Ditter M, et al. Murine features of neurogenesis in the human hippocampus across the lifespan from 0 to 100 years. PLoS One. 2010;5:e8809.

17. Boldrini M, Fulmore CA, Tartt AN, et al. Human hippocampal neurogenesis persists throughout aging. Cell Stem Cell. 2018;22(4):589–599.

18. Spalding KL, Bergmann O, Alkass K, et al. Dynamics of hippocampal neurogenesis in adult humans. Cell. 2013;153(6):1219–1227.

19. Galea LAM, McEwen BS. Sex and seasonal changes in the rate of cell proliferation in the dentate gyrus of adult wild meadow voles. Neuroscience. 1999;89(3):955–964.

20. Barnea A, Nottebohm F. Seasonal recruitment of hippocampal neurons in adult free-ranging black-capped chickadees. Proc Natl Acad Sci U S A. 1994;91(23):11217–11221.

21. Yagi S, Splinter JEJ, Tai D, Wong S, Wen Y, Galea LAM. Sex differences in maturation and attrition of adult neurogenesis in the hippocampus. eNeuro. 2020;7(4):1–14.

22. Falconer EM, Galea LAM. Sex differences in cell proliferation, cell death and defensive behavior following acute predator odor stress in adult rats. Brain Res. 2003;975(1–2):22–36.

23. Westenbroek C, Den Boer JA, Veenhuis M, Ter Horst GJ. Chronic stress and social housing differentially affect neurogenesis in male and female rats. Brain Res Bull. 2004;64(4):303–308.

24. Mahmoud R, Wainwright SR, Galea LAM. Sex hormones and adult hippocampal neurogenesis: Regulation, implications, and potential mechanisms. Front Neuroendocrinol. 2016;41:129–152.

25. Fortune JE, Armstrong DT. Androgen production by theca and granulosa isolated from proestrous rat follicles. Endocrinology. 1977;100(5):1341–1347.

26. Neville AM, O'Hare MJ. Functional activity of the adrenal cortex. In: The Human Adrenal Cortex. Berlin: Germany, Springer-Verlag. 1982; pp 68–98.

27. Corpechot C, Robel P, Axelson M, Sjovall J, Baulieu EE. Characterization and measurement of dehydroepiandrosterone sulfate in rat brain. Proc Natl Acad Sci. 1981;78:4704–4707.

28. Robel P, Synguelakis M, Halberg F, Baulieu EE. Persistence of the circadian rhythm of dehydroepiandrosterone in the brain, but not in the plasma, of castrated and adrenalectomized rats. C R Acad Sci III. 1986; 303(6):235–238.

29. Baulieu E-E, Robel P, Vatier O, Haug M, Le Goascogne C, Bourreau E. Neurosteroids: Pregnenolone and dehydroepiandrosterone in the brain. In: Receptor-Receptor Interactions. London: Palgrave Macmillan. 1987; pp 89–104.

30. Mukai H, Takata N, Ishii H-t., et al. Hippocampal synthesis of estrogens and androgens which are paracrine modulators of synaptic plasticity: Synaptocrinology. Neuroscience. 2006;138:757–764.

31. Caruso D, Pesaresi M, Abbiati F, et al. Comparison of plasma and cerebrospinal fluid levels of neuroactive steroids with their brain, spinal cord and peripheral nerve levels in male and female rats. Psychoneuroendocrinology. 2013;38:2278–2290.

32. Jalabert C, Ma C, Soma KK. Profiling of systemic and brain steroids in male songbirds: Seasonal changes in neurosteroids. J Neuroendocrinol. 2020;33(1):e12922.

33. Handelsman DJ. Androgen physiology, pharmacology, and abuse. Endocrinology. 2010:2469–2498.

34. McHenry J, Carrier N, Hull E, Kabbaj M. Sex differences in anxiety and depression: Role of testosterone. Front Neuroendocrinol. 2014;35(1): 42–57.

35. Handa RJ, Pak TR, Kudwa AE, Lund TD, Hinds L. An alternate pathway for androgen regulation of brain function: Activation of estrogen receptor beta by the metabolite of dihydrotestosterone, 5α-androstane-$3\beta,17\beta$-diol. Horm Behav. 2008;53(5):741–752.

36. Kuiper GG, Lemmen JG, Carlsson B, et al. Interaction of estrogenic chemicals and phytoestrogens with estrogen receptor β. Endocrinology. 1998;139(10):4252–4263.

37. Bennett NC, Gardiner RA, Hooper JD, Johnson DW, Gobe GC. Molecular cell biology of androgen receptor signalling. Int J Biochem Cell Biol. 2010;42(6):813–827.

38. Gatson JW, Singh M. Activation of a membrane-associated androgen receptor promotes cell death in primary cortical astrocytes. Endocrinology. 2007;148(5):2458–2464.

39. Revankar CM, Cimino DF, Sklar LA, Arterburn JB, Prossnitz ER. A transmembrane intracellular estrogen receptor mediates rapid cell signaling. Science. 2005;307(5715):1625–1630.

40. Cutress ML, Whitaker HC, Mills IG, Stewart M, Neal DE. Structural basis for the nuclear import of the human androgen receptor. J Cell Sci. 2008;121: 957–968.

41. Matsuda KI, Sakamoto H, Mori H, et al. Expression and intracellular distribution of the G protein-coupled receptor 30 in rat hippocampal formation. Neurosci Lett. 2008;441(1):94–99.

42. Mehra RD, Sharma K, Nyakas C, Vij U. Estrogen receptor α and β immunoreactive neurons in normal adult and aged female rat hippocampus: A qualitative and quantitative study. Brain Res. 2005;1056(1):22–35.

43. Solum DT, Handa RJ. Localization of estrogen receptor alpha (ERα) in pyramidal neurons of the developing rat hippocampus. Dev Brain Res. 2001;128(2):165–175.

44. Hamson DK, Wainwright SR, Taylor JR, Jones BA, Watson NV, Galea LA. Androgens increase survival of adult-born neurons in the dentate gyrus by an androgen receptor-dependent mechanism in male rats. Endocrinology. 2013;154(9):3294–3304.

45. Simerly RB, Swanson LW, Chang C, Muramatsu M. Distribution of androgen and estrogen receptor mRNA-containing cells in the rat brain: An in situ hybridization study. J Comp Neurol. 1990;294(1): 76–95.

46. Tabori NE, Stewart LS, Znamensky V, et al. Ultrastructural evidence that androgen receptors are located at extranuclear sites in the rat hippocampal formation. Neuroscience. 2005;130(1):151–163.

47. Duarte-Guterman P, Lieblich SE, Wainwright SR, et al. Androgens enhance adult hippocampal neurogenesis in males but not females in an age-dependent manner. Endocrinology. 2019;160(9):2128–2136.

48. Xiao L, Jordan CL. Sex differences, laterality, and hormonal regulation of androgen receptor immunoreactivity in rat hippocampus. Horm Behav. 2002;42(3):327–336.

49. Wu D, Lin G, Gore AC. Age-related changes in hypothalamic androgen receptor and estrogen receptor α in male rats. J Comp Neurol. 2009; 512(5):688–701.

50. Edwards A, Hammond HA, Jin L, Caskey CT, Chakraborty R. Genetic variation at five trimeric and tetrameric tandem repeat loci in four human population groups. Genomics. 1992;12(2):241–253.

51. Chamberlain NL, Driver ED, Miesfeld RL. The length and location of CAG trinucleotide repeats in the androgen receptor N-terminal domain affect transactivation function. Nucleic Acids Res. 1994;22(15):3181–3186.

52. Braun SM, Jessberger S. Adult neurogenesis: Mechanisms and functional significance. Development. 2014;141(10):1983–1986.

53. Kee N, Sivalingam S, Boonstra R, Wojtowicz JM. The utility of Ki-67 and BrdU as proliferative markers of adult neurogenesis. J Neurosci Methods. 2002;115(1):97–105.

54. Brown JP, Couillard-Després S, Cooper-Kuhn CM, Winkler J, Aigner L, Kuhn HG. Transient expression of doublecortin during adult neurogenesis. J Comp Neurol. 2003;467(1):1–10.

55. Snyder JS, Choe JS, Clifford MA, et al. Adult-born hippocampal neurons are more numerous, faster maturing, and more involved in behavior in rats than in mice. J Neurosci. 2009;29(46):14484–14495.

56. Taupin P. BrdU immunohistochemistry for studying adult neurogenesis: Paradigms, pitfalls, limitations, and validation. Brain Res Rev. 2007;53(1): 198–214.

57. von Bohlen und Halbach O. Immunohistological markers for proliferative events, gliogenesis, and neurogenesis within the adult hippocampus. Cell Tissue Res. 2011;345:1–19.

58. Sidman RL, Miale IL, Feder N. Cell proliferation and migration in the primitive ependymal zone; An autoradiographic study of histogenesis in the nervous system. Exp Neurol. 1959;1(4):322–333.

59. Gratzner H. Monoclonal antibody to 5-bromo- and 5-iododeoxyuridine: A new reagent for detection of DNA replication. Science. 1982; 218(4571):474–475.

60. Miller MW, Nowakowski RS. Use of bromodeoxyuridine-immunohisto-chemistry to examine the proliferation, migration and time of origin of cells in the central nervous system. Brain Res. 1988;457(1):44–52.

61. Galea LA, Wainwright SR, Roes MM, Duarte-Guterman P, Chow C, Hamson DK. Sex, Hormones and neurogenesis in the hippocampus: Hormonal modulation of neurogenesis and potential functional impli-cations. J Neuroendocrinol. 2013;25(11):1039–1061.

62. Wojtowicz JM, Kee N. BrdU assay for neurogenesis in rodents. Nat Pro-toc. 2006;1:1399–1405.

63. Seaberg RM, van der Kooy D. Adult rodent neurogenic regions: The ventricular subependyma contains neural stem cells, but the dentate gyrus contains restricted progenitors. J Neurosci. 2002;22(5):1784–1793.

64. Bull ND, Bartlett, PF. The adult mouse hippocampal progenitor is neu-rogenic but not a stem cell. J Neurosci. 2005;25(47):10815–10821.

65. Seri B, García-Verdugo Jose Manuel, McEwen BS, Alvarez-Buylla A. Astrocytes give rise to new neurons in the adult mammalian hippo-campus. J Neurosci. 2001;21(18):7153–7160.

66. Steiner B, Klempin F, Wang L, Kott M, Kettenmann H, Kempermann G. Type-2 cells as link between glial and neuronal lineage in adult hippo-campal neurogenesis. Glia. 2006;54(8):805–814.

67. Lagace DC, Whitman MC, Noonan MA, et al. Dynamic contribution of nestin-expressing stem cells to adult neurogenesis. J Neurosci. 2007; 27(46):12623–12629.

68. Kempermann G, Wiskott L, Gage FH. Functional significance of adult neurogenesis. Curr Opin Neurobiol. 2004;14(2):186–191.

69. Cameron HA, Woolley CS, McEwen BS, Gould E. Differentiation of newly born neurons and glia in the dentate gyrus of the adult rat. Neuro-science. 1993;56(2):337–344.

70. Seaberg RM, van der Kooy D. Stem and progenitor cells: The premature desertion of rigorous definitions. Trends Neurosci. 2003;26(3):125–131.

71. Sorrells SF, Paredes MF, Cebrian-Silla A, et al. Human hippocampal neurogenesis drops sharply in children to undetectable levels in adults. Nature. 2018;555:377–381.

72. Cipriani S, Ferrer I, Aronica E, et al. Hippocampal radial glial subtypes and their neurogenic potential in human fetuses and healthy and Alz-heimer's disease adults. Cereb Cortex. 2018;28(7):2458–2478.

73. Ponti G, Farinetti A, Marraudino M, Panzica GC, Gotti S. Sex steroids and adult neurogenesis in the ventricular-subventricular zone. Front Endo-crinol. 2018;9:156.

74. Peretto P, Paredes RG. Frontiers in neurosciencesocial cues, adult neuro-genesis, and reproductive behavior. In: Neurobiology of Chemical Communication (Mucignat-Caretta C, ed). Boca Raton, FL: CRC Press, Taylor & Francis Group. 2014; pp 367–383.

75. Jessberger S, Zhao C, Toni N, Clemenson GD, Li Y, Gage FH. Seizure-associated, aberrant neurogenesis in adult rats characterized with retrovirus-mediated cell labeling. J Neurosci. 2007;27(35):9400–9407.

76. Jakubs K, Nanobashvili A, Bonde S, et al. Environment matters: Synaptic properties of neurons born in the epileptic adult brain develop to re-duce excitability. Neuron. 2006;52(6):1047–1059.

77. Parent JM, Yu TW, Leibowitz RT, Geschwind DH, Sloviter RS, Lowenstein DH. Dentate granule cell neurogenesis is increased by seizures and contributes to aberrant network reorganization in the adult rat hippo-campus. J Neurosci. 1997;17(10):3727–3738.

78. Houser CR. Granule cell dispersion in the dentate gyrus of humans with temporal lobe epilepsy. Brain Res. 1990;535(2):195–204.

79. van Praag H, Kempermann G, Gage FH. Running increases cell prolifer-ation and neurogenesis in the adult mouse dentate gyrus. Nat Neurosci. 1999a;2:266–270.

80. van Praag H, Christie BR, Sejnowski TJ, Gage FH. Running enhances neurogenesis, learning, and long-term potentiation in mice. Proc Natl Acad Sci. 1999b;96(23):13427–13431.

81. Epp JR, Silva Mera R, Köhler S, Josselyn SA, Frankland PW. Neurogenesis-mediated forgetting minimizes proactive interference. Nat Comm. 2016; 7:10838.

82. Cameron HA, Christie BR. Do new neurons have a functional role in the adult hippocampus? Debates Neurosci. 2007;1:26–32.

83. Kempermann G. Why new neurons? Possible functions for adult hip-pocampal neurogenesis. J Neurosci. 2002;22(3):635–638.

84. Christian KM, Song H, Ming G-li. Functions and dysfunctions of adult hippocampal neurogenesis. Annu Rev Neurosci. 2014;37:243–262.

85. Zhao C, Deng W, Gage FH. Mechanisms and functional implications of adult neurogenesis. Cell. 2008;132(4):645–660.

86. Winocur G, Becker S, Luu P, Rosenzweig S, Wojtowicz JM. Adult hippo-campal neurogenesis and memory interference. Behav Brain Res. 2012; 227(2):464–469.

87. Leutgeb JK, Leutgeb S, Moser M-B, Moser EI. Pattern separation in the dentate gyrus and CA3 of the hippocampus. Science. 2007;315(5814): 961–966.

88. Clelland CD, Choi M, Romberg C, Clemenson GD, Fragniere A, Tyers P, et al. A functional role for adult hippocampal neurogenesis in spatial pattern separation. Science. 2009;325(5937):210–213.

89. Tronel S, Belnoue L, Grosjean N, et al. Adult-born neurons are necessary for extended contextual discrimination. Hippocampus. 2010;22(2):292–298.

90. França TF, Bitencourt AM, Maximilla NR, Barros DM, Monserrat JM. Hip-pocampal neurogenesis and pattern separation: A meta-analysis of be-havioral data. Hippocampus. 2017;27(9):937–950.

91. Kesner RP, Hui X, Sommer T, Wright C, Barrera VR, Fanselow MS. The role of postnatal neurogenesis in supporting remote memory and spatial metric processing. Hippocampus. 2014;24(12):1663–1671.

92. Danielson NB, Kaifosh P, Zaremba JD, et al. Distinct contribution of adult-born hippocampal granule cells to context encoding. Neuron. 2016;90(1):101–112.

93. Treves A, Tashiro A, Witter MP, Moser EI. What is the mammalian dentate gyrus good for? Neuroscience. 2008;154(4):1155–1172.

94. Saxe MD, Battaglia F, Wang J-W, et al. Ablation of hippocampal neuro-genesis impairs contextual fear conditioning and synaptic plasticity in the dentate gyrus. Proc Natl Acad Sci. 2006;103(46):17501–17506.

95. Sahay A, Scobie KN, Hill AS, et al. Increasing adult hippocampal neuro-genesis is sufficient to improve pattern separation. Nature. 2011;472: 466–470.

96. Shors TJ, Townsend DA, Zhao M, Kozorovitskiy Y, Gould E. Neurogenesis may relate to some but not all types of hippocampal-dependent learning. Hippocampus. 2002;12(5):578–584.

97. Winocur G, Wojtowicz JM, Sekeres M, Snyder JS, Wang S. Inhibition of neurogenesis interferes with hippocampus-dependent memory func-tion. Hippocampus. 2006;16(3):296–304.

98. Miller SM, Sahay A. Functions of adult-born neurons in hippocampal memory interference and indexing. Nat Neurosci. 2019;22:1565–1575.

99. Anacker C, Hen R. Adult hippocampal neurogenesis and cognitive flexibility—Linking memory and mood. Nat Rev Neurosci. 2017;18:335–346.

100. Roberts GW, Woodhams PL, Polak JM, Crow TJ. Distribution of neuro-peptides in the limbic system of the rat: The hippocampus. Neuro-science. 1984;11(1):35–77.

101. Fanselow MS, Dong H-W. Are the dorsal and ventral hippocampus functionally distinct structures? Neuron. 2010;65(1):7–19.

102. Bannerman DM, Sprengel R, Sanderson DJ, et al. Hippocampal synaptic plasticity, spatial memory and anxiety. Nat Rev Neurosci. 2014;15:181–192.

103. Snyder JS, Soumier A, Brewer M, Pickel J, Cameron HA. Adult hippo-campal neurogenesis buffers stress responses and depressive behav-iour. Nature. 2011;476:458–461.

104. Eid RS, Gobinath AR, Galea LAM. Sex differences in depression: Insights from clinical and preclinical studies. Prog Neurobiol. 2019; 176:86–102.

105. Tanti A, Westphal W-P, Girault V, et al. Region-dependent and stage-specific effects of stress, environmental enrichment, and antidepressant treatment on hippocampal neurogenesis. Hippocampus. 2013;23(9): 797–811.

106. Wainwright SR, Workman JL, Tehrani A, et al. Testosterone has antidepressant-like efficacy and facilitates imipramine-induced neuro-plasticity in male rats exposed to chronic unpredictable stress. Horm Behav. 2016;79:58–69.

107. Boldrini M, Underwood MD, Hen R, et al. Antidepressants increase neural progenitor cells in the human hippocampus. Neuropsychopharmacol-ogy. 2009;34:2376–2389.

108. Epp JR, Beasley CL, Galea LAM. Increased hippocampal neurogenesis and p21 expression in depression: Dependent on antidepressants, sex,

age, and antipsychotic exposure. Neuropsychopharmacology. 2013;38: 2297–2306.

109. Surget A, Tanti A, Leonardo ED, et al. Antidepressants recruit new neurons to improve stress response regulation. Mol Psychiatry. 2011;16: 1177–1188.

110. Ormerod BK, Galea LAM. Reproductive status influences the survival of new cells in the dentate gyrus of adult male meadow voles. Neurosci Lett. 2003;346(1–2):25–28.

111. Spritzer MD, Galea LAM. Testosterone and dihydrotestosterone, but not estradiol, enhance survival of new hippocampal neurons in adult male rats. Dev Neurobiol. 2007;67(10):1321–1333.

112. Wainwright SR, Lieblich SE, Galea LAM. Hypogonadism predisposes males to the development of behavioural and neuroplastic depressive phenotypes. Psychoneuroendocrinology. 2011;36(9):1327–1341.

113. Benice TS, Raber J. Castration and training in a spatial task alter the number of immature neurons in the hippocampus of male mice. Brain Res. 2010;1329:21–29.

114. Swift-Gallant A, Duarte-Guterman P, Hamson DK, Ibrahim M, Monks DA, Galea LA. Neural androgen receptors affect the number of surviving new neurones in the adult dentate gyrus of male mice. J Neuroendocrinol. 2018;30(4):e12578.

115. Allen KM, Fung SJ, Rothmond DA, Noble PL, Shannon Weickert C. Gonadectomy increases neurogenesis in the male adolescent rhesus macaque hippocampus. Hippocampus. 2013;24(2):225–238.

116. Allen KM, Purves-Tyson TD, Fung SJ, Shannon Weickert C. The effect of adolescent testosterone on hippocampal BDNF and TrkB mRNA expression: Relationship with cell proliferation. BMC Neurosci. 2015;16:4.

117. Spritzer MD, Ibler E, Inglis W, Curtis MG. Testosterone and social isolation influence adult neurogenesis in the dentate gyrus of male rats. Neuroscience. 2011;195:180–190.

118. Markakis EA, Gage FH. Adult-generated neurons in the dentate gyrus send axonal projections to field CA3 and are surrounded by synaptic vesicles. J Comp Neurol. 1999;406:449–460.

119. Hastings NB, Gould E. Rapid extension of axons into the CA3 region by adult-generated granule cells. J Comp Neurol. 1999;413:146–154.

120. Hatanaka Y, Mukai H, Mitsuhashi K, et al. Androgen rapidly Increases Dendritic thorns of ca3 neurons in male rat hippocampus. Biochem Biophys Res Comm. 2009;381:728–732.

121. Chaiton JA, Wong SJ, Galea LAM. Chronic aromatase inhibition increases ventral hippocampal neurogenesis in middle-aged female mice. Psychoneuroendocrinology. 2019;106:111–116.

122. Fester L, Ribeiro-Gouveia V, Prange-Kiel J, von Schassen C, Bottner M, Jarry H, et al. Proliferation and apoptosis of hippocampal granule cells require local oestrogen synthesis. J Neurochem. 2006;97(4):1136–1144.

123. Barker JM, Galea LAM. Repeated estradiol administration alters different aspects of neurogenesis and cell death in the hippocampus of female, but not male, rats. Neuroscience. 2008;152(4):888–902.

124. Tanapat P, Hastings NB, Gould E. Ovarian steroids influence cell proliferation in the dentate gyrus of the adult female rat in a dose- and time-dependent manner. J Comp Neurol. 2004;481(3):252–265.

125. Ormerod BK, Lee TT-Y, Galea LAM. Estradiol enhances neurogenesis in the dentate gyri of adult male meadow voles by increasing the survival of young granule neurons. Neuroscience. 2004;128(3):645–654.

126. Chiba S, Suzuki M, Yamanouchi K, Nishihara M. Involvement of granulin in estrogen-induced neurogenesis in the adult rat hippocampus. J Reprod Dev. 2007;53(2):297–307.

127. Barha CK, Galea LAM. Motherhood alters the cellular response to estrogens in the hippocampus later in life. Neurobiol Aging. 2011;32(11): 2091–2095.

128. Moser VA, Christensen A, Liu J, et al. Effects of aging, high-fat diet, and testosterone treatment on neural and metabolic outcomes in male brown Norway rats. Neurobiol Aging. 2019;73:145–160.

129. Ramsden M, Nyborg AC, Murphy MP, et al. Androgens modulate β-amyloid levels in male rat brain. J Neurochem. 2003;87(4):1052–1055.

130. Cheng J, Wu H, Liu H, et al. Exposure of hyperandrogen during pregnancy causes depression- and anxiety-like behaviors, and reduced hippocampal neurogenesis in rat offspring. Front Neurosci. 2019;13:436.

131. Kight KE, McCarthy MM. Androgens and the developing hippocampus. Biol Sex Differ. 2020;11(30):1–14.

132. Waddell J, Bowers JM, Edwards NS, Jordan CL, McCarthy MM. Dysregulation of neonatal hippocampal cell genesis in the androgen insensitive Tfm rat. Horm Behav. 2013;64(1):144–152.

133. Zhang J-M, Konkle AT, Zup SL, McCarthy MM. Impact of sex and hormones on new cells in the developing rat hippocampus: A novel source of sex dimorphism? Eur J Neurosci. 2008;27(4):791–800.

134. Herrera-Pérez JJ, Martínez-Mota L, Jiménez-Rubio G, et al. Dehydroepiandrosterone increases the number and dendrite maturation of doublecortin cells in the dentate gyrus of middle age male Wistar rats exposed to chronic mild stress. Behav Brain Res. 2017;321:137–147.

135. Karishma KK, Herbert J. Dehydroepiandrosterone (DHEA) stimulates neurogenesis in the hippocampus of the rat, promotes survival of newly formed neurons and prevents corticosterone-induced suppression. Eur J Neurosci. 2002;16(3):445–453.

136. Wada H, Newman AEM, Hall ZJ, Soma KK, MacDougall-Shackleton SA. Effects of corticosterone and DHEA on doublecortin immunoreactivity in the song control system and hippocampus of adult song sparrows. Dev Neurobiol. 2013;74(1):52–62.

137. Suzuki M, Wright LS, Marwah P, Lardy HA, Svendsen CN. Mitotic and neurogenic effects of dehydroepiandrosterone (DHEA) on human neural stem cell cultures derived from the fetal cortex. Proc Natl Acad Sci. 2004;101(9):3202–3207.

138. Chen F, Knecht K, Birzin E, et al. Direct agonist/antagonist functions of dehydroepiandrosterone. Endocrinology. 2005;146:4568–4576.

139. Bruder JM, Sobek L, Oettel M. Dehydroepiandrosterone stimulates the estrogen response element. J Steroid Biochem Mol Biol. 1997;62:461–466.

140. Lu S-F, Mo Q, Hu S, Garippa C, Simon NG. Dehydroepiandrosterone upregulates neural androgen receptor level and transcriptional activity. J Neurobiol. 2003;57:163–171.

141. Prough RA, Clark BJ, Klinge CM. Novel mechanisms for dhea action. J Mol Endocrinol. 2016;56(3), R139–R155.

142. Pope HG, Katz DL. Psychiatric and medical effects of anabolic-androgenic steroid use. Arch Gen Psychiatr. 1994;51(5):375.

143. Menard CS, Harlan RE. Up-regulation of androgen receptor immunoreactivity in the rat brain by androgenic-anabolic steroids. Brain Res. 1993; 622(1–2):226–236.

144. Brännvall K, Bogdanovic N, Korhonen L, Lindholm D. 19-Nortestosterone influences neural stem cell proliferation and neurogenesis in the rat brain. Eur J Neurosci. 2005;21(4):871–878.

145. Novaes Gomes FG, Fernandes J, Vannucci Campos D, et al. The beneficial effects of strength exercise on hippocampal cell proliferation and apoptotic signaling is impaired by anabolic androgenic steroids. Psychoneuroendocrinology. 2014;50:106–117.

146. Amanatkar HR, Chibnall JT, Seo BW, Manepalli JN, Grossberg GT. Impact of exogenous testosterone on mood: A systematic review and meta-analysis of randomized placebo-controlled trials. Ann Clin Psychiatry. 2014;26(1):19–32.

147. Abi-Ghanem C, Robison LS, Zuloaga KL. Androgens' effects on cerebrovascular function in health and disease. Biol Sex Differ. 2020;11:35.

148. Zitzmann M. Testosterone, mood, behaviour and quality of life. Andrology. 2020;8(6):1598–1605.

149. Rosario ER. Age-related testosterone depletion and the development of Alzheimer disease. JAMA. 2004;292(12):1431–1432.

150. Jeppesen LL, Jørgensen HS, Nakayama H, Raaschou HO, Olsen TS, Winther K. Decreased serum testosterone in men with acute ischemic stroke. Arterioscler Thromb Vasc Biol. 1996;16(6):749–754.

151. Okamoto M, Hojo Y, Inoue K, et al. Mild exercise increases dihydrotestosterone in hippocampus providing evidence for androgenic mediation of neurogenesis. Proc Natl Acad Sci. 2012;109(32):13100–13105.

152. Cuartero MI, de la Parra J, Pérez-Ruiz A, et al. Abolition of aberrant neurogenesis ameliorates cognitive impairment after stroke in mice. J Clin Investig. 2019;129(4):1536–1550.

153. Zhang W, Cheng J, Vagnerova K, et al. Effects of androgens on early post-ischemic neurogenesis in mice. Transl Stroke Res. 2014;5:301–311.

154. Elliott J, Kelly SE, Millar AC. Testosterone therapy in hypogonadal men: A systematic review and network meta-analysis. BMJ Open. 2017;7(11): e015284.

155. Zarrouf FA, Artz S, Griffith J, Sirbu C, Kommor M. Testosterone and depression. J Psychiatr Pract. 2009;15(4):289–305.

156. Carrier N, Kabbaj M. Testosterone and imipramine have antidepressant effects in socially isolated male but not female rats. Horm Behav. 2012; 61(5):678–685.

157. Moriguchi S, Shinoda Y, Yamamoto Y, et al. Stimulation of the sigma-1 receptor by DHEA enhances synaptic efficacy and neurogenesis in the

hippocampal dentate gyrus of olfactory bulbectomized mice. PLoS One. 2013;8(4):e60863.

158. Pinnock SB, Lazic SE, Wong HT, Wong IHW, Herbert J. Synergistic effects of dehydroepiandrosterone and fluoxetine on proliferation of progenitor cells in the dentate gyrus of the adult male rat. Neuroscience. 2009; 158(4):1644–1651.

159. Pesce ME, Acevedo X, Bustamante D, Miranda HF, Pinardi G. Progesterone and testosterone modulate the convulsant actions of pentylenetetrazol and strychnine in mice. Pharmacol Toxicol. 2008;87:116–119.

160. Schwartz-Giblin S, Korotzer A, Pfaff DW. Steroid hormone effects on picrotoxin-induced seizures in female and male rats. Brain Res. 1989;476: 240–247.

161. Frye CA, Reed TAW. Androgenic neurosteroids: Anti-seizure effects in an animal model of epilepsy. Psychoneuroendocrinology. 1998;23:385–399.

162. Frye CA, Rhodes ME, Walf AA, Harney JP. Testosterone reduces pentylenetetrazole-induced ictal activity of wildtype mice but not those deficient in type i 5α-reductase. Brain Res. 2001;918:182–186.

163. Reddy DS. Anticonvulsant activity of the testosterone-derived neurosteroid 3α-androstanediol. NeuroReport. 2004;15:515–518.

164. Hamed SA. The effect of epilepsy and antiepileptic drugs on sexual, reproductive and gonadal health of adults with epilepsy. Exp Rev Clin Pharmacol. 2016;9:807–819.

165. Markoula S, Siarava E, Keramida A, et al. Reproductive health in patients with epilepsy. Epilepsy Behav. 2020;113:107563.

166. Scharfman HE, MacLusky NJ. Sex differences in the neurobiology of epilepsy: A preclinical perspective. Neurobiol Dis. 2014;72:180–192.

167. Cai Z, Li H. An updated review: Androgens and cognitive impairment in older men. Front Endocrinol. 2020;11.

168. Hogervorst E, Combrinck M, Smith AD. Testosterone and gonadotropin levels in men with dementia. Neuro Endocrinol Lett. 2003;24(3–4):203–208.

169. Hogervorst E, Bandelow S, Combrinck M, Smith AD. Low free testosterone is an independent risk factor for Alzheimer's disease. Exp Gerontol. 2004;39:1633–1639.

170. Moffat SD, Zonderman AB, Metter EJ, et al. Free testosterone and risk for Alzheimer disease in older men. Neurology. 2004;62:188–193.

171. Carcaillon L, Brailly-Tabard S, Ancelin M-L, et al. Low testosterone and the risk of dementia in elderly men: Impact of age and education. Alzheimer's Dement. 2013;10.

172. Rosario ER, Chang L, Head EH, Stanczyk FZ, Pike CJ. Brain levels of sex steroid hormones in men and women during normal aging and in Alzheimer's disease. Neurobiol Aging. 2011;32:604–613.

173. Coon KD, Myers AJ, Craig DW, et al. A high-density whole-genome association study reveals that APOE is the major susceptibility gene for sporadic late-onset Alzheimer's disease. J Clin Psychiatry. 2007;68:613–618.

174. Reiman EM, Arboleda-Velasquez JF, Quiroz YT, et al. Exceptionally low likelihood of Alzheimer's dementia in Apoe2 homozygotes from a 5,000-person neuropathological study. Nat Commun. 2020;11.

175. Duarte-Guterman P, Albert AY, Barha CK, Galea LAM. Sex influences the effects of APOE genotype and Alzheimer's diagnosis on Neuropathology and memory. Psychoneuroendocrinology. 2021;129:105248.

176. Sundermann EE, Panizzon MS, Chen X, Andrews M, Galasko D, Banks SJ. Sex differences in Alzheimer's-related Tau biomarkers and a Mediating effect of testosterone. Biol Sex Differ. 2020;11.

177. Cherrier MM, Matsumoto AM, Amory JK, et al. Testosterone improves spatial memory in men with Alzheimer disease and mild cognitive impairment. Neurology. 2005;64:2063–2068.

178. Li B, Yamamori H, Tatebayashi Y, et al. Failure of neuronal maturation in Alzheimer disease dentate gyrus. J Neuropathol Exp Neurol. 2008;67: 78–84.

179. Panizzon MS, Hauger R, Dale AM, et al. Testosterone modifies the effect of APOE genotype on hippocampal volume in middle-aged men. Neurology. 2010;75:874–880.

180. Panizzon MS, Hauger R, Xian H, et al. Interaction of APOE genotype and testosterone on episodic memory in middle-aged men. Neurobiol Aging. 2014;35:1778.e1–1778.e8.

Abbreviations Used

3α-diol = 5α-androstane-3α,17β-diol
3β-diol = 5α-androstane-3β,17β-diol
AAS = androgenic anabolic steroids
AD = Alzheimer's disease
ARs = androgen receptors
BrdU = 5-bromo-2-deoxyuridine
CAG = cytosine-adenine-guanine
DCX = doublecortin
DHT = 5α-dihydrotestosterone
DHEA = dehydroepiandrosterone
ERs = estrogen receptors
GCL = granular cell layer
GFAP = glial fibrillary acidic protein
GPER = G protein-coupled ER
ML = molecular layer
NeuN = neuronal nuclei
NPC = neural progenitor cells
NSC = neural stem cell
NSERC = Natural Sciences and Engineering Research Council of Canada
p-Tau = phosphorylated Tau
SGZ = subgranular zone
SVZ = subventricular zone
TAPC = transient amplifying progenitor cell

5

Obstructive Sleep Apnea and Testosterone Replacement Therapy

Sandro La Vignera,[1,*] Aldo E. Calogero,[1] Rossella Cannarella,[1] Rosita A. Condorelli,[1] Cristina Magagnini,[1] and Antonio Aversa[2]

Abstract

The evidence on the role of obstructive sleep apnea (OSA) in the pathogenesis of hypogonadism and the impact of testosterone replacement therapy (TRT) in OSA patients are still contradictory. OSA is generally considered to be a relative contraindication as TRT is feared to worsen sleep apnea so that ventilatory capacity should be strictly investigated in advance and monitored thereafter. Few controlled studies have been released on the long-term effects of TRT in patients with OSA due to methodological limitations at study entry. Data from recent randomized placebo-controlled studies show a time-dependent influence on nocturnal hypoxia, and a positive impact after a longer time of exposure in selected patients. Since these results await further confirmation from larger studies, we suggest to use TRT cautiously in obese hypogonadal patients with hypoventilatory syndrome, especially if they are not on continuous positive airway pressure treatment.

Keywords: obstructive sleep apnea; hypogonadism; testosterone; testosterone replacement therapy

Introduction

Sleep disorders are clinical conditions that worsen the quality of life and prognosis.[1] They include a number of diseases characterized by abnormal breathing during sleep, due to a shrinkage or obstruction of the upper airways. One of the most common forms of sleep disorders is obstructive sleep apnea (OSA).[2] OSA is characterized by repetitive and intermittent, partial or complete collapse of the upper airway during sleeping, regardless of the presence of daytime symptoms. This happens because upper airway dilator muscles fail to counter the negative pressure in the airways during inspiration. This effect is present during sleep because an enhanced muscular activity is lost. If symptoms are present, this condition is called "OSA syndrome" (OSAS) and the main presentations are sleep fragmentation with breathing interruptions, decreased sleep time, shorter REM time, loud snoring, and daytime sleepiness. This leads to oxygen (O_2) desaturation with hypoxemia and hypercapnia.[3] Over 50 years, $\sim$1–2% of women and 2–4% of men have OSA.[4] OSA severity is classified by measuring the "apnea–hypopnea index" (AHI). An "apneic event" is defined by a decrease of airflow by >90% lasting for at least 10 sec; meanwhile hypopnea is defined as a decrease of airflow from 30% to 90% with 3% or more O_2 desaturation. On the basis of the number of "apnea–hypopnea" events during sleeping, three OSA levels can be identified: normal (AHI ≤5), mild (5 < AHI <15), moderate (15 ≤ AHI <30), and severe (AHI ≥30).[2] Etiopathogenesis of OSAS implies several factors, the main being obesity due to fatty deposits in the upper airways.

OSA is an independent risk factor for several diseases. These include cerebrocardiovascular diseases (hypertension, myocardial infarction, congestive heart failure, arrhythmias such as atrial fibrillation, and stroke), metabolic diseases (type 2 diabetes mellitus),

[1]Department of Clinical and Experimental Medicine, University of Catania, Catania, Italy.
[2]Department of Experimental and Clinical Medicine, "Magna Graecia" University, Catanzaro, Italy.

*Address correspondence to: Sandro La Vignera, MD, PhD, Department of Clinical and Experimental Medicine, University of Catania, Policlinico "G. Rodolico," via S. Sofia 78, Catania 95123, Italy, Email: sandrolavignera@unict.it

and depression. Recently, hypoxia has been suggested as possibly involved in the pathogenesis of pituitary–gonadal axis alterations, leading to obesity-related hypogonadotropic hypogonadism.[3] The evidence on the impact of testosterone replacement therapy (TRT) on OSAS is still contradictory. The aim of this review was to analyze the impact of OSA in the pathogenesis of hypogonadism and to critically examine the pros and cons of TRT in hypogonadal patients with OSA. To accomplish this, we performed a search on Pubmed, Science-direct, Ovid, and Scopus, using the following keywords: obstructive sleep apnea, OSA, hypogonadism, testosterone replacement therapy, and TRT. Particularly, special attention was given to evidence coming from randomized controlled study design unbiased by improperly high TRT dosages.

The Role of OSA in the Pathogenesis of Hypogonadism

A strong relationship between serum testosterone levels and sleep disorders such as OSA has been shown. Testosterone synthesis is regulated by the hypothalamic–pituitary–testicular axis and it relies on luteotropic hormone and follicle-stimulating hormone pulsatile secretion. Serum testosterone levels change during the day: they peak on the early morning upon awakening and reach the nadir at the end of the day.[5–7] Accordingly, plasma testosterone levels raise with the sleep onset, they then have a spike at the first REM sleep episode, and continue to rise until awakening. Testosterone levels decrease when REM latency is longer, such as in old age and in sleep disorders. The sleep fragmentation disrupts testosterone rhythm.[5,6]

OSAS is associated with a decreased gonadal function, because of less REM sleep episodes and major sleep fragmentation, which contribute to an alteration of gonadotrophin-releasing hormone pulsatility,[8] and this is confirmed by negative correlation between AHI score serum testosterone levels.[3] Further proof is given by the O_2 desaturation index and by O_2 nadir, both related with testosterone decrease.

Obesity may play a role in the correlation between OSAS and hypogonadism. Accordingly, the aromatase enzyme, expressed in adipocytes, converts testosterone into 17β-estradiol. The latter exerts its negative feedback on gonadotropin secretion and leads to testosterone decrease. The alteration of testosterone/17β-estradiol ratio brings to a compensatory synthesis of sex-hormone binding glubulin, which binds testosterone in the bloodstream. Intermittent hypoxia and

repetitive short cycles of desaturation and reoxygenation are all involved in white adipose tissue proliferation and pathophysiological processes, leading to OSAS, that is, overproduction of cytokines, chemokines, and adipokines. An increase of T cells, B cells, macrophages, leukocytes, mast cell, and neoangiogenesis mechanisms has been observed in fat tissue of obese patients. Macrophages infiltrate adipocytes and worsen tissue inflammation and insulin resistance. T cells and B cells change their phenotype from M2 to M1-proinflammatory, which produces proinflammatory adipokines, such as tumor necrosis factor-α, interleukin (IL)-6, IL-1β, and leptin. Local tissue hypoxia leads to the activation of hypoxia-inducible factor, which triggers the expression of vascular endothelial growth factor and plasminogen activator inhibitor-1.[8] Moreover, obesity worsens hypotestosteronemia. The body mass index is considered the primary determinant of testosterone levels in men with OSA[5,6,9] and it is associated with increased severity of the disorder. These data are further confirmed by the linear correlation shown between weight loss and increased plasma testosterone in obese men (Fig. 1).[10]

Low testosterone levels are strictly correlated with the presence both physical and mental fatigue and decreased physical capacity in OSA patients.[3] Bercea et al. found that reduced physical activity and physical fatigue are related with serum testosterone and not with O_2 saturation. Therefore, low serum testosterone is an independent predictor of this condition in OSA patients.[7] According to erectile dysfunction (ED) definition,[11] this is recognized as the main symptom that forces OSAS patients to seek help.[2,12] It is especially evident in patients with severe OSA and less evident in patients with mild or moderated OSA.[3,13,14] A recent meta-analysis showed that patients with OSA have a relative risk of 1.82 to develop ED. A study conducted by Gonçalves et al. reported a prevalence of 48% of ED in patient with severe OSA[15]; the severity of OSA is considered to be an important factor for the development of ED.[2,16] Phosphodiesterase type 5 inhibitors (PDE5is) on demand are useful as a treatment for ED in this subgroup of patients, with high satisfaction rates and no contraindication reported.[17]

TRT and OSA

Historically, TRT has been considered dangerous for patients with severe OSAS because it could exacerbate symptoms, increasing AHI, decreasing O_2 saturation, and interfering with central response to hypo- and

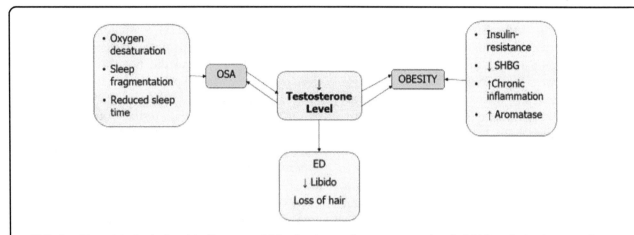

FIG. 1. Two-sided relationship between OSA, obesity, and testosterone level. OSAS and obesity contribute to reduce testosterone level in bloodstream; at the same time, lower testosterone level worsens obesity and sleep disorders. OSA, obstructive sleep apnea; OSAS, OSA syndrome.

hypercapnia.[5,6] The physiological mechanisms that are supposed to interfere with OSA are (1) reduced contraction of airway dilator muscles and subsequent collapse of the upper airways, (2) increased metabolic consumption with greater O_2 demand and subsequent hypoxia and polycythemia, and (3) reduced neural central response to hypoxia and hypercapnia, with increase in the number of apneas and hypopneas and the rela-

tive AHI. However, TRT does not influence upper airways size or the Epworth Sleepness Scale. Nevertheless, it is a cause of reduced total time slept and of increased disrupted sleeping and duration of hypoxia (Fig. 2).[18]

Current guidelines recommend TRT for adult men with severely reduced testosterone levels (<9.2 nmol/L),[19] but they suggest against its use in patients with untreated severe OSA since treating hypogonadal patients may

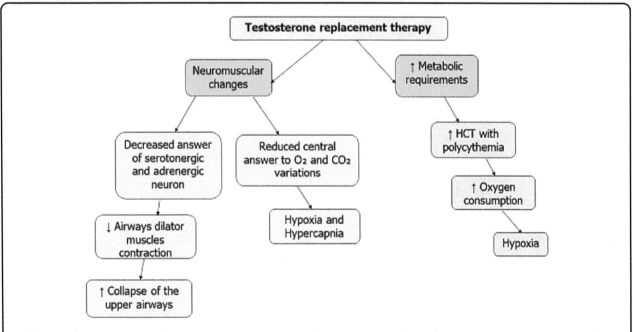

FIG. 2. Testosterone replacement therapy worsens OSA symptoms through neuromuscular changes and raised metabolic requirements. This condition causes collapse of the upper airway and onset of hypoxia.

cause an increase of apneas and hypopneas events.[2] Actually, few studies have considered the effect of TRT in patients with OSAS. In one of them, testosterone given IM was compared with placebo and it has been shown that hypoxic ventilatory drive significantly decreased in TRT patients, whereas hypercapnoic ventilatory drive did not significantly change.[20] However, this 6-week-long prospective study examined only five hypogonadal patients, reporting the development of OSA in one case and no change in respiratory parameters in the latter patients.[20] Overall, the evidence provided by this study is very low due to the small duration and sample size. Similarly, a randomized placebo-controlled double-blind study on 17 patients without OSA analyzed the effects of high testosterone dosage on the quality of sleep. Particularly, the TRT scheme consisted of 500 mg IM administered in the first week, 250 mg in the second, and 250 mg in the third week. Unsurprisingly, TRT at high doses showed to worsen total time slept and to increase the duration of hypoxia and to disrupt breathing during sleep.[21] This proved the negative effects of TRT on ventilatory function when a high dosage is chosen. However, the adverse effects of high-dose TRT have already been ascertained.[19]

A prospective cohort study carried out in 3422 male U.S. military service members, retired and dependents aged 40–64 years, analyzed the risk of developing TRT-dependent adverse events in a 17-month-long observation. Patients on TRT had a reduced risk of coronary artery disease with an improved cardiovascular event-free survival. By contrast, the risk of OSA development was higher in TRT users than in controls (16.5% vs. 12.7%).[22] Thus, starting TRT in patients with no previous sign of OSA may prompt to its development. This could be due to the exacerbation of polycythemia.[23] For this reason, TRT in OSA patients must be monitored by polysomnography and, potentially, treated with continuous positive airway pressure (CPAP); in patients who are not responsive to CPAP, TRT dosage must be lowered or withdrawn.[24,25]

But what about the effects of TRT in hypogonadal patients with OSAS? Four randomized placebo-controlled clinical trials have been performed on this matter so far. The study by Shigehara et al. has been performed in 48 OSA patients with hypogonadism who underwent TRT. Interestingly, the authors reported an improvement of sleep disturbances compared with placebo at the 12th month of TRT.[26] This represents the longest trial carried out so far, since other studies showed a duration ranging from 12 to 18 weeks. After 12 weeks, TRT (testosterone undecanoate was administered in a randomized placebo-controlled study design at the dose of 1000 mg at weeks 0, 6, and 12) and did not show to influence sleep quality in 67 obese patients with OSA.[27] Another study carried out in 21 obese patients with OSA and hypogonadism treated with testosterone undecanoate (1000 mg at weeks 0, 6, and 12) reported a positive correlation between serum testosterone levels and hyperoxic ventilator recruitment threshold, correlating with time of oxygen desaturation during sleep at 7 weeks but not at 18 weeks.[28] Similarly, another randomized placebo-controlled trial in 67 obese patients with OSA and hypogonadism found that TRT worsens oxygen saturation at week 7. No effect of TRT on sleep time with oxygen saturation <90% was observed after 18 weeks.[29] Taken together, these findings highlight that the influence of TRT on nocturnal oxygen saturation in OSA patients is time dependent.[30] Particularly, although after 7 weeks, a negative impact seems to occur, no effect has been registered after 12 and 18 weeks and even a positive effect has been described after 12 months.[31] However, further prospective studies on larger sample size and with longer duration are needed to confirm this initial evidence.

Conclusion

In summary, this review summarizes the evidence on the mechanisms involved in the pathogenesis of hypogonadism in patients with OSAS, such as abnormal circadian rhythm of gonadotrophin secretory patterns associated with obesity. TRT may represent a risk factor for OSA development and therefore, respiratory function monitoring is recommended especially in obese patients during TRT. Scanty evidence has been released on the effect of TRT in patients with OSA. Data from recent randomized placebo-controlled studies address to TRT a time-dependent influence on nocturnal hypoxia, showing a positive impact after a longer time of exposure. Also, CPAP and PDE5i can be considered safe procedures to ameliorate sexuality in hypogonadal patients with OSA. We suggest to use TRT cautiously in obese hypogonadal patients with hypoventilatory syndrome especially if they are not on CPAP. The latter aspect needs to be further confirmed by larger controlled studies.

References

1. Kazuyoshi S, Hiroyuki K, Kazuhiro S, et al. Sleep disturbance as a clinical sign for severe hypogonadism: Efficacy of testosterone replacement therapy on sleep disturbance among hypogonadal men without obstructive sleep apnea. Aging Male. 2018;21(2):99–105.

2. Cho YW, Kim KT, Moon HJ, et al. Comorbid insomnia with obstructive sleep apnea: Clinical characteristics and risk factors. J Clin Sleep Med. 2018;14(3):409–417.

3. Foti DP, Brunetti A. Editorial: "linking hypoxia to obesity." Front Endocrinol (Lausanne) 2017;8:34.

4. Maspero C, Giannini L, Galbiati G, Rosso G, Farronato G. Obstructive sleep apnea syndrome: A literature review. Minerva Stomatol. 2015;64(2):97–109.

5. Wittert G. The relatioship between sleep disorders and testosterone. Curr Opin Endocrinolo Diabetes Obes. 2014;21(3):239–243.

6. Wittert G. The relationship between sleep disorders and testosterone in men. Asian J Androl. 2014;16(2):262–265.

7. Bercea RM, Mihaescu T, Cojocaru C, Bjorvatn B. Fatigue and serum testosterone in obstructive sleep apnea patients. Clin Respir J. 2015;9(3):342–349.

8. Messineo S, Laria AE, Arcidiacono B, et al. Cooperation between HMGA1 and HIF-1 contributes to hypoxia-induced VEGF and Visfatin gene expression in 3T3-L1 adipocytes. Front Endocrinol (Lausanne) 2016;7:73.

9. Macrea MM, Martin Tj, Zagrean L. Infertility and obstructive sleep apnea: The effect of continuous positive airway pressure therapy on serum prolactin levels. Sleep Breath. 2010;14(3):253–257.

10. Donini LM, Cuzzolaro M, Gnessi L, et al. Obesity treatment: Results after 4 years of a nutritional and psycho-physical rehabilitation program in an outpatient setting. Eat Weight Disord. 2014;19(2):249–260.

11. Feldman HA, Goldstein I, Hatzichrisou DG, Krane RJ, McKinlay JB. Impotence and its medical and psychosocial correlates: Result of Massachusetts Male Aging Study. J Urol. 1994;151(1):54–61.

12. Lue FT. Erectile dysfunction. N Engl J Med. 2000;342(24):1802–18013.

13. Margel D, Cohen M, Livne PM, Pillar G. Severe, but not mild, obstructive sleep apnea syndrome is associated with erectile dysfunction. Urology. 2004;63(3):545–549.

14. Liu L, Kang R, Zhao S, et al. Sexual dysfunction in patient with obstructive sleep apnea: A systemic review and meta-analysis. J Sex Med. 2015;12(10):1992–2003.

15. Gonçalves MA, Guilleminault C, Ramos E, et al. Erectile dysfunction, obstructive sleep apnea syndrome and nasal CPAP treatment. Sleep Med. 2005;6(4):333–339.

16. Omar B, Jing W. Testosterone deficiency and sleep apnea. Sleep Med Clin. 2016;11(4):525–529.

17. Campos-Juanatey F, Fernandez-Barriales M, Gonzalez M, Portillo-Martin JA. Effects of obstructive sleep apnea and its treatment over the erectile function: A systematic review. Asian J Androl. 2017;19(3):303–310.

18. Hanafy HM. Testosterone therapy and obstructive sleep apnea: Is there a real connection? J Sex Med. 2007;4(5):1241–1246.

19. Bhasin S, Brito JP, Cunningham GR, et al. Testosterone therapy in men with hypogonadism: An Endocrine Society Clinical Practice Guideline. J Clin Endocrinol Metab. 2018;103(5):1715–1744.

20. Matsumoto AM, Sandblom RE, Schoene RB, et al. Testosterone replacement in hypogonadal men: Effects on obstructive sleep apnea, respiratory drives and sleep. Clin Endocrinol. 1985;22(6):713–721.

21. Liu PY, Yee B, Wishart SM, et al. The short-term effects of high-dose testosterone on sleep, breathing, and function in older men. J Clin Endocrinol Metab. 2003;88(8):3605–3613.

22. Cole AP, Hanske J, Jiang W, et al. Impact of testosterone replacement therapy on thromboembolism, heart disease and obstructive sleep apnoea in men. BJU Int. 2018;121(5):811–818.

23. Zelveian PA, Dgerian LG. The main pathophysiological mechanisms of kidney injury in obstructive sleep apnea syndrome. Ter Arkh. 2014;86(6):100–105.

24. Choi JB, Loredo JS, Norman D, et al. Does obstructive sleep apnea increase hematocrit? Sleep Breath. 2006;10(3):155–160.

25. Bachman E, Travison TG, Basaria S, et al. Testosterone induces erythrocitosis via increased erythropoietin/hemoglobin set point. J Gerontol A Biol Sci Med Sci. 2014;69(6):725–735.

26. Shigehara K, Konaka H, Sugimoto K, et al. Sleep disturbance as a clinical sign for severe hypogonadism: Efficacy of testosterone replacement therapy on sleep disturbance among hypogonadal men without obstructive sleep apnea. Aging Male. 2018;21(2):99–105.

27. Melehan KL, Hoyos CM, Yee BJ, et al. Increased sexual desire with exogenous testosterone administration inmen with obstructive sleep apnea: A randomized palcebo-controlled study. Andrology. 2016;4(1):55–61.

28. Killick R, Wang D, Hoyos CM, Yee BJ, Grunstein RR, Liu PY. The effects of testosterone on ventilatory responses in men with obstructive sleep apnea: A randomised, placebo-controlled trial. J Sleep Res. 2013;22(3):331–336.

29. Hoyos CM, Killick R, Yee BJ, Grunstein RR, Liu PY. Effects of testosterone therapy on sleep and breathing in obese men with severe obstructive sleep apnoea: A randomized placebo-controlled trial. Clin Endocrinol (Oxf). 2012;77(4):599–607.

30. Kim SD, Cho KS. Obstructive sleep apnea and testosterone deficiency. World J Mens Health. 2019;37(1):12–18.

31. Pastore AL, Palleschi G, Ripoli A, et al. Severe obstructive sleep apnoea syndrome and erectile dysfunction: A prospective randomised study compare sildenafil vs nasal continuous positive airway pressure. Int J Clin Pract. 2014;68(8):995–1000.

Abbreviations Used

AHI = apnea–hypopnea index
CPAP = continuous positive airway pressure
ED = erectile dysfunction
IL = interleukin
IM = intramuscular
OSA = obstructive sleep apnea
OSAS = OSA syndrome
PDE5is = phosphodiesterase type 5 inhibitors
REM = rapid eye movements
TRT = testosterone replacement therapy

6

Updated Review of Testosterone Replacement Therapy in the Setting of Prostate Cancer

Michael Polchert, Igor Voznesensky, Ayman Soubra, and Wayne J.G. Hellstrom[*]

Abstract
Since the 1940s, elevated serum testosterone (T) levels have been infamously suggested as a causal factor in the development of prostate cancer (PCa); this time was also the dawn of both surgically and pharmacologically induced castration. However, men suffering from primary or secondary hypogonadism and who are concomitantly paradoxically at risk for developing PCa cited the adverse effects of T deficiency. In the past 25 years, researchers have published on the genetic, biochemical, and clinical outcomes of testosterone replacement therapy (TRT) in hypogonadal men. The longstanding dogma of the deleterious effects of TRT has recently been challenged, and it now appears that TRT may have an important therapeutic role in the treatment of hypogonadism in those men with either low-risk, active, or previously treated PCa. This review summarizes the latest findings on the treatment of hypogonadal men with a history of PCa, emphasizing results of clinical research studies.

Keywords: testosterone; PCa; hypogonadism; androgen treatment

Introduction

Prostate cancer (PCa) is the most common cancer in men in the United States, with ~192,000 new cases in 2020.[1] This number of annual cases is expected to rise as the population ages. For patients deemed to have low-risk PCa, active surveillance (AS) is an accepted treatment option.[2–5] In cases that require treatment, surgery, radiation therapy, high-intensity focused ultrasound (HIFU), and cryotherapy are available options.

Even after successful treatment, biochemical recurrence (BCR) of PCa has been cited at a rate of 13–53% in patients after radiation therapy[6] and at 30.2% 3 years post–radical prostatectomy (RP).[7] It is estimated that up to 30% of males between 40 and 79 years of age are hypogonadal and 39% of males between the ages of 45–85 have a testosterone (T) level <300 ng/dL.[8,9] Hence, it is not uncommon for PCa patients to also be diagnosed with T deficiency at any stage in their disease, whether it is before treatment, after cure, in those who have BCR, or in those who

are on AS. Low T levels have been studied regarding their potential to increase the risk of PCa complications in diagnosed men, including higher incidence of extraprostatic metastasis,[10] seminal vesicle invasion,[11] and increased positive surgical margins.[12]

Irrespective of PCa, hypogonadal men treated with testosterone replacement therapy (TRT) experience clinical benefits through increased muscle mass, bone density, mood, and sexual health/performance.[13] Normalization of T levels is also postulated to potentially lower cardiovascular disease risk by reducing cholesterol levels, ameliorating glucose metabolism, and lessening the risk of metabolic syndrome.[14] Potential side effects of TRT include polycythemia, gynecomastia, BPH, and lowered HDL cholesterol.

The exact nature of the relationship between androgens and PCa is a particularly relevant topic given that PCa mortality has decreased by ~50% in the past two decades, resulting in a significant increase in PCa survivors with potential for experiencing symptoms

Department of Urology, Tulane University School of Medicine, New Orleans, Louisiana, USA.

*Address correspondence to: Wayne J.G. Hellstrom, MD, FACS, Department of Urology, Tulane University School of Medicine, 1430 Tulane Avenue, 8642, New Orleans, LA 70112, USA, Email: whellst@tulane.edu

of hypogonadism.[15] In this communication, the available evidence on the safety of TRT in men at risk for or with a previous or current diagnosis of PCa is reviewed.

Androgen Receptors and the Prostate

In the 1940s, Huggins and Hodgkins established a connection between androgenic hormones and PCa, laying the foundation for ADT in the treatment of PCa. They suggested that exogenous T would lead to increased cancer recurrence, measured by prostatic acid phosphatase (PAP) levels. This conclusion was based on the results of a very small study of three PCa patients who experienced a rise in PAP levels on administration of T injections, which was followed by a subsequent drop in enzyme levels after cessation of treatment. PAP has since been observed to be much less reliable than prostate-specific antigen (PSA) in the diagnosis of PCa (45% sensitivity for PAP vs. 96% for PSA) and in monitoring disease recurrence (25% of patients with metastatic disease presented with normal PAP levels[16,17]).

In 1996, Morgentaler et al. observed a high prevalence of PCa confirmed by biopsy in men with low total or free T levels, regardless of normal PSA levels.[18] Ten years later, Morgentaler and Rhoden documented additional results wherein, in 345 hypogonadal men with a PSA of ≤4.0 ng/mL, PCa was detected in 21% of men with T levels ≤250 ng/mL,[19] compared with 12% of men with a T level >250 ng/mL.

Morgentaler and Traish have proposed a saturation model to describe the varying sensitivity of the androgen receptor (AR) to either physiologically low or high T concentrations. They postulate that maximum AR activity is achieved at low T concentrations and saturation is responsible for less AR activity at higher T concentrations.[20] In human prostatic tissue, the AR is reported to become saturated and unreceptive to further increases in activity at T concentrations of 120 ng/dL *in vitro* and 240 ng/dL *in vivo*.[21,22] Separately, Rastrelli et al. identified the T AR saturation at a concentration of ~8 nmol/L (231 ng/dL).[23]

In one study, healthy men injected with 250 and 500 mg T per week had prostate volumes measured after 15 weeks. Despite significant elevations in free and total T, no increase in PSA or prostate volume was observed, thereby supporting the androgen saturation theory.[24] A randomized, double blind, placebo-controlled study also concluded that a 6-month TRT trial did not cause a significant increase in prostate tissue androgen concentrations.[25] The T saturation model also has interesting implications in the development of castration-resistant prostate cancer (CRPC). It has been postulated that supraphysiologic androgen levels may even paradoxically inhibit the growth of AR expressing human PCa cells, and similar antitumor activity has been observed in breast cancer patients exposed to high concentrations of estrogen.[26]

TRT and Risk of Developing PCa

Researchers have evaluated whether TRT increases the risk of developing newly diagnosed PCa. We review several pertinent studies with large sample sizes and new data in this section. Although many of these reports are limited by their study design, variability of inclusion criteria, and uncertainty regarding the length of TRT, and although the RCTs have reported data with mean and median follow-up less than 5 years, it appears that TRT is safe and does not increase the incidence of PCa.

A UK-based retrospective database review published in 2019 identified 12,779 patients with "late-onset hypogonadism.[27]" The mean follow-up period was 4.6 years, though 37.3% and 9.2% of patients received follow-up for at least 5 and 10 years, respectively. The use of TRT in that population did not result in increased risk of PCa (hazard ratio [HR] = 0.97 [95% confidence interval; CI 0.71–1.32) in an overall analysis, nor when propensity score matching was applied (HR = 0.87, 95% CI 0.56–1.36).[27]

In another longer-term study of T therapy in 1023 hypogonadal men, with a mean follow-up of 5 years, there were 11 cases of PCa (1.08%)—a prevalence figure lower than that reported by two large screening studies—the Prostate, Lung, Colorectal, and Ovarian (PLCO) Cancer Screening Trial (7.35%) and the European Randomized Study of Screening for PCa (ERSPC) (9.6%). An important limitation of this study was that younger men were included, unlike the PLCO and ERSPC trials.[28]

In a case–control study in the United States, using a Surveillance, Epidemiology and End Results (SEER) Medicare-linked database, patients with a diagnosis of PCa and with history of T use (574 men) were compared with PCa patients without history of T use (51,945). Those patients who had received TRT in the 5 years before diagnosis were found not to have an increased risk of high-grade disease at diagnosis (odds ratio [OR] 0.84, 95% CI 0.67–1.05). A multivariable analysis to assess a dose–response association among T users also did not reveal any correlation (OR 1.00, 95% CI 0.99–1.01).[29]

Another retrospective study evaluated 247 patients in Texas who commenced T therapy for a mean follow-up period of 6.5 years and compared them with 211 patients who did not receive TRT. By the end of the study, 47 men developed cancer: 27 (12.8%) not on TRT and 20 (8.1%) on TRT. No significant difference in PCa risk was found to be associated with TRT (HR 1.2, 95% CI 0.54–2.50).

In a similar report, from Sweden, Loeb et al. reported the results of a nested case–control study using the National PCa Registry of Sweden. From a multivariate analysis, no significant difference was demonstrated in PCa risk in patients with TRT exposure (OR 1.03; 95% CI 0.90–1.17). The authors went on to report that patients who had received TRT were observed to have more favorable-outcome PCa (OR 1.35; 95% CI 1.16–1.56) and a lower risk of aggressive cancer (OR 0.50; 95% CI 0.37–0.67) (28447913).[30]

In their study of 776 hypogonadal men with negative PCa screening at enrollment, Zhang et al. argued that TRT may accelerate the diagnosis of occult cancer, but not affect the overall prevalence at 7-year follow-up. They studied two groups of hypogonadal men with negative PCa screenings according to the European Association of Urology (EAU) guidelines. No significant difference was observed between the TRT group and the non-TRT group in cancer incidence at the end of the study period (9/398 vs. 5/230 respectively, $p = 0.9999$), even after performing propensity score matching to account for differences in baseline characteristics, most notably age and PSA. Of note, all cases in the TRT group were diagnosed within 18 months of treatment initiation, as compared with all cases diagnosed in the non-TRT group after 24 months of enrollment.[31] The authors concluded that TRT may speed up the diagnosis of occult cancer already present at initiation of treatment, but the therapy had a protective effect from the end of their predefined latency period until the end of the study.[31] Limitations of the study included a small subject number and aggressive lab testing/screening of the treatment group. Indeed, ongoing tri-annual transrectal ultrasound and digital rectal exam could be a potential explanation for the earlier cancer diagnosis.

In a recent meta-analysis of 26 placebo-controlled trials studying the effect of TRT on PCa, there was minimal absolute change of PSA between the beginning and end of the trial (0.1 ng/mL, 95% CI −0.28 to 0.48).[32] A major limitation of this result was the short median trial duration of 196 days. The same

group reviewed 11 trials to estimate the risk of PCa diagnosis while on TRT, and they concluded that there was no significant increase in risk measured by pooled OR (0.87, 95% CI 0.3–2.5). They also did not find evidence for heterogeneity or publication bias when assessing the quality of the results.[32]

In a similar analysis, data were pooled from random-controlled trials (RCTs) but divided into two groups: short-term follow-up (less than 12 months) and long-term follow-up (12–36 months). Pooling data from the RCTs with short-term follow-up did not show an increased PCa diagnosis rate, with OR of 0.39 (95% CI 0.06–2.45; P 1/4 0.32) for the study using injectable T and 1.10 (95% CI 0.26–4.65; P 1/4 0.90) for the study using transdermal T. However, these studies did find a rise in PSA with a standard mean difference of 0.52 (95% CI 0.00–1.05, $p = 0.05$) in studies using injectable T and a standard mean difference of 0.33 (95% CI 0.21–0.45, $p = 0.00001$) for studies using transdermal T. For RCTs with a longer-term follow-up, no difference in PCa diagnosis between the treatment and placebo group 0.99 (95% CI 0.24–4.02; $p = 0.99$) was determined.[33]

TRT in Patients with Untreated PCa

Several recent retrospective studies described in this sub-section have evaluated the risk associated with TRT in hypogonadal men with untreated PCa undergoing AS.[34–38] In general, these studies are limited by their retrospective design, few participants, and short follow-up periods (Table 1).

Two trials have demonstrated that a subset of men presenting with PCa had both an improvement in symptomatic hypogonadism and PCa characteristics after T administration.[39,40] Researchers from one 2009 study treated 15 PCa patients with three progressively increasing doses of transdermal T. Three patients saw a decline in PSA, though a total of 12 patients were taken off the study after possible disease progression, as evaluated through either PSA increases or findings on imaging studies.[39]

In an analysis of SEER Medicare data, Kaplan et al. estimated that, between 1991 and 2007, 0.79% (1181/149,354 men) of men received exogenous T after a PCa diagnosis. Several statistically significant findings were presented: Men on AS were noted to be less likely to receive TRT overall (6.9 vs. 5.4 events per 100-person years, $p = 0.0001$), and cancer-related mortality was higher in the non-TRT groups when compared with the TRT group (1.6 vs. 0.9 events per 100-person years, $p < 0.0001$).[41] Limitations of the study included

Table 1. Published Studies on Testosterone Replacement Therapy in Men Treated for Prostate Cancer on Active Surveillance

References	Patients	Stage/risk category	GG/Grade Group	Pre-TRT PSA median (ng/mL)	Post-TRT PSA median (ng/mL)	Median follow-up (months)	Cancer progression definition	Comments
Morgentaler[34]	1	NR	6 (1)	8.3	3.8	24	NR	Decline in PSA in man with untreated PCa who received TRT for 2 years.
Morales[35]	7	T1 (6)	6 (5); 8 (1)	4.8	NR	24	PSA >1 ng/mL quarterly or doubling within 12 months	Observational study without substantial discussion of patient follow-up after TRT. Study asserts that TRT candidates "should be willing and able to adhere to a strict follow-up (quarterly for the first 2 years and bi-annually thereafter if they are stable)."
Morgentaler et al.[36]	13	NR	6 (12) 7 (1)	5.0 (mean)	3.6 (mean)	30	NR	Researchers concluded that TRT in patients with untreated PCa was not associated with PCa progression in the short to medium term—citing consistency with the saturation model—or maximal PCa growth at low androgen concentrations.
Kacker et al.[37]	28	NR	6 (22) 7 (6)	• 3.21 (3+3 GG TRT cohort) • 2.58 (3+4 GG TRT cohort) • 4.46 (no TRT cohort)	• 1.04 (3+3 group increase) • 0.54 (3+4 group increase) • 0.22 (no TRT group increase)	42.9	Increase in GG upon biopsy	Retrospective chart review of 28 men who underwent TRT vs. 96 men on AS for PCa who did not receive TRT. Researchers concluded: "Biopsy progression rates were similar for both groups and historical controls. Biopsy progression in men on AS appears unaffected by T therapy over 3 years. Prospective placebo-controlled trials of T therapy in T-deficient men on AS should be considered given the symptomatic benefits experienced by treated men."
Ory et al.[38]	8	Low risk	6 (6)	3.9	5.2	33	Increase in GG on biopsy	No patients on AS put on TRT were observed to show clinical or pathological PCa progression. Researchers concluded: "In the absence of randomized, placebo controlled trials our study supports the hypothesis that testosterone therapy may be oncologically safe in hypogonadal men after definitive treatment or in those on active surveillance for prostate cancer."

AS, active surveillance; GG, Gleason Grade; NR, not reported; PCa, prostate cancer; PSA, prostate-specific antigen; T, testosterone; TRT, testosterone replacement therapy only evaluating a 5-year follow-up period and potentially unreliable clinical information available in a claims-based database.

Morgentaler et al. reported the results of prostate biopsies, serum PSA, and prostate volume in 13 hypogonadal men on AS who received TRT for 6 months for untreated PCa for 2.5 years.[36] Although the men experienced a 2.8-fold increase in serum T levels (238–664 ng/dL; $p < 0.001$), there was no significant change in mean PSA (5.5 ± 6.4 at initial biopsy vs. 3.6 ± 2.6 ng/mL after TRT, $p = 0.29$). These researchers noted that all men receiving TRT also experienced symptomatic improvement in libido, sexual performance, mood, and energy.

TRT in Patients with Treated PCa

Tables 2 and 3 summarize the published series on TRT after PCa treated with RP and radiotherapy modalities, respectively.[42–49] Recent studies have confirmed that TRT after definitive treatment for localized PCa appears safe and does not lead to increased disease recurrence.

In a large cohort analysis utilizing the Veterans Affairs Informatics and Computing Infrastructure (VINCI) database, Sarkar et al. identified 69,984 men with localized PCa, of whom 28,651 underwent RP and 41,333 received radiation. Of this total number, 469 RP (1.64%) and 543 radiation (1.31%) patients received TRT with a median follow-up of almost 7 years.[50] The investigators found that comparing those men who received TRT with those who did not, there were no between-group differences in BCR, PCa-specific mortality, or overall mortality after surgery (HR: 1.07; HR: 0.72 [$p = 0.43$]; and HR: 1.11 [$p = 0.43$], respectively) or radiation (HR: 1.07; HR: 1.02 [$p = 0.95$]; and HR: 1.02 [$p = 0.86$], respectively). One strength of this study was that it pooled a large, multi-ethnic, nationwide cohort with a high prevalence of African American men (24% prostatectomy, 28% radiation).

Ahlering et al. examined the rates of BCR in 850 patients who underwent RP for localized PCa, of whom 152 (18%) were started on TRT compared with 419 (82%) proportionally matched controls. After a median follow-up of 3.5 years, BCR occurred in 11 out of 152 (7.2%) and 53 out of 419 (12.6%) patients in the TRT and control groups, respectively. In adjusted time-to-event analysis, TRT was an independent predictor of recurrence-free survival. After accounting for the Gleason grade (GG) group, pathological stage, preoperative PSA level, and calculated free T, the authors determined that patients prescribed TRT were

~54% less likely to recur (HR 0.54, 95% CI 0.292–0.997).[51] Among those men who would eventually recur, TRT appeared to delay time to recurrence by an average of 1.5 years. Importantly, this study reported that by 2 years post-RP, 96% of patients had re-gained erectile function.

Specifically regarding hypogonadal men who underwent curative treatment for high-risk PCa, Teeling et al. conducted a single-arm meta-analysis to determine the relationship between TRT and risk of BCR. In this analysis of 13 studies and 109 men, the BCR rate was 0.00% (0.00–0.05%), lower than the expected rate for high-risk PCa survivors, suggesting that T therapy may not increase BCR risk in this patient population. The authors strongly cautioned against over interpretation, seeing that the available body of evidence was of very low quality.[52]

Another meta-analysis sought to evaluate the association between TRT in nonmetastatic PCa patients after definitive local therapy and the rate of BCR. Twenty-one studies were included with an overall pooled BCR rate of 0.01 (95% CI 0.00 − 0.02), suggesting a lack of association between TRT and BCR.[53] In subgroup analyses, pooled BCR rates were 0.00% (95% CI 0.00 − 0.02) in patients treated with RP and 0.02% (95% CI 0.00 − 0.04) in patients treated with external beam radiotherapy, brachytherapy (BT), cryotherapy, or HIFU. No heterogeneity was observed among included studies or in the subgroup analyses. A meta-analysis of 21 studies of BCR of PCa in men prescribed TRT after initiation of cancer therapy revealed that TRT in the setting of definitive PCa treatment did not increase BCR risk. Although studies varied in their PSA cutoff point for BCR, the majority (13/21) used the Phoenix definition of nadir +2 ng/mL as the end point. The researchers supported their conclusions with an identified BCR rate of 0.01% after TRT.[54]

Another study monitored PCa in 13 hypogonadal men who received TRT after previous BT or external beam radiotherapy treatment between 2006 and 2011.[55] After a median follow-up time of 29.7 months, no significant increases in PSA were observed during the study period (0.16–1.35 ng/mL, $p = 0.345$), and no reported cases of BCR were reported. Pastuszak et al. also organized a multicenter study that identified 98 men diagnosed with PCa and treated with radiation therapy. While on TRT for a median follow-up of 40.8 months, the men experienced a statistically significant median rise of 211 ng/mL in T levels and a nonsignificant increase in PSA from 0.08 ng/mL at baseline

Table 2. Published Studies on Testosterone Replacement Therapy in Men Treated for Prostate Cancer with Radical Prostatectomy

References	Patients	Stage/Risk category	GG/Grade Group	Pretreatment PSA, mean/median (ng/mL)	Treatment	Pre-TRT PSA (ng/mL)	Post-TRT PSA (ng/mL)	Median follow-up, months	BCR definition	BCR rate
Kaufman and Graydon[42]	7	NR	6 (6), 7 (1)	5.2	RP	<0.1	<0.1	19	PSA >0.1 ng/mL	0
Agarwal et al.[54]	10	NR	6 (2), 7 (7), 8 (1)	7	RP	<0.1	<0.1	24	PSA >0.1 ng/mL	0
Nabulsi et al.[49]	22	T2 (21), >T2 (1)	≤6 (58%), 7 (32%)	5.9	RP	NR	NR	20	NR	0.05
Khera et al.[45]	57	≤T2	6 (24), 7 (26), ≥8 (4)	5.58	RP	<0.1	<0.1	13	PSA >0.1 ng/mL	0
Sathyamoorthy et al.[47]	21	High risk	≥8 (21)	NR	RP	0.003	0.01	12	NR	0.00
Matsushita et al.[48]	71	≤T2 (84%), T3a (13%), T3b (3%)	7 (Median)	4.5	RP	NR	NR	19	PSA >0.1 ng/mL	0.014
Pastuszak et al.[55]	103	Not high risk (77), high risk (26)	<6 (1), 6–7 (74), >8 (9), NR (19)	5.2	RP	0.004	NR	27.5	PSA ≥0.2 ng/mL	0.04
Ahlering et al.[51]	152	T2 (86), ≥T3 (21)	GG1 (43), GG2 (77), GG3 (23), GG4 (2), GG5 (7)	7.2	RP	<0.05	NR	42	PSA ≥0.2 ng/mL	0.072

BCR, biochemical recurrence; ; PSA, prostate-specific antigen; RP, radical prostatectomy.

Table 3. Published Studies on Testosterone Replacement Therapy in Men Treated for Prostate Cancer with Radiotherapy or Radical Prostatectomy

References	Number of patients	Stage/Risk category	GG	Pretreatment PSA, mean/median (ng/mL)	Treatment	Pre-TRT PSA (ng/mL)	Post-TRT PSA (ng/mL)	Median follow-up, months	BCR definition	BCR rate
Sarosdy[43]	31	T1b (1), T1c (20), T2a (8), T2c (2)	≤6 (22), 7 (6), ≥8 (3)	5.3	BT	5.3	<1	60	NR	0
Davila et al.[46]	20	NR	Mean Gleason 6.2 (RP), 5 (EBRT)	6.05 (RP), 3.5 (EBRT)	14 RP, 6 EBRT	0.1 (RP), 0.15 (EBRT)	0.1 (RP), 0.1 (EBRT)	12 (RP), 9 (EBRT)	NR	0
Morales et al.[44]	5	NR	6 (2), 7 (1), 8 (2)	11.96	EBRT	0.3	0.47	14.6	NR	0
Pastuszak et al.[55]	13	NCCN low (4), intermediate (7), high (2)	6 (4), 7 (7), 8 (2)	5.8	BT/EBRT	0.3	0.66	29.7	Two consecutive increases of PSA of >0.5 ng/ml	0
Ory et al.[38]	74	D'Amico low (14), intermediate (30), high (30)	6 (24), 7 (39), 8 (7), 9 (4)	NR	22 RP, 50 RT, 1 BT, 1 HIFU			48 (RP), 36.5 (RT), 9 (BT), 42 (HIFU)	PSA ≥0.2 ng/mL (RP), nadir +2 ng/mL (RT)	0.06 (RT)

BT, brachytherapy; HIFU, high-intensity focused ultrasound; NCCN, National Comprehensive Cancer Network; RT, radiotherapy.

to 0.09 ng/mL ($p = 0.05$). Six men (6.1%) experienced BCR and three of these men underwent BT before PSA levels consequently normalized.[56]

In 20 men (49–74 age range) who underwent BT for PCa (6.2 ng/mL PSA at time of diagnosis), there was a decrease in mean PSA level, from 0.7 ng/mL before TRT to 0.1 ng/mL after TRT (TRT not initiated before at least 3 months of treatment) at the time of last follow-up (median time of 31 months).[57] Patients received long-acting 1000 mg T injections and subsequent adjusted T concentration injections to meet a free T concentration >11.7 ng/dL. Another small study of five patients also identified benefits of TRT administration in hypogonadal patients following external beam radiotherapy for localized PCa. Patients began TRT once their PSA levels reached their nadir and only one patient had a transitory PSA level increase, not more than 1.5 ng/mL.[35] All men reported improvements in symptoms associated with hypogonadism.

TRT in Patients with Advanced PCa

In the setting of metastatic castration-resistant PCa (mCRPC), an emerging body of literature supports the use of supraphysiologic levels of androgens as an adjunctive therapeutic treatment. Although the exact mechanism remains under active investigation, it appears that high-dose androgen may act by inducing double-strand DNA breaks, inhibiting relicensing of DNA in cells expressing high levels of AR repressing genes in DNA repair, downregulating AR splice variants (e.g., AR-V7), and delaying restoration of damaged DNA.[26,58–62] Both continuous and intermittent administration of high-dose testosterone (HDT) has been described, with a greater body of literature available for the latter. This intermittent HDT strategy, where T levels are quickly raised to supraphysiologic levels and then brought down to near-castration levels over ~ 1 month, is termed bipolar androgen therapy (BAT).

Multiple recent Phase I and II studies have been conducted to investigate TRT in the CRPC setting. The first Phase I trial evaluated the effect of increasing doses of transdermal T (2.5, 5, or 7.5 mg/day) in 15 men with low-risk CRPC. The authors observed that one patient had symptomatic progression, and three patients had a decrease in PSA (maximums decrease of 43%).[39] Those men receiving the highest dose of TRT demonstrated a longer time to progression, which was not noted to be statistically significant. No grade 3 or 4 toxicities were reported apart from one patient with cardiac toxicity at week 53.

Table 4. Published Studies on Testosterone Replacement Therapy in Men with Castration-Resistant Prostate Cancer

References	Patients	Stage/risk category	GG/Grade Group	Pretreatment PSA, mean/median (ng/mL)	Post-TRT PSA (ng/mL)	Median follow-up, mo	BCR definition	Comments
Szmulewitz et al.[39]	15	CRPC, 6 of 15 patients evidence of bone metastasis	NR	11.1	NR	2	PSA >3 × nadir PSA	One patient was removed from the study due to grade 4 cardiac toxicity. The majority of patients were taken off the study due to the progression of disease by either PSA ($n = 9$) criteria or for both imaging and PSA ($n = 3$). No significant improvement in QOL identified—with further QOL improvement results pending from a larger clinical trial being performed. Researchers concluded that TRT was a "feasible and well-tolerated therapy for men with early CRPC."
Morris et al.[40]	12	CRPC metastatic cancer (soft tissue and/or bone)	8 (Median)	91	NR	2	25% increase in PSA over 3 tests	One patient was removed from the study due to epidural disease—subsequently treated with radiation. Nine of 12 patients exhibited biochemical or radiographic progression. One patient exhibited a > 50% decrease in PSA from baseline measurement. Researchers concluded that "patients with CRPC can be safely treated in clinical trials using high-dose exogenous testosterone."

The second Phase I study examined 12 men with CRPC administered transdermal TRT (7.5 mg/day) for 1 week, 1 month, or until disease progression.[40] Despite the goal of reaching supraphysiologic levels of T during the study, average serum T levels were within normal limits. Although no objective responses were observed, 33% of patients had declines of PSA of at least 20% and one reached $a > 50\%$ decline in PSA (PSA50). There were no grade 3 or 4 toxicities. Results from these aforementioned Phase I studies are presented in Table 4.

Subsequently, the Phase II TRANSFORMER trial examined 30 asymptomatic mCRPC patients with disease progression on abiraterone/enzalutamide who were treated with BAT and then re-challenged with enzalutamide.[63] The study reported a 30% PSA50 response to BAT. Twenty-one patients proceeded to enzalutamide re-challenge with a 52% PSA50 response. This study appears to support the use of BAT as a means of targeting the AR in patients who have disease progression on second-line AR signaling inhibitors.

The currently ongoing RESTORE Phase II trial has enrolled 59 asymptomatic mCRPC patients with disease progression on abiraterone ($n = 29$) or enzalutamide ($n = 30$) who were then treated with BAT and re-challenged with their most recent androgen receptor-targeted therapy.[62] After BAT, the postenzalutamide cohort showed a 30% PSA50 response versus 17% PSA50 in the postabiraterone cohort, a difference that was not statistically significant. After AR targeted therapy re-challenge, PSA50 response was significantly higher in the postenzalutamide cohort (68% vs. 16%). Median progression free survival (PFS) was longer in the postenzalutamide versus postabiraterone re-challenge cohort (12.8 months vs. 8.1 months). The authors also noted that men with detectable AR-V7 mutations in circulating-tumor DNA had worse PFS (10.3 months vs. 7.1 months). From the currently reported data, BAT appears to demonstrate clinical benefit in pretreated mCRPC patients with a greater re-sensitization seen in men treated with enzalutamide compared with abiraterone and that the presence of certain splice variants such as AR-V7 may prognose a worse response to BAT.[62]

Conclusion

The TRT for patients who have a history of untreated or treated PCa remains a debated practice, given the long-established dogma that T could act as "fuel on the fire" for PCa recurrence and growth. As previously described, this paradigm has shifted since the introduction of the saturation model hypothesis. Since then, a growing body of published case series appear to support TRT in this clinical setting. Researchers currently recommend that patients be prescribed the lowest necessary T dose to achieve serum androgen normalization and then be screened at regular intervals, depending on the administration method.

The American Urological Association (AUA) TRT guidelines recognize the lack of evidence linking TRT to the development of PCa, as well as insufficient evidence to quantify a risk–benefit ratio of TRT in patients with a history of PCa.[64] As such, hypogonadal patients should make an informed consent before initiating TRT, after a thorough conversation with their provider of the risks and benefits. Until definitive evidence from long-term prospective or placebo-controlled RCTs becomes available, patients under AS, or with a history of PCa must understand the importance of strict compliance with increased T, PSA, and digital rectal exam monitoring frequency.

Currently, neither the AUA nor EAU provides guidelines on monitoring intervals for TRT patients on AS or after RP or radiation therapy. Data from available studies indicate that serum T, PSA, and digital rectal exam findings should be evaluated at least every 3–6 months, according to a physician's best judgment given a patient's goals, medical history, and perceived PCa risk.[65] For patients on AS, it has been suggested that a patient's relative risk be evaluated by a multidisciplinary medical team, including a urologist, endocrinologist, and oncologist.[66] In all cases, serum T levels should be kept as low as possible to meet a patient's replacement needs.

Future studies, in addition to focusing on specific PCa risk with TRT in populations stratified by factors such as GG group, treatment during AS, or history of prior definitive treatment for localized PCa, should also focus on providing results of quality-of-life metrics to help enumerate the risk–benefit ratio for patients when making health care decisions.

Authors' Contributions

Conception and design: W.J.G.H.; Data acquisition and analysis: M.P. and I.V.; Drafting article: M.P. and I.V.; Revising article: A.S. and W.J.G.H.; Approval: All authors.

References

1. American Cancer Society. Cancer Facts & Figures 2020. https://www.cancer.org/research/cancer-facts-statistics/all-cancer-facts-figures/cancer-facts-figures-2020.html. Accessed August 15, 2020.

2. Klotz L, Vesprini D, Sethukavalan P, et al. Long-term follow-up of a large active surveillance cohort of patients with prostate cancer. J Clin Oncol. 2015;33(3):272–277.

3. Soloway MS, Soloway CT, Williams S, Ayyathurai R, Kava B, Manoharan M. Active surveillance; a reasonable management alternative for patients with prostate cancer: The Miami experience. BJU Int. 2008;101(2):165–169.

4. Roemeling S, Roobol MJ, de Vries SH, et al. Active surveillance for prostate cancers detected in three subsequent rounds of a screening trial: Characteristics, PSA doubling times, and outcome. Eur Urol. 2007;51(5):1244–1250; discussion 1251.

5. Khatami A, Aus G, Damber JE, Lilja H, Lodding P, Hugosson J. PSA doubling time predicts the outcome after active surveillance in screening-detected prostate cancer: Results from the European randomized study of screening for prostate cancer, Sweden section. Int J Cancer. 2007;120(1):170–174.

6. Pastuszak AW, Pearlman AM, Lai WS, et al. Testosterone replacement therapy in patients with prostate cancer after radical prostatectomy. J Urol. 2013;190(2):639–644.

7. Arcangeli G, Strigari L, Arcangeli S, et al. Retrospective comparison of external beam radiotherapy and radical prostatectomy in high-risk, clinically localized prostate cancer. Int J Radiat Oncol Biol Phys. 2009;75(4):975–982.

8. Mulligan T, Frick MF, Zuraw QC, Stemhagen A, McWhirter C. Prevalence of hypogonadism in males aged at least 45 years: The HIM study. Int J Clin Pract. 2006;60(7):762–769.

9. Traish AM, Miner MM, Morgentaler A, Zitzmann M. Testosterone deficiency. Am J Med. 2011;124(7):578–587.

10. Kim HJ, Kim BH, Park CH, Kim CI. Usefulness of preoperative serum testosterone as a predictor of extraprostatic extension and biochemical recurrence. Korean J Urol. 2012;53(1):9–13.

11. Salonia A, Gallina A, Briganti A, et al. Preoperative hypogonadism is not an independent predictor of high-risk disease in patients undergoing radical prostatectomy. Cancer. 2011;117(17):3953–3962.

12. Teloken C, Da Ros CT, Caraver F, Weber FA, Cavalheiro AP, Graziottin TM. Low serum testosterone levels are associated with positive surgical margins in radical retropubic prostatectomy: Hypogonadism represents bad prognosis in prostate cancer. J Urol. 2005;174(6):2178–2180.

13. Kaplan AL, Lenis AT, Shah A, Rajfer J, Hu JC. Testosterone replacement therapy in men with prostate cancer: A time-varying analysis. J Sex Med. 2015;12(2):374–380.

14. Umbas R, Sugiono M. Testosterone replacement therapy in prostate cancer patients: Is it safe? Acta Med Indones. 2010;42(3):171–175.

15. Nguyen TM, Pastuszak AW. Testosterone therapy among prostate cancer survivors. Sex Med Rev. 2016;4(4):376–388.

16. Oesterling JE. Prostate specific antigen: A critical assessment of the most useful tumor marker for adenocarcinoma of the prostate. J Urol. 1991;145(5):907–923.

17. Johnson DE, Prout GR, Scott WW, Schmidt JD, Gibbons RP. Clinical significance of serum acid phosphatase levels in advanced prostatic carcinoma. Urology. 1976;8(2):123–126.

18. Morgentaler A, Bruning CO, III, DeWolf WC. Occult prostate cancer in men with low serum testosterone levels. JAMA. 1996;276(23):1904–1906.

19. Morgentaler A, Rhoden EL. Prevalence of prostate cancer among hypogonadal men with prostate-specific antigen levels of 4.0 ng/mL or less. Urology. 2006;68(6):1263–1267.

20. Levine LA, Estrada CR, Morgentaler A. Mechanical reliability and safety of, and patient satisfaction with the Ambicor inflatable penile prosthesis: Results of a 2 center study. J Urol. 2001;166(3):932–937.

21. Traish AM, Williams DF, Hoffman ND, Wotiz HH. Validation of the exchange assay for the measurement of androgen receptors in human and dog prostates. Prog Clin Biol Res. 1988;262:145–160.

22. Traish AM, Muller RE, Wotiz HH. A new procedure for the quantitation of nuclear and cytoplasmic androgen receptors. J Biol Chem. 1981;256(23):12028–12033.

23. Rastrelli G, Corona G, Vignozzi L, et al. Serum PSA as a predictor of testosterone deficiency. J Sex Med. 2013;10(10):2518–2528.

24. Cooper CS, Perry PJ, Sparks AE, MacIndoe JH, Yates WR, Williams RD. Effect of exogenous testosterone on prostate volume, serum and semen prostate specific antigen levels in healthy young men. J Urol. 1998;159(2):441–443.

25. Marks LS, Mazer NA, Mostaghel E, et al. Effect of testosterone replacement therapy on prostate tissue in men with late-onset hypogonadism: A randomized controlled trial. JAMA. 2006;296(19):2351–2361.

26. Chatterjee P, Schweizer MT, Lucas JM, et al. Supraphysiological androgens suppress prostate cancer growth through androgen receptor-mediated DNA damage. J Clin Invest. 2019;129(10):4245–4260.

27. Santella C, Renoux C, Yin H, Yu OHY, Azoulay L. Testosterone replacement therapy and the risk of prostate cancer in men with late-onset hypogonadism. Am J Epidemiol. 2019;188(9):1666–1673.

28. Haider A, Zitzmann M, Doros G, Isbarn H, Hammerer P, Yassin A. Incidence of prostate cancer in hypogonadal men receiving testosterone therapy: Observations from 5-year median followup of 3 registries. J Urol. 2015;193(1):80–86.

29. Baillargeon J, Kuo YF, Fang X, Shahinian VB. Long-term exposure to testosterone therapy and the risk of high grade prostate cancer. J Urol. 2015;194(6):1612–1616.

30. Loeb S, Folkvaljon Y, Damber JE, Alukal J, Lambe M, Stattin P. Testosterone replacement therapy and risk of favorable and aggressive prostate cancer. J Clin Oncol. 2017;35(13):1430–1436.

31. Zhang X, Zhong Y, Saad F, Haider K, Haider A, Xu X. Clinically occult prostate cancer cases may distort the effect of testosterone replacement therapy on risk of PCa. World J Urol. 2019;37(10):2091–2097.

32. Boyle P, Koechlin A, Bota M, et al. Endogenous and exogenous testosterone and the risk of prostate cancer and increased prostate-specific antigen (PSA) level: A meta-analysis. BJU Int. 2016;118(5):731–741.

33. Cui Y, Zong H, Yan H, Zhang Y. The effect of testosterone replacement therapy on prostate cancer: A systematic review and meta-analysis. Prostate Cancer Prostatic Dis. 2014;17(2):132–143.

34. Morgentaler A. Two years of testosterone therapy associated with decline in prostate-specific antigen in a man with untreated prostate cancer. J Sex Med. 2009;6(2):574–577.

35. Morales A. Effect of testosterone administration to men with prostate cancer is unpredictable: A word of caution and suggestions for a registry. BJU Int. 2011;107(9):1369–1373.

36. Morgentaler A, Lipshultz LI, Bennett R, Sweeney M, Avila D, Jr, Khera M. Testosterone therapy in men with untreated prostate cancer. J Urol. 2011;185(4):1256–1260.

37. Kacker R, Hult M, San Francisco IF, et al. Can testosterone therapy be offered to men on active surveillance for prostate cancer? Preliminary results. Asian J Androl. 2016;18(1):16–20.

38. Ory J, Flannigan R, Lundeen C, Huang JG, Pommerville P, Goldenberg SL. Testosterone therapy in patients with treated and untreated prostate cancer: Impact on oncologic outcomes. J Urol. 2016;196(4):1082–1089.

39. Szmulewitz R, Mohile S, Posadas E, et al. A randomized phase 1 study of testosterone replacement for patients with low-risk castration-resistant prostate cancer. Eur Urol. 2009;56(1):97–103.

40. Morris MJ, Huang D, Kelly WK, et al. Phase 1 trial of high-dose exogenous testosterone in patients with castration-resistant metastatic prostate cancer. Eur Urol. 2009;56(2):237–244.

41. Kaplan AL, Trinh QD, Sun M, et al. Testosterone replacement therapy following the diagnosis of prostate cancer: Outcomes and utilization trends. J Sex Med. 2014;11(4):1063–1070.

42. Kaufman JM, Graydon RJ. Androgen replacement after curative radical prostatectomy for prostate cancer in hypogonadal men. J Urol. 2004;172(3):920–922.

43. Sarosdy MF. Testosterone replacement for hypogonadism after treatment of early prostate cancer with brachytherapy. Cancer. 2007;109(3):536–541.

44. Morales A, Black AM, Emerson LE. Testosterone administration to men with testosterone deficiency syndrome after external beam radiotherapy for localized prostate cancer: Preliminary observations. BJU Int. 2009;103(1):62–64.

45. Khera M, Grober ED, Najari B, et al. Testosterone replacement therapy following radical prostatectomy. J Sex Med. 2009;6(4):1165–1170.

46. Davila HH AC, Hall MK, Salup R, Lockhart JM, Carrion RE. Analysis of the PSA response after testosterone supplementation in patients who have previously received management for their localized prostate cancer. J Urol. 2008;(179):428.

47. Sathyamoorthy K, Stein M, Lipshultz L, Khera M. Follow-up series of testosterone replacement therapy following radical prostatectomy: The Baylor experience. J Sex Med. 2010;7:10–11.

48. Matsushita K, Katz D, Stember D, Nelson C, Mulhall J. Analysis of the safety and efficacy of testosterone suplementation following radical prostatectomy. J Sex Med. 2012;9:205.

49. Nabulsi O, Tal R, Gotto G, Narus J, Goldenberg L, Mulhall JP. Outcomes analysis of testosterone supplementation in hypogonadal men following radical prostatectomy. J Urol. 2008(179):426–427.

50. Sarkar RR, Patel SH, Parsons JK, et al. Testosterone therapy does not increase the risks of prostate cancer recurrence or death after definitive treatment for localized disease. Prostate Cancer Prostatic Dis. 2020;23(4): 689–695.

51. Ahlering TE, My Huynh L, Towe M, et al. Testosterone replacement therapy reduces biochemical recurrence after radical prostatectomy. BJU Int. 2020;126(1):91–96.

52. Teeling F, Raison N, Shabbir M, Yap T, Dasgupta P, Ahmed K. Testosterone therapy for high-risk prostate cancer survivors: A systematic review and meta-analysis. Urology. 2019;126:16–23.

53. Kardoust Parizi M, Abufaraj M, Fajkovic H, et al. Oncological safety of testosterone replacement therapy in prostate cancer survivors after definitive local therapy: A systematic literature review and meta-analysis. Urol Oncol. 2019;37(10):637–646.

54. Agarwal PK, Oefelein MG. Testosterone replacement therapy after primary treatment for prostate cancer. J Urol. 2005;173(2):533–536.

55. Pastuszak AW, Pearlman AM, Godoy G, Miles BJ, Lipshultz LI, Khera M. Testosterone replacement therapy in the setting of prostate cancer treated with radiation. Int J Impot Res. 2013;25(1):24–28.

56. Pastuszak AW, Khanna A, Badhiwala N, et al. Testosterone therapy after radiation therapy for low, intermediate and high risk prostate cancer. J Urol. 2015;194(5):1271–1276.

57. Balbontin FG, Moreno SA, Bley E, Chacon R, Silva A, Morgentaler A. Long-acting testosterone injections for treatment of testosterone deficiency after brachytherapy for prostate cancer. BJU Int. 2014;114(1):125–130.

58. Murthy S, Wu M, Bai VU, et al. Role of androgen receptor in progression of LNCaP prostate cancer cells from G1 to S phase. PLoS One. 2013;8(2):e56692.

59. D'Antonio JM, Vander Griend DJ, Isaacs JT. DNA licensing as a novel androgen receptor mediated therapeutic target for prostate cancer. Endocr Relat Cancer. 2009;16(2):325–332.

60. Litvinov IV, Vander Griend DJ, Antony L, et al. Androgen receptor as a licensing factor for DNA replication in androgen-sensitive prostate cancer cells. Proc Natl Acad Sci U S A. 2006;103(41):15085–15090.

61. Haffner MC, Aryee MJ, Toubaji A, et al. Androgen-induced TOP2B-mediated double-strand breaks and prostate cancer gene rearrangements. Nat Genet. 2010;42(8):668–675.

62. Markowski MC, Wang H, Sullivan R, et al. A Multicohort Open-label Phase II Trial of Bipolar Androgen Therapy in Men with Metastatic Castration-resistant Prostate Cancer (RESTORE): A Comparison of post-abiraterone versus post-enzalutamide cohorts. Eur Urol. 2020. [Epub ahead of print]; DOI: 10.1016/j.eururo.2020.06.042.

63. Teply BA, Wang H, Luber B, et al. Bipolar androgen therapy in men with metastatic castration-resistant prostate cancer after progression on enzalutamide: An open-label, phase 2, multicohort study. Lancet Oncol. 2018;19(1):76–86.

64. Mulhall JP, Trost LW, Brannigan RE, et al. Evaluation and management of testosterone deficiency: AUA Guideline. J Urol. 2018;200(2):423–432.

65. Gray H, Seltzer J, Talbert RL. Recurrence of prostate cancer in patients receiving testosterone supplementation for hypogonadism. Am J Health Syst Pharm. 2015;72(7):536–541.

66. Lenfant L, Leon P, Cancel-Tassin G, et al. Testosterone replacement therapy (TRT) and prostate cancer: An updated systematic review with a focus on previous or active localized prostate cancer. Urol Oncol. 2020; 38(8):661–670.

Abbreviations Used

AR = androgen receptor
AS = active surveillance
AUA = American Urological Association
BAT = bipolar androgen therapy
BCR = biochemical recurrence
BT = brachytherapy
CRPC = castration-resistant prostate cancer
EAU = European Association of Urology
ERSPC = European Randomized Study of Screening for PCa
HDT = high-dose testosterone
HIFU = high-intensity focused ultrasound
HR = hazard ratio
mCRPC = metastatic castration-resistant PCa
PAP = prostatic acid phosphatase
PCa = prostate cancer
PLCO = Prostate, Lung, Colorectal, and Ovarian
PSA = prostate-specific antigen
RCT = random-controlled trial
RP = radical prostatectomy
RT = radiotherapy
SEER = Surveillance, Epidemiology and End Results
T = testosterone
TRT = testosterone replacement therapy

7

Testosterone Implant Therapy in Women with and without Breast Cancer: Rationale, Experience, Evidence

Rebecca Glaser[1,2,*,i] and Constantine Dimitrakakis[3,4]

Abstract

Testosterone (T) is the most abundant biologically active hormone in women. It has a direct effect at the androgen receptor in every major organ system. Local aromatization of T is a major source of bioavailable estradiol. Adequate amounts of bioavailable T are essential for optimal health, immune function, and disease prevention. More than 80% of bioavailable T in women is from the local intracrine production of T from the adrenal precursor steroids androstenedione and dehydroepiandrosterone (sulfate). Serum T levels reflect <20% of the total androgen pool in women, which limits its usefulness in diagnosing or treating androgen deficiency. The gradual decline of androgens associated with aging is responsible for many of the adverse signs and symptoms of aging, including mental and physical deterioration. Decades of evidence support the safety and efficacy of T therapy in women. We have found that subcutaneous T implant therapy relieves symptoms of hormone deficiency in women with and without breast cancer, improves their quality of life, and maintains overall health and well-being. T does not increase and may lower the risk of breast cancer. The combination of T with an aromatase inhibitor prevents the conversion of androgens to estrogens, limiting their stimulatory effect in estrogen-sensitive diseases, including breast cancer. Adequate doses of T therapy should provide adequate levels of bioavailable T in the target organs—determined by clinical response (benefits) versus adverse side effects (risks). Pharmacological dosing of T implants in women is safe and necessary for physiological effect.

Keywords: androgens in women; testosterone therapy; pellet implants; aromatase; breast cancer

Introduction

Androgens are critical for immune function and overall health in both sexes. Androgens decline with age, adversely affecting mental and physical health. Replacing (declining) androgens with the consistent and continuous release of testosterone (T) from the subcutaneous implant significantly improves women's health, sexuality, and quality of life (QoL).[1–6]

Many controversies surround the use of T therapy in women. Recent pharmaceutical sponsored studies have focused on topical T formulations and recent narratives have argued against the use of T pellet implants.[7] However, T implant therapy has been (safely) used in female patients since 1937 in doses of 50–400 mg without excessive androgenic effects.[3–6,8,9] In addition, significantly higher doses (500–1800 mg) have been safely used to treat breast cancer patients.[3,10]

Understanding the physiology of androgens in women is the foundation for understanding the extent of T's clinical effects; the rationale behind 'T dosing'

[1]Millennium Wellness Center, Dayton, Ohio, USA.
[2]Department of Surgery, Wright State University Boonshoft School of Medicine, Dayton, Ohio, USA.
[3]First Department of Ob-Gyn, Athens University Medical School, Athens, Greece.
[4]NICHD, National Institutes of Health, Bethesda, Maryland, USA.
[i]ORCID ID (https://orcid.org/0000-0001-5747-3448).

*Address correspondence to: Rebecca Glaser, MD, Millennium Wellness Center, 228 E. Spring Valley Road, Dayton, OH 45458, USA, Email: rglaser@woh.rr.com; rglasermd@gmail.com

and 'serum levels on therapy'; the significance of local aromatase production and its role in estrogen-sensitive diseases; and the therapeutic effects of T alone (no estrogen). In a series of studies, we provide decades of experience and evidence supporting the safety and efficacy of T implant therapy in women, including breast cancer patients.[1,11–25] The therapeutic potential of T combined with an aromatase inhibitor (AI) is discussed and supported by clinical evidence.

Androgens in Women

T is the most abundant biologically active hormone in women. It is produced in the ovaries, adrenal gland, and locally at the cellular level in target organs from androgen precursors. The major portion of serum T is bound to albumin and sex hormone-binding globulin. T has a direct effect at the androgen receptor (AR). It is metabolized through the enzyme 5α-reductase to the more potent androgen, dihydrotestosterone. T is also aromatized to estradiol (E2) in the ovaries and locally in all peripheral tissues, thereby having a secondary effect through the estrogen receptor (ER). Many physicians are not aware that serum T levels are markedly (10- to more than 15-fold) higher than E2 levels throughout the female lifespan, barring pregnancy (Fig. 1).[26]

The major source of androgenic activity in both pre- and postmenopausal women is the local intracrine production of T from the adrenal precursor steroids dehydroepiandrosterone-sulfate (DHEAS), dehydroepiandrosterone (DHEA), and androstenedione (Fig. 2).

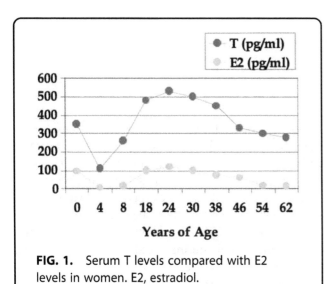

FIG. 1. Serum T levels compared with E2 levels in women. E2, estradiol.

Androstenedione, the direct precursor to T, is found in more than fivefold higher concentrations than serum T in women.[27,28] Circulating DHEA and DHEAS are present in 20- to 1000-fold higher concentrations than T. Interestingly, men and women produce similar amounts of adrenal androgens. The preandrogens contribute >75–80% of biologically active T to the AR in premenopausal women and near 100% in postmenopausal women—versus 50% in men.[29–31]

Serum levels of T are *not* a valid marker of tissue exposure in women, reflecting <20% of the total androgen activity. Accordingly, serum T levels would not be expected to correlate with androgen deficiency symptoms or clinical conditions caused by androgen deficiency.[30] This concept is extremely important to comprehend. Serum T levels should *not* be relied on to diagnose T deficiency or manage T dosing in women.[5–9]

It is well recognized that T has a profound effect on lean muscle mass, bone density, and confidence as well as sex drive and performance in both sexes. It is beyond the scope of this article to provide a detailed review of the physiological effects of androgens. Excellent reviews have been previously published on the clinical significance of T in women.[32]

It is important to recognize that there are active ARs located in every major organ system throughout the body.[33–38] Adequate amounts of (local) bioavailable T at the AR are *critical* for overall health, immune function, and preventing inflammation, as well as cardiovascular, neurological, gastrointestinal, pulmonary, endocrine, breast, and genitourinary health (Supplementary Table S1).[32–42] Thus, clinical indications for T therapy include many signs and symptoms caused by T deficiency (Table 1).[1,43]

T is the direct precursor for E2 in every major organ system, including the ovaries. The enzyme aromatase (P450) catalyzes the biosynthesis of estrogens from androgens. Tissue-specific aromatase and other steroidogenic enzymes are located in every organ system—supplying estrogens locally to the ER from T and androgen precursors (Fig. 2).[44–46] The main source of estrogen in postmenopausal women is the local conversion (paracrine/intracrine) of T to biologically active E2. Unlike adipose tissue, which can contribute to the circulating pool of estrogens, E2 from local aromatization would not be measurable in serum.[31,46,47] Therefore, similar to serum T levels, serum levels of E2 should be interpreted with caution and taken into context with clinical evaluation.

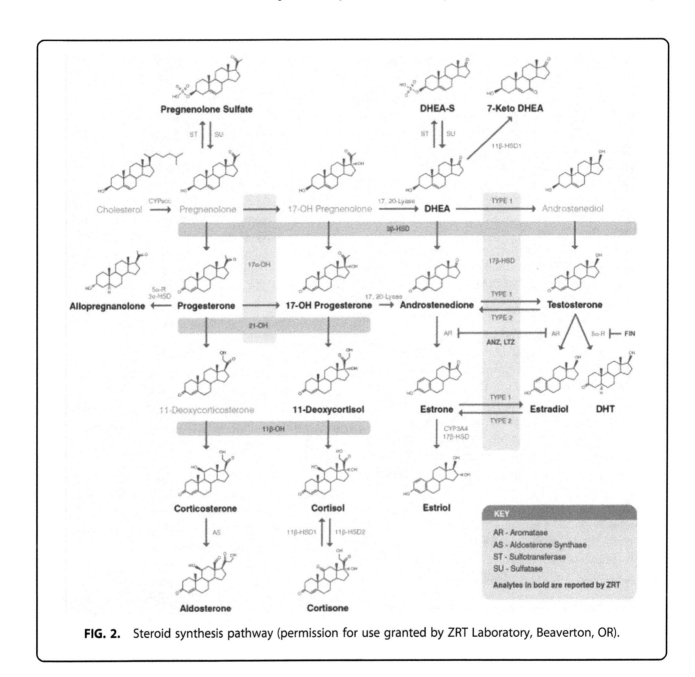

FIG. 2.   Steroid synthesis pathway (permission for use granted by ZRT Laboratory, Beaverton, OR).

Table 1. Signs and Symptoms of Aging Related to Androgen Deficiency

A diminished sense of well-being
Dysphoric mood, anxiety, and irritability
Fatigue
Decreased libido, sexual activity, and pleasure
Vasomotor instability
Bone loss
Decreased muscle strength
Insomnia
Changes in cognition and memory loss
Urinary symptoms and incontinence
Vaginal dryness and atrophy
Joint and muscular pain

Obesity, medications, xenoestrogens, certain disease states (endometriosis and fibroids) and cancers (breast and endometrial) upregulate aromatase resulting in excess intracellular (local) E2 production. Increased aromatase activity and excess estrogen relative to T can stimulate breast and uterine tissues and remains an underappreciated cofactor in the etiology of endometriosis, dysfunctional uterine bleeding, uterine fibroids, as well as breast and uterine cancers.[44–53]

A marked decline of T and the adrenal precursor steroids (DHEA and androstenedione) occurs in women between their late 20s and 50s, which has a significant impact on their health, sexuality, and QoL.[32,54,55] Symptoms of androgen deficiency can occur before menopause and are not related to estrogen levels.[1,3–6,43] In fact, many premenopausal women have symptoms of estrogen excess in addition to androgen deficiency.[1,3–6] As evidenced earlier, serum T testing would not be reliable in diagnosing androgen deficiency. The gradual decline of (all) androgens is associated with signs, symptoms, and disease states associated with aging (Supplementary Table S1). In addition, T deficiency has a negative impact on cardiovascular and neurological health in women.[32,56]

T implant therapy in women and treatment controversies

T implant therapy has been safely used in women since 1937[3–6,8,9]—which may be a reason there are a limited number of recent controlled studies, which can be overwhelmingly costly—yet necessary for Food and Drug Administration (FDA) approval. Well-designed randomized controlled trials (RCTs) are valuable in assessing the effectiveness of drug treatments. However, by nature they obscure individual variability seen in clinical practice. Evidence-based personalized medicine promotes integrating the best research evidence, the physician's clinical expertise, and the patient's values, preferences, and expectations. Decades of clinical experience and evidence (original data) support the long-term safety and efficacy of T therapy in women.[1,11–25]

Since 2005, >2500 women have been treated with subcutaneous T implants, including >230 breast cancer patients. In 2020, 3331 T pellet insertions were performed in 1022 female patients, 105 of whom had a diagnosis of breast cancer. All patient's initial severity of symptoms and subsequent hormone-related changes are evaluated using the validated Health-Related QoL questionnaire, Menopause Rating Scale (MRS) (Fig. 3). Additional symptom-specific validated questionnaires are administered if clinically applicable. T implants are not regulated.

All patients are required to sign a consent informing them of the "off-label" use, benefits, and risks of T implants in women (Supplementary Data S1). Patients are informed of (expected) elevated serum T levels on therapy and the stimulation of red blood cell production. Patients are monitored for secondary polycythemia.

In the United States, androgens are listed as a "class X" teratogen and premenopausal patients are instructed that they "must use birth control" (listed on the consent) with the "warning" that T could masculinize a female fetus.

However, there are no reports in the literature evidencing that T delivered by subcutaneous implants (i.e., a daily dose/release rate of 1–3 mg per day)[2,11] has any adverse effect on a fetus—even in animal studies.[57] Although 400–800 mg of danazol (a potent synthetic androgen) results in clitoromegaly and fused labia in some female fetuses,[58] animal studies have shown that virilization of a female fetus requires >30 times normal maternal levels or >50–500 times human T doses.[57,59] In addition, the placenta buffers hormone diffusion and is a significant source of aromatase, which metabolizes maternal T to E2.

In our clinic, a 38-year-old nulliparous patient treated with T pellets (two insertions) became pregnant after a decade of not having menstrual cycles and not using birth control for 4 years; she subsequently delivered a healthy baby girl. The author is aware of several other unexpected pregnancies with similar results (RL Glaser, personal communications). Nevertheless, contraception should be mandated.

Original data

Glaser and Dimitrakakis have shown that T implant therapy successfully relieves symptoms of hormone deficiency improving QoL in both pre- and postmenopausal patients.[1] Three hundred female patients were evaluated; 36% were premenopausal and 64% were postmenopausal. Pre- and postmenopausal women had similar baseline T levels.

As expected, there was no relationship between baseline T levels and presenting symptoms (other than sexual complaints) or response to therapy. Premenopausal women reported a higher incidence of psychological complaints (depressive mood, anxiety, and irritability), which may be contributed to by higher—or fluctuating—levels of estrogen relative to declining T levels.[3,60] Postmenopausal women reported more hot flashes, vaginal dryness, and urological symptoms, which may be contributed to by lower levels of estrogen. T alone (no estrogen) delivered subcutaneously resulted in statistically significant improvement ($p < 0.0001$) in *all* 11 MRS symptom categories (Fig. 3).

Both groups demonstrated similar improvement in the total score, as well as psychological, somatic, and urogenital subscale scores. Higher doses of T correlated with greater improvement in symptoms. There were no adverse drug events reported in 285 patients treated for

Menopause Rating Scale (MRS)

Which of the following symptoms apply to you at this time? Please, mark the appropriate box for each symptom. For symptoms that do not apply, please mark 'none'.

Symptoms:	none	mild	moderate	severe	very severe
Score =	0	1	2	3	4
1. Hot flushes, sweating (episodes of sweating)	☐	☐	☐	☐	☐
2. Heart discomfort (unusual awareness of heart beat, heart skipping, heart racing, tightness)	☐	☐	☐	☐	☐
3. Sleep problems (difficulty in falling asleep, difficulty in sleeping through, waking up early)	☐	☐	☐	☐	☐
4. Depressive mood (feeling down, sad, on the verge of tears, lack of drive, mood swings)	☐	☐	☐	☐	☐
5. Irritability (feeling nervous, inner tension, feeling aggressive)	☐	☐	☐	☐	☐
6. Anxiety (inner restlessness, feeling panicky)	☐	☐	☐	☐	☐
7. Physical and mental exhaustion (general decrease in performance, impaired memory, decrease in concentration, forgetfulness)	☐	☐	☐	☐	☐
8. Sexual problems (change in sexual desire, in sexual activity and satisfaction)	☐	☐	☐	☐	☐
9. Bladder problems (difficulty in urinating, increased need to urinate, bladder incontinence)	☐	☐	☐	☐	☐
10. Dryness of vagina (sensation of dryness or burning in the vagina, difficulty with sexual intercourse)	☐	☐	☐	☐	☐
11. Joint and muscular discomfort (pain in the joints, rheumatoid complaints)	☐	☐	☐	☐	☐

FIG. 3. Health-related QoL, MRS-validated questionnaire: indications for T therapy in pre- and postmenopausal women. MRS, Menopause Rating Scale; QoL, quality of life.

>1 year (mean 28.1 ± 10.4 months). These benefits are consistently seen in clinical practice (Supplementary Table S1).

T therapy in premenopausal women has not been evaluated in controlled trials. However, clinical studies have reported positive effects in conditions caused by excess estrogen, including hypermenorrhea, uterine fibroids, endometriosis, premenstrual tension, dysmenorrhea, breast pain, and chronic mastitis.[3,5,6] We have also published a case report on T implant therapy during breastfeeding—a 100-mg subcutaneous T pellet was effective in relieving maternal symptoms of depression, anxiety, fatigue, decreased libido, memory problems, and pain—T was not measurably increased in breast milk or infant serum.[61]

Evidence supports that T is neuroprotective (Supplementary Table S1).[32,41,42] T's neuroprotective effect is consistent with our experience in clinical practice, where "self-reported" memory issues are improved on therapy, returning toward the end of the T implant cycle. Essential tremors are also improved on T therapy (Fig. 4).

A significant finding noted in the past 15 years is the consistent relief of migraine headaches in pre- and postmenopausal women, which we documented in a small pilot study.[15] Hormonal stabilization may improve headaches and other conditions, including epilepsy.[62–64]

Currently in clinical practice, premenopausal women with migraine headaches, seizures, dysfunctional uterine bleeding, and endometriosis—are treated

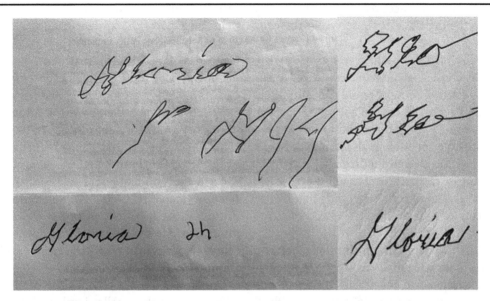

FIG. 4. Left: a 65-year-old patient's attempted signature (top) and initials (middle) before her first T pellet implant and 2 h post-160-mg T implants (bottom). The patient also reported being able to drink from a water bottle without spilling, blow dry her hair, eat soup in a restaurant for the first time in 4 years, and use automated teller machines. Right: the same patient overdue for implants. Two attempted signatures before T implant therapy (top) and 24 h post-300-mg T implants (bottom). T, testosterone.

with an AI (anastrozole [A]) combined with T in the implant—as these conditions are affected by excess or fluctuating estrogens.[44-53,62-64] Since serum levels of E2 do not reflect the local production of estrogen, the clinical signs and symptoms of *excess* estrogen should be monitored, including breast pain, fluid retention, anxiety, emotional disturbances, irritability, aggression, and lack of effect from T therapy.[1,18-20]

Some women discontinue T therapy for cosmetic and skin side effects, including facial hair growth, acne, mild clitoromegaly, and hirsutism. Some women choose to lower their T dose, whereas others prefer the benefits of higher T doses and choose to treat the side effects.

We have previously addressed some common myths and misconceptions surrounding T therapy in women.[12] In a questionnaire study on 285 patients, 48 of 76 (63%) patients who complained of age-related hair loss before therapy reported hair regrowth on T pellet therapy.[13] Interestingly, baseline serum T levels were *lower* in women who reported age-related hair thinning compared with women who reported "no hair thinning."[13] T does increase red blood cell production, which can lower iron levels and contribute to iron deficiency—indirectly affecting hair. Thyroid, iron, and ferritin levels are monitored.

A prospective study specifically designed to investigate the effect of T implant therapy on the female voice demonstrated that therapeutic doses of T—resulting in "supraphysiological" T levels—had no adverse effect on the female voice, including lowering or deepening of the voice.[14] Interestingly, two of three patients with "lower than expected" fundamental frequencies at baseline improved on T therapy, which may be due to T's anti-inflammatory effects.[14,39]

Androgens and breast cancer

Although some epidemiological studies have shown an "association" between endogenous T levels and breast cancer risk, there is no evidence that T treatment causes breast cancer.[7,17-19,32]

Almost two decades ago, it was surmised that it is the balance (ratio) of T to E2 that prevents breast tissue from oncogenesis.[26] Subsequently, in an experimental *in vivo* primate model, we showed that the addition of T to "conventional" hormone replacement therapy attenuated the proliferative effects of estrogens on breast tissue.[65] The same effect was reported in women from Australia: "The addition of testosterone to conventional hormone therapy for postmenopausal women does not increase and may reduce the hormone therapy-associated breast cancer risk, thereby returning the incidence to the normal rates observed in the general untreated population."[66]

We measured salivary hormone levels in 357 newly diagnosed breast cancer patients and compared them with a matched "control" group. Steroid concentrations measured in saliva represent bioavailable hormone levels, excluding the fraction tightly bound to serum proteins (i.e., unavailable for biological action) and thus more accurately reflect steroid (androgenic) activity.[67] We found that breast cancer patients had lower T levels and a lower ratio of T to estrone, suggesting that higher bioavailable T counters the proliferative effects of estrogen in the breast.[67]

In March 2008, a prospective Institutional Review Board-approved cohort study was initiated, which was specifically designed to investigate the incidence of breast cancer in women ($n = 1267$) treated with T implant therapy. Ten-year results revealed a reduced incidence of invasive breast cancer in women treated with T therapy.[19,20] A total of 11 (vs. 18 expected)

cases of infiltrating breast cancer were diagnosed in patients on T pellet therapy equating to an incidence rate of 165/100,000 person-years (p-y), which was significantly less than the age-matched "Surveillance, Epidemiology, and End Results" expected incidence rate of 271/100,000 p-y ($p < 0.001$) and historical controls.

Withdrawal of T therapy led to an increasing trend toward diagnosis of clinically active tumors over time (Fig. 5)—suggesting that T may reduce the progression of undetected cancers.[19] Data reported at year 5 showed that—unlike adherence to estrogen/progestin therapy (increased events)[68]—adherence to T therapy decreased the incidence of breast cancer, signifying a protective effect.[18] The reduced incidence of breast cancer in our cohort of women treated with T implants continues into 2021 (13 years).

The innovative yet obvious use of an AI combined with T in a solitary pellet implant (T+AI) has revolutionized the use of T therapy in breast cancer patients. The combination T+AI subcutaneous implant enables the simultaneous and continuous delivery of both

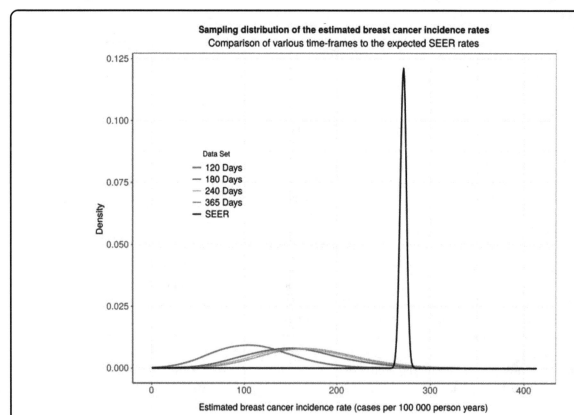

FIG. 5. Bootstrap results confirm a significant reduction in the incidence of invasive breast cancers on T therapy (≤120 day) compared with SEER incidence rates—with an increasing incidence after withdrawal of T therapy—number of days since last insert.[19]. SEER, Surveillance, Epidemiology, and End Results.

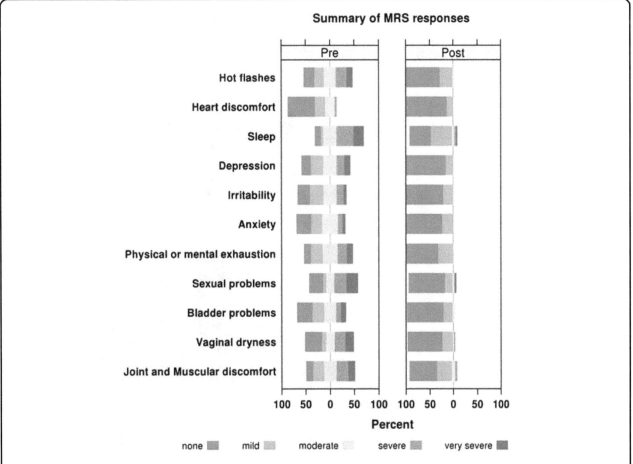

FIG. 6. Summary of the distribution of severity scores in each of the 11 symptom categories at baseline (pretherapy) and post-T+A implant therapy.[41] A, anastrozole.

pharmaceutical active ingredients while avoiding the first pass effect.[69] The combined use of T and an AI provides women with the beneficial effects of T without compromising these results with the conversion of T to estrogens and their possible adverse effects in estrogen-dependent diseases, for example, hormone receptor-positive breast cancer.

Subcutaneous delivery (T+AI) has also proven useful in patients unable to tolerate oral AI therapy. There are no gastrointestinal side effects, including nausea and gastritis, abdominal or stomach pain, and vomiting. Subcutaneous delivery also bypasses the liver avoiding the enterohepatic circulation and hepatic metabolism, which is significant in patients with mild or moderate liver impairment or on oral medications that have a high "hepatic adverse drug reaction" potential.[70]

Data presented at the American Society of Clinical Oncology conference demonstrated the beneficial effects of T on the relief of severe hormone deficiency symptoms

in breast cancer survivors (stage 0–4) using the validated MRS questionnaire (Fig. 3).[23] Survivors were treated with the combination of T with A combined in the pellet implant. T doses and levels on therapy were followed. E2 levels were monitored and remained low. Statistically significant ($p < 0.0001$) improvement in all 11 symptom categories was reported (Fig. 6), supporting the *direct effect* of T at the AR in the relief of symptoms. In addition, there was (and continues to be) a reduced incidence of breast cancer recurrence in patients treated with subcutaneous T + A implants.[23]

In clinical practice, T+AI implants (anastrozole or letrozole) used to treat symptoms of hormone deficiency in breast cancer patients, have also significantly reduced tumor size, including complete clinical and complete radiological responses (Fig. 7). Multiple case reports on the *in vivo* tumor responses to T+AI therapy have been published demonstrating the unarguable direct beneficial effect of T on invasive breast cancers.[17,22,23]

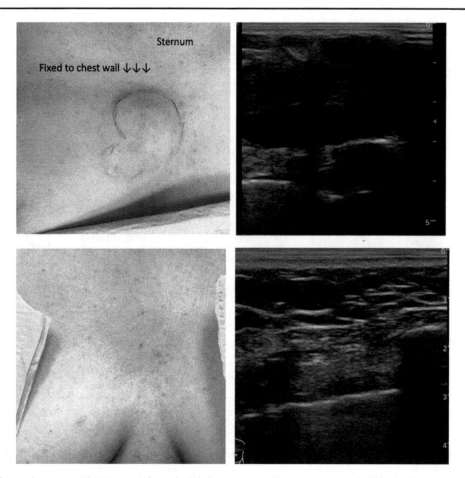

FIG. 7. Fifty-eight-year-old patient referred with large immobile breast cancer fixed to sternum. Refused conventional therapy. She was treated with T 180–240 mg +12 mg letrozole combination pellet implants at baseline, weeks 6, 14, and 26. She also implemented dietary changes. Top left: baseline, 6-cm tumor fixed to chest wall (sternum) UIQ R breast, skin discoloration. Top right: baseline ultrasound, tumor invading periosteum (sternum) and skin—too large to be measured (extends off screen). Bottom left: week 14, complete clinical response, mass no longer palpable. Note indentation/shadow where tumor had stretched skin. Bottom right: week 26, complete radiographic response confirmed on ultrasound. Patient continues on T + A pellets and remains healthy and disease free at 2 years. UIQ, upper inner quadrant.

There is pre-clinical evidence suggesting that T may attenuate some side effects from chemotherapy, which is consistent with T's protective effects (neurological and cardiac) and with what we have experienced in clinical practice.[22] Subcutaneous T+AI therapy has been "life-changing" in the palliative treatment of women with metastatic breast cancer. T therapy significantly improves patient's QoL while simultaneously controlling disease—alone or along with conventional therapy (Figs. 8 and 9).

One of us (R.G.) was a clinical consultant to the Mayo Clinic for the "Alliance Trial A221102, a

Randomized Double-Blind Placebo Controlled Study of Subcutaneous Testosterone (pellets) in the Adjuvant Treatment of Postmenopausal Women with Aromatase Inhibitor Induced Arthralgias."[71] Patients receiving subcutaneous T + A implants reported statistically significant improvements in hot flashes, fatigue, mood swings, urinary incontinence, and skin appearance, tone, and texture.[71]

However, the 120-mg T implant dose (with 8 mg anastrozole) did not (significantly) relieve arthralgias in patients on oral AIs. The investigators surmised that the dose of subcutaneous T was too low.

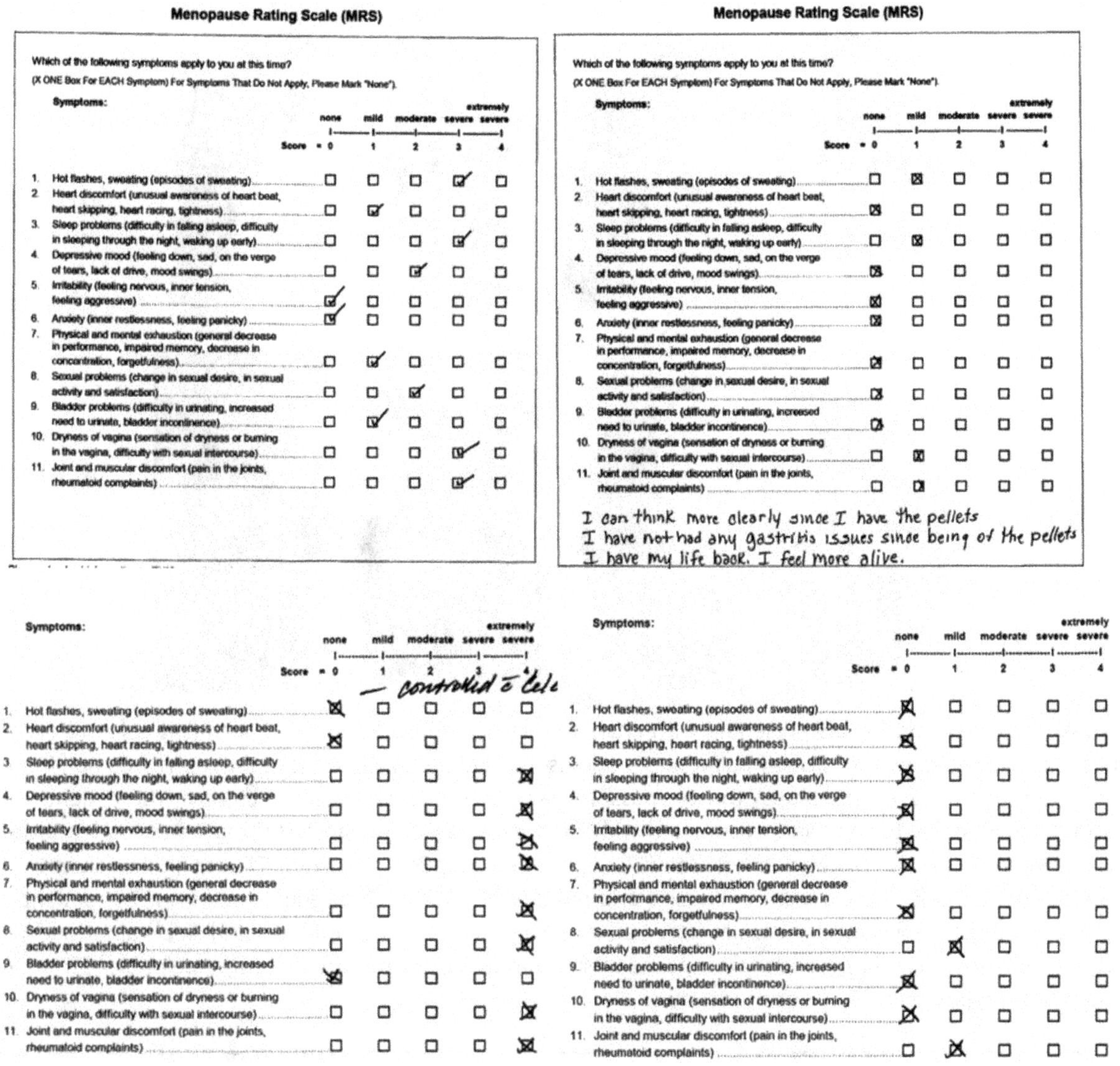

FIG. 8. Significant improvement in QoL documented by MRS in two patients with metastatic breast cancer. Left side, baseline. Right side, on T+AI implant therapy. Top: 58-year-old patient with metastatic breast cancer, 4.5-cm palpable right breast mass, severe abdominal pain, weight loss, incontinence, malnutrition, unable to tolerate oral letrozole therapy. Refused chemotherapy. Patient treated with T + A alone. Breast tumor is responding to therapy. Bottom: 60-year-old patient presented (2015) with metastatic breast cancer (on conventional therapy), extremely severe bone pain, severe menopausal symptoms, and required assistance to walk. Currently 5-years out (65-year-old), alive, and well (thriving) on T+AI therapy. Continues conventional therapy. AI, aromatase inhibitor.

Consistent with T's dose-dependent effects,[1,11,72,73] a previous observational study using higher doses of subcutaneous T (169 ± 32 mg) in breast cancer survivors (not on oral AI therapy) reported significant improvements in somatic symptoms, including joint pain and muscular discomfort.[23] Unfortunately no RCTs using higher doses of subcutaneous T have been performed.

Pharmacological dosing for a physiological effect

Controversial topics in treating women with T include the following: the diagnosis of androgen deficiency, T dosing, and T levels on therapy.[7,43,74]

Some guidelines recommend against treating women with T because serum levels do not correlate with symptoms.[7,43,74] We have shown that neither symptoms of

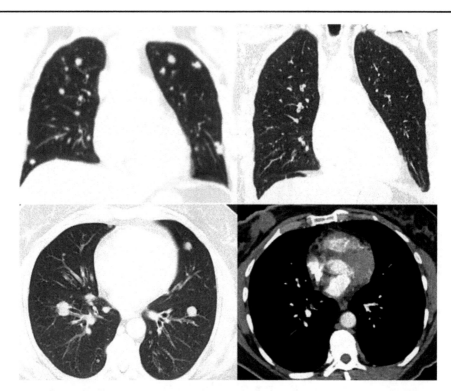

FIG. 9. A 67-year-old female presented with acute respiratory failure. Baseline CT scan (left column) of the chest showed multiple noncalcified pulmonary nodules—bilateral and throughout the lungs—compatible with metastatic disease. Core biopsy (breast mass) revealed ER+ invasive ductal carcinoma. The patient refused conventional therapy and was treated with T+letrozole pellet implants (320 mg T + 24 mg letrozole every 9 weeks). She also began a "whole food" low glycemic diet. One year later, CT scan (right column) showed considerable improvement in the size and number of nodules throughout the lungs. The patient lost 13.6 kg (note significant decrease in fatty tissue on CT), remains asymptomatic, and "feels amazing." The large 8-cm breast mass has markedly decreased in size and axillary nodes are no longer palpable. CT, computed tomography; ER, estrogen receptor.

androgen deficiency (with the exception of sexual complaints) nor response to therapy correlate with baseline T levels, which is consistent with other studies and the physiology of androgens in women.[1,11]

The decision to initiate T therapy is a clinical decision between the doctor and patient based on the patient's symptomatology.[1,11] This assessment is in agreement with the American College of Obstetricians and Gynecologists (ACOG) Committee Opinion, which states that "Individualized testing is only indicated when a narrow therapeutic window exists for a drug or drug class. Steroid hormones do not meet these criteria and do not require individualized testing" *and* "If treatment is initiated for symptom control, subjective improvement in symptoms is the therapeutic end-point, and there is no need to assess hormone

levels. Hormone therapy should not be titrated to hormone levels."[75] This opinion differs from statements and guidelines that recommend baseline testing and monitoring hormone therapy with serum levels.[7,74]

Recent guidelines use the terms "physiological dosing" and "physiological levels" when making recommendations for T therapy.[7] However, this is counterintuitive to physiology—the major source of bioavailable T in women is *unmeasurable* and not reflected in serum T levels. "Physiological dosing" may be why T therapy—effectively raising T levels into the mid to high physiological range—has proven clinically ineffective in some studies.[76] T's effect is dose dependent, and there is no evidence (i.e., drug concentration in blood studies), or documented adverse events, supporting the "opinion" that serum T

Table 2. Testosterone Doses and Serum Levels on Therapy

Year published Study	Mean T dose (mg)	n (time postdose)	T levels ng/dL Mean ± SD (CV)	Study results
2013[11] PK	133.3 ± 26.8	n = 154 (4 weeks) n = 261 (trough/end)	300 ± 107 (CV 35.9%) 171 ± 73 (CV 42.6%)	Pharmacological dosing of T implants (resulting in serum levels above endogenous physiological ranges) proved safe and clinically effective
2014[23] ASCO (T+A)	168.9 ± 32.3	n = 73 (4 weeks)	354 ± 149 (CV 42.1%)	T+A implant therapy safely relieved clinical symptoms, improving QoL in breast cancer survivors
2016[14] Voice	138.0 ± 22.7	n = 10 (variable)	472 ± 148	Therapeutic T levels had no adverse effect on the female voice, including lowering or deepening of the voice
2019[20] Prevention 10-year data	198.7 ± 55.8	n = 398 (variable)	490 ± 210 (CV 42.6%)	Long-term T therapy was associated with a reduced incidence of invasive breast cancer

Trough/end levels were drawn when patient symptoms returned. Of note, trough levels were several-fold higher than endogenous T ranges.

A, anastrozole; ASCO, American Society of Clinical Oncology, CV, coefficient of variation, PK, pharmacokinetic; QoL, quality of life; SD, standard deviation; T, testosterone.

levels on therapy should remain within endogenous or "physiological" ranges—concentration/dose–response studies support the opposite.[1,11,72,73]

True "physiological" T dosing must deliver adequate amounts of T to the AR (tissue level) to replace the minor contribution (<20%) from circulating T (measurable in serum)—and most importantly—to replace the major contribution (>80%) to T from the preandrogens, which also decline with age.[27–31] *Severe T deficiency* occurs in conditions that affect production of adrenal precursor steroids—further supporting the major contribution of DHEAS, DHEA, and androstenedione to the peripheral production of T in target organs.[77]

Doses and therapeutic ranges for exogenous therapy with T pellet implants have been published in the peer-reviewed literature (Table 2).[11,14,20,23] Trough (nadir) levels, measured when symptoms returned,[11] support that T levels on exogenous therapy cannot be compared with, monitored by, or dosed based on endogenous T ranges in serum.[8,9,77] In addition, there is a significant interindividual variation (coefficient of variation [CV] >40%) as well an intraindividual variation (CV 25%) in T levels on therapy suggesting that a single T level is extremely variable and of little or no value in clinical decision making, further supporting ACOG's position on hormone testing.[11,75]

Of note, salivary T levels may be more accurate than serum for assessing *bioavailable T* in patients treated with T implant therapy (Supplementary Data S2). However, serum is readily available and commonly used in clinical practice.

Additional data

Between March 2017 and January 2021, we collected 1106 data points on 667 female patients treated with T implants. These data points do not represent all patients receiving T pellets, only those who had laboratory data collected during this time frame. Of note, breast cancer patients are monitored (E2 levels) more frequently (month 1 and nadir)—and may represent a higher proportion of patients in this series.

Patient's age, body mass index (BMI), weight, T dose, interval of insertion, and blood count on therapy are listed in Table 3. T stimulates erythropoietin and increases red blood cell production. Patients sign a consent informing them that T therapy can raise "red blood counts" and that "high blood counts have been associated with blood clots." Hemoglobin (Hb) and hematocrit (Hct) are monitored in patients treated with T implant therapy. Four of 667 female patients had Hb >17 g/dL and two patients had a Hct >52%. One patient had a Hb of 18.8 and a Hct of 53.4%. It was recommended that she must consult with a hematologist and discontinue T therapy.

In the past 15 years, no female or male patient in our clinical practice has had any adverse events (cardiac or thrombotic) due to secondary polycythemia.[1,11,25,78] Although some studies show an association between elevated Hct and thrombosis, thrombosis does not accompany most types of erythrocytosis.[79] True erythrocytosis

Table 3. Patient Demographics

	Mean ± SD	Minimum	Maximum
Age at insert (years)	59.1 ± 9.2	28.6	93.2
BMI	26.1 ± 4.9	15.4	50.0
Weight (kg)	71.0 ± 13.6	43.1	140.6
T dose (mg)	207.1 ± 46.0	60	380
Interval of insertion (days)	91.9 ± 25.0	47	182
Hemoglobin (gm/dL)	14.5 ± 1.07	8.1	18.8
Hematocrit (%)	43.0 ± 3.12	29.1	53.4

BMI, body mass index.

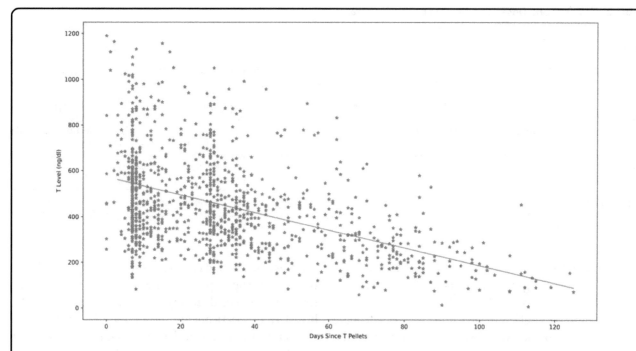

FIG. 10. T levels on subcutaneous implants throughout the implant cycle. $n = 1106$ data points. Intercept 572.49 ng/dL. Slope −3.86 (ng/dL per day).

is defined as a packed red blood cell volume >125% of predicted for an individual's height and weight or a Hct >56% in a female.[80]

Secondary polycythemia from T therapy or other nonmedical conditions (e.g., high altitude) does not have the same risk of thrombotic events compared with polycythemia due to medical conditions (e.g., chronic lung disease/hypoxia), which are associated with many confounding health problems.[79,81,82] This lack of adverse events is consistent with the lack of adverse thrombotic and cardiovascular events reported in transgender men and male patients treated with T therapy.[78,82–89]

T levels over time (days since implantation) are shown in Figure 10. In this particular data set, we were interested in T levels at week 1. Note the cluster of levels at week 1 and at month 1, which is a frequent collection time frame. T levels peak at insertion. There was a gradual decline of serum T levels, at a rate of 3.86 ng/dL per day. The intercept was 572.5 (ng/dL): week 1 levels (collected between day 4 and 10) were 518.6 ng/dL ±215.2 (CV 0.41) (Fig. 10).

Trough (nadir) serum T levels were drawn when "symptoms returned" and obtained within ≤7 days before the patients subsequent T insertion procedure. Mean serum T levels at the end of the implant cycle, that

is, when symptoms returned, was 236.9 ± 108.0 ng/dL (CV 45.6). However, in some circumstances (e.g., meta-static breast cancer, multiple sclerosis, and memory loss) patients return before the onset of clinical symptoms for optimal disease control.

Correlations between patient demographics and T doses and levels on therapy are presented in Table 4. T dosing is weight based and there was a moderate positive correlation between weight/BMI and T dose. There was also a small positive correlation between age and T dose. The total androgen pool declines with age and we have found that some women benefit from increasing doses of T as they age.

Serum T levels were collected throughout the implant cycle, which makes correlations with T levels

Table 4. Pearson Correlations

	Weight	T dose	T level	Hb	Hct	BMI	Age
Weight	1	0.43	−0.15	0.17	0.18	0.92	−0.09
T dose	0.43	1	0.26	0.26	0.26	0.4	0.13
T level	−0.15	0.26	1	0.06	0.06	−0.14	0.24
Hb	0.17	0.26	0.06	1	0.95	0.16	0.04
Hct	0.18	0.26	0.06	0.95	1	0.18	0.05
BMI	0.92	0.4	−0.14	0.16	0.18	1	−0.06
Age	−0.09	0.13	0.24	0.04	0.06	−0.06	1

Hb, hemoglobin; Hct, hematocrit.

on therapy difficult to interpret. However, there was a small negative correlation between BMI/weight and T levels on therapy. This is consistent with what we reported in male patients: men with lower BMI had higher serum T levels on therapy (all time frames) despite lower dosing.[25] There were small (<0.29) positive correlations between Hb/Hct and body weight, BMI, T dose, and T level on therapy—the strongest correlation with T dose (Table 4).

Adequate dosing of T is critical for optimal therapeutic effect. Symptom response and control of disease should guide therapy rather than arbitrary serum T levels. T therapy is continued or adjusted based on the patient's response to therapy (benefits) versus side effects, not on a single T level, which is inherently unreli-
                    Pellets are (re) inserted when symptoms return. The T dose and/or the interval of insertion are adjusted based on an individual's disease state, response to therapy, goals, and preferences.

Additional data supporting the safety of pharmacological T dosing include long-term studies on transgender men, which have shown that significantly higher (male) doses of T do *not* increase the risk of cardiovascular events, stroke, cancer—and increase insulin sensitivity.[84–89] The increase in insulin sensitivity may be surprising as women with polycystic ovarian syndrome and insulin resistance also have high T levels. However, evidence suggests that hyperandrogenism is secondary to hyperinsulinemia—insulin stimulates the production of androgens and treating hyperinsulinemia ameliorates hyperandrogenism.[90,91] The absence of significant "therapy-related" adverse health events is consistent with our long-term experience.

We have provided clinical evidence supporting indications for, safety of, and benefits of androgen therapy in women, which extends beyond hypoactive sexual desire disorder/dysfunction. This is in contrast to the Global Consensus Position Statement on the Use of Testosterone Therapy for Women—which was widely publicized by specialty societies—and lists hypoactive sexual desire disorder/dysfunction as the "only evidence-based" indication for T therapy.[7] However, relying solely on industry-sponsored RCTs (which many of the authors have been involved with)[7] as the only "evidence," could lead to biased recommendations (Supplementary Data S3).[92,93]

Although we recognize that other studies on T and T implant therapy often include heterogeneous popula-

tions, have variable dosing, and have different outcome measurements, they should not be totally omitted or disparaged by guideline authors.[92,93] Although guidelines are a valuable source of information, there are "concerns" regarding their integrity and, in particular, recommendations based on "opinion" as the level of evidence (Supplementary Data S3).[7,92–96]

Although unregulated, T pellets have been safely used for >80 years in clinical practices around the world. We presented original data supporting the efficacy and safety of T implant therapy in clinical practice and detailed an unmet and urgent need in breast cancer patients. Understanding the physiology of androgens in women enables one to comprehend the rationale behind T implant therapy (indications and dosing), and counters disingenuous arguments against the use of "T preparations that result in supraphysiological concentrations."[7]

Conclusion

T is not a "new" drug. It is an endogenous steroid hormone with a wide margin of safety—high therapeutic index.[a] Adequate amounts of bioavailable T at the AR are critical for optimal physical and mental health. T therapy in women should be dosed based on clinical efficacy and response to therapy. There is no evidence that T therapy should be monitored by serum T levels or managed based on arbitrary ranges.

In >15 years of clinical experience, T implant therapy has proven invaluable, dramatically improving the health, sexuality, and QoL of thousands of women. T combined with an AI should be considered in patients with symptoms of estrogen excess or a history of ER-positive breast cancer.

The values and goals of the individual patient should be paramount in decision making. Decades of evidence support both the safety and efficacy of T therapy in women, including breast cancer patients. Withholding adequate doses of T therapy could be detrimental to an individual's health, QoL, and survival.

Authors' Contributions

Both authors contributed to the conception and design of the article, critical revisions, and final approval of the article. Both authors agree to be accountable for all aspects of the study.

---

[a]LD 50 (500–1000 mg/kg, ≅ 50,000 mg per 70 kg patient). T dose release from a 200 mg pellet implant dose is ~2 mg/day.

Acknowledgments

We thank Jennifer Dichito, MA, and Shayna Smith, BS, for data collection and diligent patient follow-up, and Michael Glaser-Garbrick, BS, MS, for his technical assistance and statistical analysis.

Supplementary Material

Supplementary Table S1
Supplementary Data S1
Supplementary Data S2
Supplementary Data S3

References

1. Glaser R, York AE, Dimitrakakis C. Beneficial effects of testosterone therapy in women measured by the validated Menopause Rating Scale (MRS). Maturitas. 2011;68:355–361.
2. Kelleher S, Howe C, Conway AJ, Handelsman DJ. Testosterone release rate and duration of action of testosterone pellet implants. Clin Endocrinol. 2004;60:420–428.
3. Loeser A. Male hormone in gynaecology and obstetrics and in cancer of the female breast. Obst Gynecol Surv. 1948;3:363–381.
4. Greenblatt R, Hair L. Testosterone propionate pellet absorption in the female. J Clin Endocrinol. 1942;2:315–317.
5. Greenblatt RB. Testosterone propionate pellet implantation in gynecic disorders. J Am Med Assoc. 1943;121:17–24.
6. Greenblatt RB, Suran RR. Indications for hormonal pellets in the therapy of endocrine and gynecic disorders. Am J Obst Gynecol. 1949;57:294–301.
7. Davis SR, Baber R, Panay N, et al. Global consensus position statement on the use of testosterone therapy for women. J Clin Endocrinol Metab. 2019;104:4660–4666.
8. Cardozo L, Gibb DMF, Tuck SM, Thom MH, Studd JWW, Cooper DJ. The effects of subcutaneous hormone implants during the climacteric. Maturitas. 1984;5:177–184.
9. Brincat M, Studd JWW, O'Dowd T, et al. Subcutaneous hormone implants for the control of climacteric symptoms: A prospective study. Lancet. 1984;323:16–18.
10. Loeser A. Mammary carcinoma response to implantation of male hormone and progesterone. Lancet. 1941;238:698–700.
11. Glaser R, Kalantaridou S, Dimitrakakis C. Testosterone implants in women: Pharmacological dosing for a physiologic effect. Maturitas. 2013;74:179–184.
12. Glaser R, Dimitrakakis C. Testosterone therapy in women: Myths and misconceptions. Maturitas. 2013;74:230–234.
13. Glaser RL, Dimitrakakis C, Messenger AG. Improvement in scalp hair growth in androgen-deficient women treated with testosterone: A questionnaire study. Br J Dermatol. 2012;166:274–278.
14. Glaser R, York A, Dimitrakakis C. Effect of testosterone therapy on the female voice. Climacteric. 2016;19:198–203.
15. Glaser R, Dimitrakakis C, Trimble N, Martin V. Testosterone pellet implants and migraine headaches: A pilot study. Maturitas. 2012;71:385–388.
16. Glaser R, Dimitrakakis C. Beneficial effects of subcutaneous testosterone therapy on lipid profiles in women. Maturitas. 2013;71:S41.
17. Glaser R, Dimitrakakis C. Testosterone and breast cancer prevention. Maturitas. 2015;82:291–295.
18. Glaser RL, Dimitrakakis C. Reduced breast cancer incidence in women treated with subcutaneous testosterone, or testosterone with anastrozole: A prospective, observational study. Maturitas. 2013;76(4):342–349.
19. Glaser RL, York AE, Dimitrakakis C. Reduced incidence of breast cancer with testosterone implant therapy: A 10-year cohort study. Proceedings of the 2018 San Antonio Breast Cancer Symposium. AACR; Cancer Res. 2019;79(4 Suppl.):Abstract nr P6-13-02.
20. Glaser RL, York AE, Dimitrakakis C. Incidence of invasive breast cancer in women treated with testosterone implants: A prospective 10-year cohort study. BMC Cancer. 2019;19:1–10.
21. Glaser RL, Dimitrakakis C. Rapid response of breast cancer to neoadjuvant intramammary testosterone-anastrozole therapy: Neoadjuvant hormone therapy in breast cancer. Menopause (New York, NY). 2014;21:673.
22. Glaser RL, York AE, Dimitrakakis C. Subcutaneous testosterone-letrozole therapy before and concurrent with neoadjuvant breast chemotherapy: Clinical response and therapeutic implications. Menopause. 2017;24:859–864.
23. Glaser RL, York AE, Dimitrakakis C. Efficacy of subcutaneous testosterone on menopausal symptoms in breast cancer survivors. J Clin Oncol. 2014;10(32):109.
24. Glaser R, Marinopoulos S, Dimitrakakis C. Breast cancer treatment in women over the age of 80: A tailored approach. Maturitas. 2018;110:29–32.
25. Glaser RL, York AE. Subcutaneous testosterone anastrozole therapy in men: Rationale, dosing, and levels on therapy. Int J Pharm Compd. 2019;23:325–339.
26. Dimitrakakis C, Zhou J, Bondy CA. Androgens and mammary growth and neoplasia. Fertil Steril. 2002;77:26–33.
27. Labrie F. DHEA and the intracrine formation of androgens and estrogens in peripheral target tissues: Its role during aging. Steroids. 1997;11:733.
28. Longcope C. Adrenal and gonadal androgen secretion in normal females. Clin Endocrinol Metab. 1986;15(2):213–228.
29. Labrie F, Bélanger A, Luu-The V, et al. DHEA and the intracrine formation of androgens and estrogens in peripheral target tissues: Its role during aging. Steroids. 1998;63:322–328.
30. Labrie F, Martel C, Belanger A, Pelletier G. Androgens in women are essentially made from DHEA in each peripheral tissue according to intracrinology. J Steroid Biochem Mol Biol. 2017;168:9–18.
31. Labrie F, Martel C, Balser J. Wide distribution of the serum dehydroepiandrosterone and sex steroid levels in postmenopausal women: Role of the ovary. Menopause. 2011;18:30–43.
32. Davis SR, Wahlin-Jacobsen S. Testosterone in women—The clinical significance. Lancet Diabetes Endocrinol. 2015;3:980–992.
33. Chang C, Yeh S, Lee SO, Chang T-m. Androgen receptor (AR) pathophysiological roles in androgen related diseases in skin, metabolism syndrome, bone/muscle and neuron/immune systems: Lessons learned from mice lacking AR in specific cells. Nucl Recept Signal. 2013;11:nrs.11001.
34. Hickey TE, Robinson JLL, Carroll JS. Minireview: The androgen receptor in breast tissues: Growth inhibitor, tumor suppressor, oncogene. Mol Endocrinol. 2013;26(8):1252–1267.
35. Matsumoto T, Sakari M, Okada M, et al. The androgen receptor in health and disease. Ann Rev Physiol. 2013;75:201–224.
36. Jones TH, Saad F. The effects of testosterone on risk factors for, and the mediators of, the atherosclerotic process. Atherosclerosis. 2009;207(2):308–327.
37. Traish AM, Vignozzi L, Simon JA, Goldstein I, Kim NN. Role of androgens in female genitourinary tissue structure and function: Implications in the genitourinary syndrome of menopause. Sex Med Rev. 2018;6:558–571.
38. SYu K, Tyuzikov IA, Vorslov LO, Tishova YA. Testosterone functions in women. Part 1. General and age-specific endocrine and other physiological functions of testosterone in women. Doctor Ru. 2015;14:59–64.
39. Traish A, Bolanos J, Nair S, Saad F, Morgentaler A. Do androgens modulate the pathophysiological pathways of inflammation? Appraising the contemporary evidence. J Clin Med. 2018;7:549.
40. Traish AM, Feeley RJ, Guay AT. Testosterone therapy in women with gynecological and sexual disorders: A triumph of clinical endocrinology from 1938 to 2008. J Sex Med. 2009;6:334–351.
41. Bialek M, Zaremba P, Borowicz KK, Czuczwar SJ. Neuroprotective role of testosterone in the nervous system. Pol J Pharmacol. 2004;56:509–518.
42. Fargo KN, Foecking EM, Jones KJ, Sengelaub DR. Neuroprotective actions of androgens on motoneurons. Front Neuroendocrinol. 2009;30:130–141.
43. Bachmann G, Bancroft J, Braunstein G, et al. Female androgen insufficiency: The Princeton consensus statement on definition, classification, and assessment. Fertil Steril. 2002;77:660–665.
44. Blakemore J, Naftolin F. Aromatase: Contributions to physiology and disease in women and men. Physiology. 2016;31:258–269.
45. Czajka-Oraniec I, Simpson ER. Aromatase research and its clinical significance. Endokrynol Polska. 2010;61:126–134.
46. Simpson ER. Sources of estrogen and their importance. J Steroid Biochem Mol Biol. 2003;86:225–230.
47. Nelson LR, Bulun SE. Estrogen production and action. J Am Acad Dermatol. 2001;45:S116–S124.

48. Williams GP. The role of oestrogen in the pathogenesis of obesity, type 2 diabetes, breast cancer and prostate disease. Eur J Cancer Prev. 2010;19:256–271.

49. Santen RJ, Brodie H, Simpson ER, Siiteri PK, Brodie A. History of aromatase: Saga of an important biological mediator and therapeutic target. Endocr Rev. 2009;30:343–375.

50. Bulun SE, Noble LS, Takayama K, et al. Endocrine disorders associated with inappropriately high aromatase expression. J Steroid Biochem Mol Biol. 1997;61:133–139.

51. Cohen PG. Aromatase, adiposity, aging and disease. The hypogonadal-metabolic-atherogenic-disease and aging connection. Med Hypotheses. 2001;56:702–708.

52. Wang X, Simpson ER, Brown KA. Aromatase overexpression in dysfunctional adipose tissue links obesity to postmenopausal breast cancer. J Steroid Biochem Mol Biol. 2015;153:35–44.

53. Zhao H, Zhou L, Shangguan AJ, Bulun SE. Aromatase expression and regulation in breast and endometrial cancer. J Mol Endocrinol. 2016;57:R19.

54. Labrie F, Bélanger A, Cusan L, Gomez J-L, Candas B. Marked decline in serum concentrations of adrenal C19 sex steroid precursors and conjugated androgen metabolites during aging. J Clin Endocrinol Metab. 1997;82:2396–2402.

55. Davison SL, Bell R, Donath S, Montalto JG, Davis SR. Androgen levels in adult females: Changes with age, menopause, and oophorectomy. J Clin Endocrinol Metab. 2005;90:3847–3853.

56. Davis SR. Cardiovascular and cancer safety of testosterone in women. Curr Opin Endocrinol Diabetes Obes. 2011;18:198–203.

57. Tarttelin MF. Early prenatal treatment of ewes with testosterone completely masculinises external genitalia of female offspring but has no effects on early body weight changes. Eur J Endocrinol. 1986;113:153–160.

58. Brunskill P. The effects of fetal exposure to danazol. BJOG Int J Obst Gynaecol. 1992;99:212–215.

59. Wolf CJ, Hotchkiss A, Ostby JS, LeBlanc GA, Gray Jr LE. Effects of prenatal testosterone propionate on the sexual development of male and female rats: A dose-response study. Toxicol Sci. 2002;65:71–86.

60. Payne JL. The role of estrogen in mood disorders in women. Int Rev Psychiatry. 2003;15(03):280–290.

61. Glaser R, Newman M, Parsons M, Zava D, Glaser-Garbrick D. Safety of maternal testosterone therapy during breast feeding. Int J Pharm Compd. 2009;13:314–317.

62. Vetvik KG, MacGregor EA. Sex differences in the epidemiology, clinical features, and pathophysiology of migraine. Lancet Neurol. 2017;16:76–87.

63. Finocchi C, Strada L. Sex-related differences in migraine. Neurol Sci. 2014;35:207–213.

64. Harden CL, Pennell PB. Neuroendocrine considerations in the treatment of men and women with epilepsy. Lancet Neurol. 2013;12:72–83.

65. Dimitrakakis C, Zhou J, Wang J, et al. A physiologic role for testosterone in limiting estrogenic stimulation of the breast. Menopause. 2003;10:292–298.

66. Dimitrakakis C, Jones RA, Liu A, Bondy CA. Breast cancer incidence in postmenopausal women using testosterone in addition to usual hormone therapy. Menopause. 2004;11:531–535.

67. Dimitrakakis C, Zava D, Marinopoulos S, Tsigginou A, Antsaklis A, Glaser R. Low salivary testosterone levels in patients with breast cancer. BMC Cancer. 2010;10:547.

68. Chlebowski RT, Kuller LH, Prentice RL, et al. Breast cancer after use of estrogen plus progestin in postmenopausal women. N Engl J Med. 2009;360:573–587.

69. Glaser RL. Pharmaceutical compositions containing testosterone and an aromatase inhibitor. U.S. Patent 10,792,290 B2.—declaration (data available upon request).

70. Weng Z, Wang K, Li H, Shi Q. A comprehensive study of the association between drug hepatotoxicity and daily dose, liver metabolism, and lipophilicity using 975 oral medications. Oncotarget. 2015;6(19):17031–17038.

71. Cathcart-Rake E, Novotny P, Leon-Ferre R, et al. A randomized, double-blind, placebo-controlled trial of testosterone for treatment of postmenopausal women with aromatase inhibitor-induced arthralgias: Alliance study A221102. Support Care Cancer. 2021;29:387–396.

72. Huang G, Basaria S, Travison TG, et al. Testosterone dose-response relationships in hysterectomized women with and without oophorectomy: Effects on sexual function, body composition, muscle performance and physical function in a randomized trial. Menopause (New York, NY). 2014;21:612.

73. Gray PB, Singh AB, Woodhouse LJ. Dose-dependent effects of testosterone on sexual function, mood, and visuospatial cognition in older men. J Clin Endocrinol Metab. 2005;90(7):3338–3840.

74. Wierman ME, Arlt W, Basson R, et al. Androgen therapy in women: A reappraisal: An Endocrine Society clinical practice guideline. J Clin Endocrinol Metab. 2014;99(10):3489–3510.

75. Practice COG. Compounded bioidentical menopausal hormone therapy. Committee opinion no. 532. American College of Obstetricians and Gynecologists. Obstet Gynecol. 2012;120:411–415.

76. Choi HH, Gray PB, Storer TW, et al. Effects of testosterone replacement in human immunodeficiency virus-infected women with weight loss. J Clin Endocrinol Metab. 2005;50(3):1531–1541.

77. Burger HG. Androgen production in women. Fertil Steril. 2002;77:3–5.

78. Glaser RL. Oral presentation and abstract. Testosterone, anastrozole and venous thrombosis. Maturitas. 2017;103:P91.

79. Gordeuk VR, Key NS, Prchal JT. Re-evaluation of hematocrit as a determinant of thrombotic risk in erythrocytosis. Haematologica. 2019;104(4):653–658.

80. McMullin MF. The classification and diagnosis of erythrocytosis. Int J Lab Hematol. 2008;30:447–459.

81. Jones S, Dukovac T, Sangkum P, Yafi FA. Erythrocytosis and polycythemia secondary to testosterone replacement therapy in the aging male. Sex Med. 2015;3(2):101–112.

82. Schreijer AJM, Reitsma PH, Cannegieter SC. High hematocrit as a risk factor for venous thrombosis. Cause or innocent bystander. Haematologica. 2010;95:182.

83. Corona G, Rastrelli G, Maseroli E, et al. Testosterone replacement therapy and cardiovascular risk: A review. World J Mens Health. 2015;33(3):130–142.

84. Sharma R, Oni OA, Chen G, et al. Association between testosterone replacement therapy and the incidence of DVT and pulmonary embolism: A retrospective cohort study of the Veterans Administration Database. Chest. 2016;150(3):563–571.

85. Jones TH, Kelly DM. Randomized controlled trials–mechanistic studies of testosterone and the cardiovascular system. Asian J Androl. 2018;20(2):120–130.

86. Gooren LJ, t'Sjoen G. Endocrine treatment of aging transgender people. Rev Endocr Metab Disord. 2018;19:253–262.

87. Irwig MS. Cardiovascular health in transgender people. Rev Endocr Metab Disord. 2018;19:243–251.

88. Shadid S, Abosi-Appeadu K, De Maertelaere A-S, et al. Effects of gender-affirming hormone therapy on insulin sensitivity and Incretin responses in transgender people. Diabetes Care. 2020;43:411–417.

89. Traish AM, Gooren LJ. Safety of physiological testosterone therapy in women: Lessons from female-to-male transsexuals (FMT) treated with pharmacological testosterone therapy. J Sex Med. 2010;7:3758–3764.

90. Nestler JE. Insulin regulation of human ovarian androgens. Human Reprod. 1997;12(1):53–62.

91. Nestler JE, Jakubowicz DJ. Insulin stimulates testosterone biosynthesis by human thecal cells from women with polycystic ovary syndrome by activating its own receptor and using inositolglycan mediators as the signal transduction system. J Clin Endocrinol Metab. 1998;83(6):2001–2005.

92. Traish A, Guay AT, Spark RF, Group TTIWS. COMMENTARY: Are the endocrine society's clinical practice guidelines on androgen therapy in women misguided? A commentary. J Sex Med. 2007;4:1223–1235.

93. Woolf S, Schünemann J. Eccles, M. et al. Developing clinical practice guidelines: Types of evidence and outcomes; values and economics, synthesis, grading, and presentation and deriving recommendations. BMC Implement Sci. 2012;7(61):1–12.

94. Lenzer J, Hoffman JR, Furberg CD, Ioannidis JPA. Ensuring the integrity of clinical practice guidelines: A tool for protecting patients. BMJ. 2013;347:f5535, 1–10.

95. Institute of Medicine. Clinical Practice Guidelines We Can Trust. Washington, DC: The National Academies Press, 2011.

96. Steinbrook R, Kassirer JP, Angell M. Justifying conflicts of interest in medical journals: A very bad idea. BMJ. 2015;350:h2942.

Abbreviations Used

A = anastrozole
AI = aromatase inhibitor
ASCO = American Society of Clinical Oncology
BMI = body mass index
CT = computed tomography
CV = coefficient of variation
E2 = estradiol
ER = estrogen receptor
Hb = hemoglobin
Hct = hematocrit
MRS = Menopause Rating Scale
PK = pharmacokinetic
QoL = quality of life
SD = standard deviation
SEER = Surveillance, Epidemiology, and End Results
T = testosterone
UIQ = upper inner quadrant

8

Testosterone Therapy: Increase in Hematocrit is Associated with Decreased Mortality

Richard C. Strange,[1] Carola S. König,[2] Adeeba Ahmed,[3] Geoff Hackett,[4,i] Ahmad Haider,[5] Karim S. Haider,[5,ii] Pieter Desnerck,[6] Farid Saad,[7,8,iii] Nathan Lorde,[9] Amro Maarouf,[9] and Sudarshan Ramachandran[1,2,9,10,*,iv]

Abstract

Objective: Testosterone therapy (TTh) may reduce morbidity/mortality in men with adult-onset testosterone deficiency (TD), though some cardiovascular safety concerns remain. Increased hematocrit (HCT), a recognized effect of therapy, may be associated with cardiovascular disease and mortality. We examined HCT change (Δ) in men prescribed/not prescribed testosterone, and associations with mortality.

Methods: We analyzed data from a prospective registry study with adult-onset TD patients: 353 men given testosterone undecanoate (TU) and 384 opting against TTh. Change in HCT after 12, 48, 72, and 96 months of TU and at final assessment was compared (nonparametric tests). The association between baseline HCT, Δ HCT, and mortality was studied using logistic and Cox regression.

Results: HCT increased significantly (median change at final assessment: +5.0%) in men on TTh. HCT was higher ($p = 0.021$, rank-sum test) in those alive than in those who died, although median values were identical (49.0%). Baseline HCT and Δ HCT were inversely associated with mortality after adjustment for age in both logistic and Cox regression models. Men with final HCT >49.0% (median) suffered lower mortality than men with HCT ≤49.0%.

Conclusions: A median HCT increase of 5.0% was associated with TTh, mostly within 48 months of commencing therapy. An increase in HCT (up to 52.0% at final assessment) was independently associated with reduced mortality, indicating current guidelines using a HCT value of 54.0% as a threshold for management change are appropriate until further study.

Keywords: testosterone therapy; hematocrit; hemoglobin; adult-onset hypogonadism; mortality

[1]Institute for Science and Technology in Medicine, Keele University, Staffordshire, United Kingdom.
[2]Department of Mechanical and Aerospace Engineering, Brunel University London, United Kingdom.
[3]Department of Diabetes, University Hospitals Birmingham NHS Foundation Trust, West Midlands, England, United Kingdom.
[4]School of Health and Life Sciences, Aston University, Birmingham, United Kingdom.
[5]Praxis Dr. Haider, Bremerhaven, Germany.
[6]Department of Engineering, University of Cambridge, Cambridge, United Kingdom.
[7]Medical Affairs Andrology, Bayer AG, Berlin, Germany.
[8]Gulf Medical University School of Medicine, Ajman, UAE.
[9]Department of Clinical Biochemistry, University Hospitals Birmingham, United Kingdom.
[10]Department of Clinical Biochemistry, University Hospitals of North Midlands, Staffordshire, United Kingdom.
[i]ORCID ID (https://orcid.org/0000-0003-2274-111X).
[ii]ORCID ID (https://orcid.org/0000-0003-4396-9324).
[iii]ORCID ID (https://orcid.org/0000-0002-0449-6635).
[iv]ORCID ID (https://orcid.org/0000-0003-2299-4133).

*Address correspondence to: Sudarshan Ramachandran, FRCPath, Department of Clinical Biochemistry, University Hospitals Birmingham NHS Foundation Trust, Good Hope Hospital, Rectory Road, Sutton Coldfield, West Midlands B75 7RR, United Kingdom, E-mail: sud.ramachandran@heartofengland.nhs.uk

Introduction

Adult-onset testosterone deficiency (TD) (also known as late-onset TD, age-related TD, and functional TD) describes, after exclusion of primary (testicular) and secondary (pituitary/hypothalamic) pathology, a combination of low serum testosterone and associated symptoms that include reduced bone mineral density, muscular strength, cognition, and sexual dysfunction.[1-3] Prevalence is estimated at 6–12%[4,5] with levels as high as 40% reported in men with type 2 diabetes (T2DM).[6,7] The diagnosis is important as adult-onset TD is also associated with increased mortality.[8] The belief that low serum testosterone is key in the causation of increased morbidity and mortality is supported by the finding that testosterone therapy (TTh) results in significant improvements in associated symptoms including sexual function, depression, physical performance, anemia, and bone mineral density[9] in men with adult-onset TD as well as reduction in mortality in men with T2DM.[10-13]

However, concerns remain regarding the safety of TTh. Although most studies demonstrate benefit or no change in cardiovascular disease (CVD), a few have reported higher CVD in men prescribed TTh.[14-17] An explanation for these discrepant findings is that the population of men with adult-onset TD is heterogeneous[18]; thus, subgroups with different lifestyles, genetic, and environmental factors may influence clinical outcomes. Hematocrit (HCT) is a possible candidate in determining outcome as an increase in this variable is the commonest effect of TTh.[19-21] Different guidelines have set varying HCT percentage thresholds above which they recommend withholding/discontinuing TTh and/or phlebotomy. For example, the British Society of Sexual Medicine,[4] Endocrine Society,[22] American Urological Association,[23] and European Association of Urology[24] have all adopted a threshold of 54%. The International Society for the Study of the Aging Male has adopted an HCT threshold of 52%,[25] whereas the International Consultation for Sexual Medicine[26] has recommended an even more conservative HCT threshold of just 50%.

HCT levels have been associated with changes in morbidity and mortality, although findings vary.[19] A meta-analysis of 16 studies has shown that the highest HCT tertile (>0.463) was associated with increased CVD compared with the lowest tertile (<0.417).[27] Similarly, in the Framingham cohort (of >34 years follow-up), the highest HCT quintile was associated with increased CVD as well as all-cause mortality.[28]

However, the European Prospective Investigation into Cancer and Nutrition-Netherlands study found no difference in CVD between the tertile distributions (>0.47 vs. <0.45) in CVD-free individuals.[29] In the Scottish Heart Health Extended Cohort Study, HCT (mean ± SD: 0.4381 ± 0.0394) was significantly associated with CVD events and mortality, although this association was lost when the analysis was adjusted for the following confounders: lipids, blood pressure (BP), diabetes, smoking status, family history of CVD, and fibrinogen.[30]

Boffetta et al. suggested that this lack of consensus may result from a nonlinear relationship between HCT, CVD, and mortality.[31] Thus, a U-shaped relationship between categories of HCT and mortality was found in Iranian adults of both genders, with low and high HCT values associated with increased overall mortality.[31] Locatelli et al. found, after erythropoietin therapy in patients with end-stage renal disease and low baseline HCT (0.301 ± 0.045), that mortality was inversely proportional to the increase in HCT, also suggesting that the association between morbidity/mortality and HCT is nonlinear.[32]

The clinical impact of increased HCT during TTh requires further understanding. In this study, we report baseline characteristics of the men prescribed/not prescribed TTh and compare changes in HCT (intra- and intergroup), though our focus is primarily on men prescribed TTh. This is because of the current uncertainty regarding clinical outcomes associated with change in HCT after TTh. We studied the relationship between HCT and all-cause mortality in men on TTh. HCT is associated with hemoglobin (Hb) level[33,34] and BP,[35-37] both of which are predictors of mortality.[38-42] Hence, these and other established risk factors such as waist circumference (WC), HbA1c, total cholesterol (TC), and triglycerides (TG) at the final assessment were included (if found to be significantly associated with mortality) as confounding variables.

Materials and Methods

We describe analysis of an observational prospective cumulative registry study comprising 737 men diagnosed with adult-onset TD in view of a serum total testosterone (TT) ≤12.1 nmol/L and symptoms of TD. In total, 737 men were recruited from 823 men presenting with urological symptoms and diagnosed with TD, after exclusion of primary hypogonadism (n = 39) and Klinefelter syndrome (n = 47) (Fig. 1). All the men were offered TTh. Testosterone undecanoate (TU)

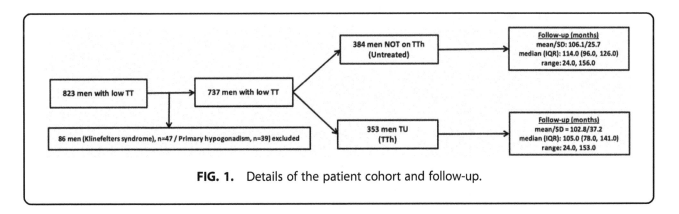

FIG. 1. Details of the patient cohort and follow-up.

1000 mg per 12 weeks after an initial 6-week interval was commenced in 353 men [median age (IQR): 60.0 (55, 64) years, median follow-up (IQR): 105.0 (78, 141) months] whereas the remaining 384 men [median age (IQR): 64.0 (60.0, 67.0) years, median follow-up (IQR): 114.0 (96, 126) months] opted against TTh (untreated) due to financial constraints and/or negative perceptions of TTh (Fig. 1 and Table 1). Data were gathered regularly (at least 6 monthly) during follow-up in all men. The German Medical Association's ethical guidelines for observational studies were followed and every participant consented to be included and have their data analyzed after being provided study details. Ethics committees (Germany and England) reviewed the study and stated that formal approval was not required. Institutional review board approval was received from University Hospitals Birmingham NHS Foundation Trust.

Study measurements

Serum TT (trough levels) was measured using an immunoassay (Abbott Architect). Hb levels were determined using photometry (CELL DYN Ruby/Abbott) and HCT was calculated using Microhaematocrit (Mindray 3000 Plus). HbA1c was measured using a high-performance liquid chromatography method on a TOSOH G7 (HLC-723-Series), whereas TC and TG concentrations were measured using a colorimetric assay on the Abbott Alinity c-Module (colorimetric analysis). BP was taken with the patient seated with his left arm resting at heart level using a sphygmomanometer according to protocol. Systolic and diastolic Korotkoff sounds were assessed twice to increase precision. Once all the requirement measurements were completed, Nebido® was administered intramuscularly and BP was again determined after a few minutes. The two values were usually the same, but if there was a dif-

ference of <5 mmHg, an average was taken, if there was a difference of >5 mmHg, a third measurement was made, and the mean of the closer values was accepted. WC was measured midway between the upper hip bone and the uppermost border of the right iliac crest.

Statistical methods

The baseline HCT in the total cohort was not normally distributed with both skewness ($p < 0.0001$) and kurtosis ($p < 0.0001$) evident, hence nonparametric tests were carried out when comparing HCT distributions. Baseline factors in men on TTh and those untreated were compared using rank-sum and chi square tests. Change during follow-up in the former group was analyzed through sign-rank tests. Risk factor prevalence between survivors/nonsurvivors in TTh-treated men was compared using rank-sum (univariate) and logistic regression (multivariate) analyses. Cox regression analyses were used to additionally study the association between HCT at final assessment (stratified) and survival, with these data presented as a Kaplan–Meier plot.

Results

Table 1 shows baseline data from both groups: men commencing ($n = 353$) and opting against ($n = 384$) TTh. Baseline HCT and Hb were significantly ($p < 0.0001$) lower in men in the TTh group. Metabolic indices also differed significantly with those about to commence TTh having higher baseline HbA1c, BP, TC, and TG levels, but lower WC (Table 1). No difference was observed in the frequency of T2DM or smoking status (Table 1 footnote). Table 1 also shows the differences between data at baseline and final assessment in men prescribed TTh: median change (Δ) in HCT (IQR) was 5.0 (3.0, 7.0)% and median Δ Hb levels (IQR) were 0.6 (0.3, 0.7) g/dL. Apart from the expected increase in trough levels of serum TT, significant

Table 1. Baseline Data of Testosterone Therapy-Treated and Untreated Men, and Changes at Final Assessment in Testosterone Therapy-Treated Men

	Baseline			Final assessment	
	Untreated		TTh (TU)	TTh (TU)	
No. of men	384		353		
		p (intergroup)		Change in values	p (intragroup)
	Median (IQR)		Median (IQR)	Median (IQR)	(Baseline vs. final)
Follow-up (months)	114.0 (96, 126)	0.52	105.0 (78, 141)		
Age (years)	64.0 (60.0, 67.0)	<0.0001	60.0 (55.0, 64.0)		
TT (nmol/l) (trough)	9.7 (9.4, 10.4)	0.079	10.1 (9.4, 10.7)	9.0 (7.6, 10.4)	<0.0001
HCT (%)	46.0 (45.0, 47.0)	<0.0001	44.0 (43.0, 46.0)	5.0 (3.0, 7.0)	<0.0001
Hb (g/dL)	14.7 (14.3, 15.1)	<0.0001	14.5 (14.1, 14.9)	0.5 (0.3, 0.7)	<0.0001
WC (cm)	109.0 (102.5, 116.0)	0.022	108.0 (100.0, 114.0)	−10.0 (−13.0, −6.0)	<0.0001
HbA1c (%)	5.4 (5.1, 7.7)	<0.0001	8.2 (5.8, 8.9), n = 270	−2.1 (−3.2, −0.7)	<0.0001
Systolic BP (mmHg)	137.5 (131.5, 154.0)	<0.0001	158.0 (141.0, 167.0)	−25.0 (−37.0, −13.0)	<0.0001
Diastolic BP (mmHg)	78.0 (75.0, 88.0)	<0.0001	94.0 (83.0, 98.0)	−17.0 (−24, −9.0)	<0.0001
TC (mmol/L)	6.5 (5.6, 7.4)	<0.0001	7.7 (7.2, 8.6)	−2.6 (−3.3, −2.1)	<0.0001
TG (mmol/L)	2.9 (2.6, 3.3)	<0.0001	3.2 (2.8, 3.5)	−0.1 (−1.3, −0.6)	<0.0001

Rank-sum and sign-rank nonparametric tests were carried out to determine differences between baseline data (intergroup: untreated vs. TTh) and changes seen at final assessment in men on TTh (intragroup) respectively. No significant differences (chi square) were observed between the two groups regarding T2DM (untreated: 42.7%, TTh: 41.9%, $p = 0.83$), smoking status (untreated: 36.8%, TTh: 38.2%, $p = 0.69$).

BP, blood pressure; Hb, hemoglobin; HCT, hematocrit; T2DM, type 2 diabetes; TC, total cholesterol; TG, triglyceride; TT, total testosterone; TTh, testosterone therapy; TU, testosterone undecanoate; WC, waist circumference.

improvements in WC, HbA1c, BP (systolic and diastolic), TC, and TG were associated with TTh. In men not given TTh, median Δ HCT (IQR) was 0.0 (−1.0, 2.0) at final assessment (however, sign-rank test suggested a higher HCT at final assessment, $p = 0.0003$).

Change in HCT at fixed time points during follow-up

Figure 2 shows median Δ HCT at 12, 48, 72, and 96 months in men prescribed/not prescribed TTh. There was a small but significant increase in HCT distribution (although the median change was 0%) in untreated men ($n = 294$) after 96 months compared with baseline, but not at 12, 48, or 72 months (median Δ HCT was 0% at all the time points). In contrast median HCT increased significantly after 12 months in men given TTh with the median Δ HCT subsequently increasing. The median Δ HCT (+4%) was identical at 48, 72, and 96 months of follow-up. At each time point, Δ HCT was greater in the TTh group (rank-sum test) than in untreated men (Fig. 2).

Association between HCT and all-cause mortality

All-cause mortality was significantly higher ($p < 0.0001$, Chi Sq) in men not prescribed TTh [74/384 men (19.3%)] than in men on TTh [20/353 men (5.7%)]. Table 2 shows that in men given TTh, HCT was significantly higher ($p = 0.021$, rank-sum test) in

men alive [median (IQR): 49.0 (48.0, 50.0)%] than in those who died [median (IQR): 49.0 (48.0, 49.0)%]. Table 2 also shows that age, diastolic BP, and TC at final assessment were significantly higher, whereas TT was lower in the men who died. Accordingly, the association between HCT (baseline and Δ) and mortality was confirmed with logistic regression analyses after adjusting for the mentioned confounding variables (Table 3: Model 1). Importantly, Table 2 shows that Hb was not associated with mortality and was not included as a confounding variable in the logistic regression analyses described in Table 3. Both baseline HCT and Δ HCT were inversely associated with mortality, and age at final assessment (baseline age+follow-up) was positively associated with mortality (Table 3: Model 1). Serum TT, diastolic BP, and TC were not associated with mortality. Interestingly, higher baseline HCT and greater Δ HCT were associated with lower mortality and with similar odds ratios (ORs). Table 3 (Model 2) gives the logistic regression analyses with baseline HCT, Δ HCT, and age at final assessment as independent variables, with all three conferring a significant association with mortality. We then replaced baseline HCT and Δ HCT with its sum (HCT at final assessment), and this, as expected from the previous logistic regression models, remained significantly associated with mortality (Table 3: Model 3). To further characterize the relationship between

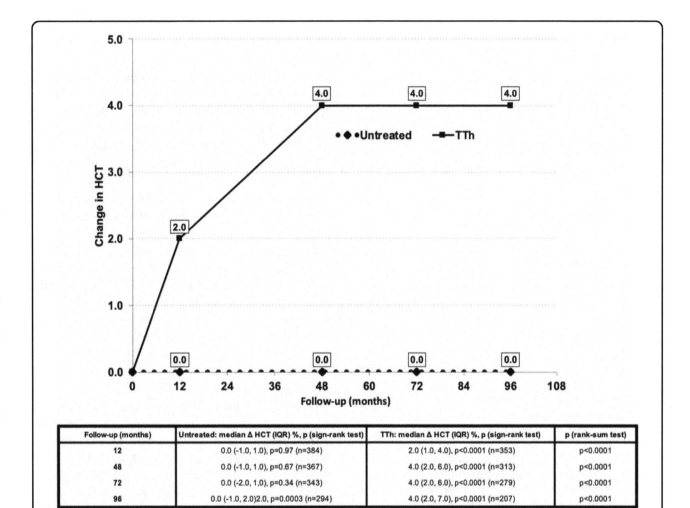

Follow-up (months)	Untreated: median Δ HCT (IQR) %, p (sign-rank test)	TTh: median Δ HCT (IQR) %, p (sign-rank test)	p (rank-sum test)
12	0.0 (-1.0, 1.0), p=0.97 (n=384)	2.0 (1.0, 4.0), p<0.0001 (n=353)	p<0.0001
48	0.0 (-1.0, 1.0), p=0.67 (n=367)	4.0 (2.0, 6.0), p<0.0001 (n=313)	p<0.0001
72	0.0 (-2.0, 1,0), p=0.34 (n=343)	4.0 (2.0, 6.0), p<0.0001 (n=279)	p<0.0001
96	0.0 (-1.0, 2.0)2.0, p=0.0003 (n=294)	4.0 (2.0, 7.0), p<0.0001 (n=207)	p<0.0001

Sign-rank test: compared to baseline values (within group).
Rank-sum test: between group comparison at that time point.

FIG. 2. Change in HCT at fixed time points (12, 48, 72 and 96 months) in untreated and TTh groups. HCT, hematocrit; TTh, testosterone therapy.

HCT at final assessment and mortality, we stratified the cohort by the median HCT (49%) at final assessment and found that men with HCT (50–52%) at final visit were at lower risk of mortality (Table 3: Model 4) than their counterparts (HCT: 46–49%). It was noted that the median HCT at final assessment of 49% was observed in a large proportion of men (*n* = 123), hence a further logistic regression analysis (not shown in Table 3) was carried out, adjusted for age at final assessment and excluding these 123 men. Men with HCT at final assessment of 50–52% (*n* = 122) were once again associated with lower mortality (OR:

0.083, 95% CI: 0.010–0.69, *p* = 0.021) than their counterparts with HCT at final assessment of 46–48% (*n* = 108). Table 3 (footnote) provides the unadjusted mortality rates by HCT at final assessment [46–48% HCT: 8/108 (7.4%), 49% HCT: 11/123 (8.9%), 50–52% HCT: 1/122 (0.8%)].

To graphically demonstrate the difference in survival in men on TTh stratified by the median HCT at final assessment, we plotted a Kaplan–Meier survival curve (Fig. 3) based on a Cox regression analysis (Fig. 3 footnote: Model 2), which, like the previous logistic regression analyses, also demonstrated that men with final

Table 2. Comparison of Variables at Final Assessment in Men Given Testosterone Therapy, Stratified by Mortality

	Men on TTh (n=353)		
	Alive	Dead	
No. of men	333	20	
	Median (IQR)		p (rank-sum)
Baseline age (years)	59.0 (55.0, 63.0)	66.0 (62.0, 68.0)	0.0001
Follow-up (months)	102.0 (78.0, 141.0)	130.5 (94.5, 135.0)	0.35
	Data at final assessment		
HCT (%)	49.0 (48.0, 50.0)	49.0 (48.0, 49.0)	0.021
Hb (g/dL)	14.9 (14.7, 15.3)	15.0 (14.7, 15.3)	0.89
Age (years)	68.5 (64.0, 71.5)	77.5 (69.3, 78.8)	<0.0001
TT (nmol/L)	19.1 (17.7, 19.8)	17.9 (16.8, 18.7)	0.0050
WC (cm)	97.0 (94.0, 101.0)	98.5 (93.5, 103.0)	0.66
HbA1c (%) (n=269)	5.4 (5.2, 5.8) n=255	5.7 (5.4, 6.1) n=14	0.089
Systolic BP (mmHg)	128.0 (123.0, 133) n=332	130.0 (126.0, 135.0)	0.12
Diastolic BP (mmHg)	75.0 (73.0, 77.0)	77.0 (74.0, 82.0)	0.017
TC (mmol/L)	5.2 (4.9, 5.4)	5.3 (5.1, 5.4)	0.019
TG (mmol/L)	2.2 (2.1, 2.3)	2.2 (2.1, 2.2)	0.99

Intragroup differences were determined using rank-sum nonparametric tests.

Table 3. Logistic Regression Analyses Studying the Association Between Baseline Hematocrit, Δ Hematocrit, Hematocrit at Final Assessment, and Mortality, the Analyses Adjusted for Confounders (Factors Significantly Associated with Mortality in Table 2) in Men on Testosterone Therapy

	OR (95% CI)	p
Model 1		
Baseline HCT	0.50 (0.31–0.79)	0.004
Δ HCT	0.55 (0.35–0.88)	0.012
Age at final assessment (years)	1.26 (1.13–1.41)	<0.001
TT at final assessment (nmol/L)	0.88 (0.74–1.04)	0.13
Diastolic BP at final assessment (mmHg)	1.07 (0.95–1.21)	0.24
Total cholesterol at final assessment (mmol/L)	1.56 (0.36–6.85)	0.55
Model 2		
Baseline HCT	0.49 (0.31–0.79)	0.003
Δ HCT	0.54 (0.34–0.86)	0.009
Age at final assessment (years)	1.26 (1.13–1.40)	<0.001
Model 3		
HCT at final assessment	0.53 (0.33–0.83)	0.006
Age at final assessment (years)	1.27 (1.14–1.41)	<0.001
Model 4 (factorized HCT)		
HCT at final assessment >49 (50–52)%	0.091 (0.012–0.70)	0.006
HCT at final assessment ≤49 (46–49)%	reference	
Age at final assessment (years)	1.27 (1.14–1.41)	<0.001

Adding T2DM into the regression models did not change the association between HCT indices, age, and mortality. Unadjusted mortality rates by HCT at final assessment (median: 49%). HCT (46–48%): mortality=8/108 (7.4%), HCT (49%): mortality=11/123 (8.9%), HCT (50–52%): mortality=1/122 (0.8%).

ORs, odds ratios.

assessment HCT >49% were at lower risk of mortality (Fig. 3 footnote: Model 1), even when adjusted for age at final assessment.

Although this article is mainly focused on men given TTh, we also present data on the association between HCT at final assessment and mortality in 384 men opting against TTh. At final assessment, HCT was significantly higher ($p=0.0001$, rank-sum test) in men alive [median (IQR): 46.0 (45.0, 47.0)%, $n=310$] than in those deceased [median (IQR): 45.0 (44.0, 46.0)%, $n=74$]. However, a logistic regression analysis revealed that HCT at final assessment was not associated with mortality (OR: 0.92, 95% CI: 0.81–1.04, $p=0.20$) when adjusting for the confounding variables (TT, WC, HbA1c, BP, and lipid values) at final assessment. This was the case when baseline HCT (OR: 0.88, 95% CI: 0.68–1.14, $p=0.32$) and Δ HCT (OR: 0.92, 95% CI: 0.81–1.05, $p=0.23$) were substituted for HCT at final assessment as independent variables.

Discussion

Increased HCT is a common consequence of TTh and clinical guidelines set action thresholds for discontinuing treatment that are not based on clear outcome evidence.[4,22–26] Longitudinal studies suggest that HCT influences CVD morbidity and mortality, although the association may not be linear. We used an ongoing registry database to demonstrate the pattern of Δ HCT associated with TTh, and study putative associations with all-cause mortality. Although HCT was not significantly changed in men not prescribed TTh, it was significantly higher (median: +5.0%) in men on TTh at the end of follow-up. Increased values were observed at 12, 48, 72, and 96 months after TTh compared with baseline, although most of the increase was evident before 48 months (Fig. 2). Down-titrating/discontinuing TU was not required as HCT did not exceed 52% in the 353 men given TTh.

It is tempting to state that the TTh-associated increase in HCT could be a reversal of low HCT values associated with low testosterone in adult-onset TD. However, the distribution of baseline values in both untreated (mean HCT: 45.8%, 95% distribution: 44–48%) and treated men (mean: 43.8%, 95% distribution: 37–47%) was within the reference range (38.3–48.6%) for males quoted by the Mayo Clinic.[43] Furthermore, HCT at final assessment in men on TTh (mean: 49.1%, 95% distribution: 47–51%) appears higher than the Mayo Clinic reference range (only 30.6% of

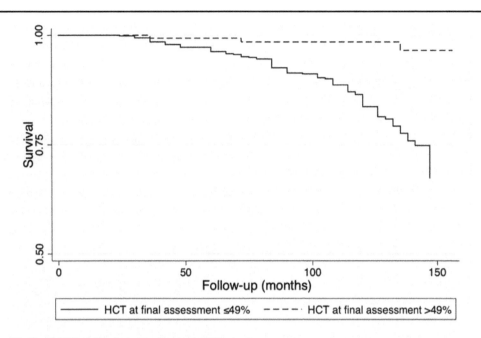

Median HCT at final assessment = 49%
The above plot is based on model 2 of the Cox regression analysis.

	HR (95% CI)	p
Model 1		
HCT at final assessment >49 (50 - 52)	0.11 (0.015 / 0.84)	0.033
HCT at final assessment ≤49 (46 - 49)	reference	
Age at final assessment (years)	1.15 (1.04 / 1.26)	0.006
Model 2		
HCT at final assessment >49 (50 - 52)	0.095 (0.013 / 0.71)	0.022
HCT at final assessment ≤49 (46 - 49)	reference	

FIG. 3. Kaplan-Meier survival curves of men on TTh, stratified by the median HCT at final assessment.

men having values within this distribution). Thus, it is unlikely to be a return to higher normal levels from a previously low level associated with TD, unless the quoted reference range is subject to a lowering of values due to a high proportion of men with adult-onset TD (prevalence considered to be 6–12%).[4]

Baseline and Δ HCT were inversely associated with mortality in men on TTh with similar ORs, independent of age, serum TT, WC, HbA1c, BP, and lipids. The greater the baseline value and increase in HCT after TTh, the lower the risk of mortality. This association remained evident when HCT at final assessment (as a continuous variable and stratified by median value

and used in a logistic regression model as a factorized variable) was substituted for baseline and Δ HCT. Our data suggest that mortality risk reduction is evident with an upper end of HCT distribution at 52% (50–52%) compared with a lower HCT (46–49%); thus, we recommend the HCT action threshold remains at 54% in well-hydrated men as dehydration can raise HCT.[44] At this moment, HCT could be considered a marker associated with mortality risk. Oxygen content in the blood is related linearly to HCT and increased HCT could plausibly increase tissue oxygenation.[45,46] However, increased HCT will exponentially increase blood viscosity, thereby potentially reducing blood flow.[47,48] Thus, an ideal HCT should allow optimized tissue oxygenation and blood flow, adding credence to the concept of a U- or J-shaped association between HCT and morbidity/mortality.[19,31,32] We did not observe a U- or J-shaped association with mortality, with the upper limit of the HCT distribution in our cohort reaching 52%, the inverse association appeared to continue to this point.

HCT at final assessment was not related with mortality in men not given TTh, when adjusted for other confounding variables. Hence, our focus remained with men on TTh. Interestingly, although many of the metabolic risk factors such as WC, HbA1c, BP, and TC were significantly decreased in men on TTh (Table 1), they were not related to intragroup mortality (Table 2).

The clinical impact of TTh-associated elevated HCT is currently in focus after the 24-month T4DM randomized controlled trial, which showed that TU/lifestyle measures (504 obese/overweight men aged 50–74 years with impaired glucose tolerance or newly diagnosed T2DM) were associated with significantly lower glucose values, compared with 503 men on placebo/lifestyle measures.[49] In contrast to our study where no man was seen to have an HCT >52%, 22% (106 men) of the men on TU had at least a single HCT ≥54% compared with 1% (6 men) treated with placebo, although it is emphasized that TU was discontinued in only 23 men due to two HCT values ≥54%.[49]

This longitudinal registry study has strengths and weaknesses. Treatment compliance was not an issue as TU was administered in clinic. Follow-up was long and we had an almost complete data set (except HbA1c). The nature of the study resulted in patients not being randomized into TTh-treated and untreated groups and differences in baseline factors were evident. To counter this, most of the analyses describe intragroup comparisons. Furthermore, our analyses using mortality as the outcome centered on the TTh group as Δ HCT only significantly changed in this cohort (Table 1), hence the disparity of risk factor levels between the two groups was not an issue. The results obtained were not affected when the cohort was stratified by T2DM (Tables 1 and 3).

Conclusions

Our study, characterizing increase in HCT associated with TTh, shows a median increase in HCT of 5.0%, mostly occurring in the initial 48 months of treatment. Our data show that benefit in mortality extended to HCT values of 52%, the HCT distribution did not allow us to extend this value further. Although it is premature to speculate whether the change in HCT is causative or a surrogate affecting the association between TTh and mortality, the data indicate current guidance suggesting only HCT >54% should trigger changes in TTh treatment, appears reasonable.[4]

Randomized controlled trials are needed to further investigate our findings regarding entry and exit thresholds and also on the association between HCT and mortality to evaluate a possible causative role using the current modified versions of the Bradford Hill criteria.[50,51]

Authors' Contributions

R.C.S. designed the study and prepared the article. C.S.K. designed the study, analyzed data, and prepared the article. A.A. designed the study and prepared the article. G.H. prepared the article. A.H. and K.S.H. recruited patients, collected data, and prepared the article. P.D. transposed data and maintained the database. F.S. maintained the database, designed the study, and prepared the article. N.L. analyzed data and prepared the article. A.M. analyzed data and prepared the article. S.R. designed the study, analyzed data, and prepared the article.

References

1. Harman SM, Metter EJ, Tobin JD, Pearson J, Blackman MR. Longitudinal effects of aging on serum total and free testosterone levels in healthy men. Baltimore longitudinal study of aging. J Clin Endocrinol Metab. 2001;86(2):724–731.
2. Araujo AB, Esche GR, Kupelian V, et al. Prevalence of symptomatic androgen deficiency in men. J Clin Endocrinol Metab. 2007;92(11):4241–4247.
3. Livingston M, Kalansooriya A, Hartland AJ, Ramachandran S, Heald A. Serum testosterone levels in male hypogonadism: Why and when to check-A review. Int J Clin Pract. 2017;71(11):e12995.

4. Hackett G, Kirby M, Edwards D, et al. British Society for Sexual Medicine Guidelines on adult testosterone deficiency, with statements for UK practice. J Sex Med. 2017;14(12):1504–1523.

5. Kapoor D, Aldred H, Clark S, Channer KS, Jones TH. Clinical and biochemical assessment of hypogonadism in men with type 2 diabetes: Correlations with bioavailable testosterone and visceral adiposity. Diabetes Care. 2007;30(4):911–917.

6. Hackett G, Cole N, Deshpande A, Popple M, Kennedy D, Wilkinson P. Biochemical hypodonadism and type 2 diabetes in primary care. Br J Diabetes Vasc Dis. 2009;9(5):226–231.

7. Holmboe SA, Jensen TK, Linneberg A, et al. Low testosterone: A risk marker rather than a risk factor for type 2 diabetes. J Clin Endocrinol Metab. 2016;101(8):3180–3190.

8. Pye SR, Huhtaniemi IT, Finn JD, et al.; EMAS Study Group. Late-onset hypogonadism and mortality in aging men. J Clin Endocrinol Metab. 2014;99(4):1357–1366.

9. Snyder PJ, Bhasin S, Cunningham GR, et al.; Testosterone Trials Investigators. Effects of testosterone treatment in older men. N Engl J Med. 2016;374(7):611–624.

10. Shores MM, Smith NL, Forsberg CW, Anawalt BD, Matsumoto AM. Testosterone treatment and mortality in men with low testosterone levels. J Clin Endocrinol Metab. 2012;97(6):2050–2058.

11. Muraleedharan V, Marsh H, Kapoor D, Channer KS, Jones TH. Testosterone deficiency is associated with increased risk of mortality and testosterone replacement improves survival in men with type 2 diabetes. Eur J Endocrinol. 2013;169(6):725–733.

12. Hackett G, Heald AH, Sinclair A, Jones PW, Strange RC, Ramachandran S. Serum testosterone, testosterone replacement therapy and all-cause mortality in men with type 2 diabetes: Retrospective consideration of the impact of PDE5 inhibitors and statins. Int J Clin Pract. 2016;70(3):244–253.

13. Hackett G, Jones PW, Strange RC, Ramachandran S. Statin, testosterone and phosphodiesterase 5-inhibitor treatments and age related mortality in diabetes. World J Diabetes. 2017;8(3):104–111.

14. Vigen R, O'Donnell CI, Barón AE, et al. Association of testosterone therapy with mortality, myocardial infarction, and stroke in men with low testosterone levels. JAMA. 2013;310(17):1829–1836. Erratum in: JAMA. 2014; 311(9):967.

15. Finkle WD, Greenland S, Ridgeway GK, et al. Increased risk of non-fatal myocardial infarction following testosterone therapy prescription in men. PLoS One. 2014;9(1):e85805.

16. Basaria S, Coviello AD, Travison TG, et al. Adverse events associated with testosterone administration. N Eng J Med. 2010;363(2):109–122.

17. Morgentaler A, Zitzmann M, Traish AM, et al. Fundamental concepts regarding testosterone deficiency and treatment: international expert consensus resolutions. Mayo Clin Proc. 2016;91(7):881–896.

18. Ramachandran S, König CS, Hackett G, Livingston M, Strange RC. Managing clinical heterogeneity: An argument for benefit based action limits. J Med Diagn Ther. 2018;1(3):034701.

19. König CS, Balabani S, Hackett GI, Strange RC, Ramachandran S. Testosterone therapy: An assessment of the clinical consequences of changes in hematocrit and blood flow characteristics. Sex Med Rev. 2019;7(4):650–660.

20. Calof OM, Singh AB, Lee ML, et al. Adverse events associated with testosterone replacement in middle-aged and older men: A meta-analysis of randomized, placebo-controlled trials. J Gerontol A Biol Sci Med Sci. 2005; 60(11):1451–1457.

21. Ohlander SJ, Varghese B, Pastuszak AW. Erythrocytosis following testosterone therapy. Sex Med Rev. 2018;6(1):77–85.

22. Bhasin S, Brito JP, Cunningham GR, et al. Testosterone therapy in men with hypogonadism: An Endocrine Society Clinical Practice Guideline. J Clin Endocrinol Metab. 2018;103(5):1715–1744.

23. Mulhall JP, Trost LW, Brannigan RE, et al. Evaluation and management of testosterone deficiency: AUA guideline. J Urol. 2018;200(2):423–432.

24. Dohle G, Arver S, Bettocchi C, Jones T, Kliesch S. EAU guidelines on male hypogonadism. 2018. Available from: http://uroweb.org/guideline/male-hypogonadism/

25. Lunenfeld B, Mskhalaya G, Zitzmann M, et al. Recommendations on the diagnosis, treatment and monitoring of hypogonadism in men. Aging Male. 2015;18(1):5–15.

26. Khera M, Adaikan G, Buvat J, et al. Diagnosis and treatment of testosterone deficiency: recommendations from the Fourth International Consultation for Sexual Medicine (ICSM 2015). J Sex Med. 2016;13(12): 1787–1804.

27. Danesh J, Collins R, Peto R, Lowe GD. Haematocrit, viscosity, erythrocyte sedimentation rate: Meta-analyses of prospective studies of coronary heart disease. Eur Heart J. 2000;21(7):515–520.

28. Gagnon DR, Zhang TJ, Brand FN, Kannel WB. Hematocrit and the risk of cardiovascular disease—The Framingham study: A 34-year follow-up. Am Heart J. 1994;127(3):674–682.

29. Lassale C, Curtis A, Abete I, et al. Elements of the complete blood count associated with cardiovascular disease incidence: Findings from the EPIC-NL cohort study. Sci Rep. 2018;8(1):3290.

30. Peters SA, Woodward M, Rumley A, Tunstall-Pedoe HD, Lowe GD. Plasma and blood viscosity in the prediction of cardiovascular disease and mortality in the Scottish Heart Health Extended Cohort Study. Eur J Prev Cardiol. 2017;24(2):161–167.

31. Boffetta P, Islami F, Vedanthan R, et al. A U-shaped relationship between haematocrit and mortality in a large prospective cohort study. Int J Epidemiol. 2013;42(2):601–615.

32. Locatelli F, Conte F, Marcelli D. The impact of haematocrit levels and erythropoietin treatment on overall and cardiovascular mortality and morbidity—The experience of the Lombardy Dialysis Registry. Nephrol Dial Transplant. 1998;13(7):1642–1644.

33. Al-Ryalat N, AlRyalat SA, Malkawi LW, Abu-Hassan H, Samara O, Hadidy A. The haematocrit to haemoglobin conversion factor: A cross-sectional study of its accuracy and application. N Z Med Lab Sci. 2018;72(1):18–21.

34. Quintó L, Aponte JJ, Sacarlal J, et al. Haematological and biochemical indices in young African children: In search of reference intervals. Trop Med Int Health. 2006;11(11):1741–1748.

35. Cinar Y, Demir G, Paç M, Cinar AB. Effect of hematocrit on blood pressure via hyperviscosity. Am J Hypertens. 1999;12(7):739–743.

36. Salazar-Vazquez BY, Intaglietta M, Rodríguez-Morán M, Guerrero-Romero F. Blood pressure and hematocrit in diabetes and the role of endothelial responses in the variability of blood viscosity. Diabetes Care. 2006;29(7): 1523–1528.

37. Cinar Y, Senyol AM, Duman K. Blood viscosity and blood pressure: Role of temperature and hyperglycemia. Am J Hypertens. 2001;14(5 Pt 1):433–438.

38. Mamas MA, Kwok CS, Kontopantelis E, et al. Relationship between anemia and mortality outcomes in a national acute coronary syndrome cohort: Insights from the UK Myocardial Ischemia National Audit Project Registry. J Am Heart Assoc. 2016;5(11):e003348.

39. Wouters HJCM, van der Klauw MM, de Witte T, et al. Association of anemia with health-related quality of life and survival: A large population-based cohort study. Haematologica. 2019;104(3):468–476.

40. Arima H, Barzi F, Chalmers J. Mortality patterns in hypertension. J Hypertens. 2011;29(Suppl 1):S3–S7.

41. Armas Rojas N, Dobell E, Lacey B, et al. Burden of hypertension and associated risks for cardiovascular mortality in Cuba: A prospective cohort study. Lancet Public Health. 2019;4(2);e107–e115. Erratum in: Lancet Public Health. 2019;4(2):e88.

42. Makridakis S, DiNicolantonio JJ. Hypertension: Empirical evidence and implications in 2014. Open Heart. 2014;1(1):e000048.

43. Mayo Clinic. Hematocrit test [Internet]. 2021 [cited 17.06.21]. Available from: https://www.mayoclinic.org/tests-procedures/hematocrit/about/pac-2038472817

44. The Association for Clinical Biochemistry and Laboratory Medicine. Lab Tests on Line. PCV [Internet]. 2020 [cited 17.06.21]. Available from: https://labtestsonline.org.uk/tests/pcv

45. Lenz C, Rebel A, Waschke KF, Koehler RC, Frietsch T. Blood viscosity modulates tissue perfusion: Sometimes and somewhere. Transfus Altern Transfus Med. 2008;9(4):265–272.

46. Salazar Vázquez BY, Martini J, Chávez Negrete A, Cabrales P, Tsai AG, Intaglietta M. Microvascular benefits of increasing plasma viscosity and maintaining blood viscosity: Counterintuitive experimental findings. Biorheology. 2009;46(3):167–179.

47. Reinhart WH. The optimum hematocrit. Clin Hemorheol Microcirc. 2016; 64(4):575–585.

48. Apostolidis AJ, Beris AN. Modeling of the blood rheology in steady-state shear flows. J Rheol. 2014;58(3):607–633.

49. Wittert G, Bracken K, Robledo KP, et al. Testosterone treatment to prevent or revert type 2 diabetes in men enrolled in a lifestyle programme

(T4DM): A randomised, double-blind, placebo-controlled, 2-year, phase 3b trial. Lancet Diabetes Endocrinol. 2021;9(1):32–45.

50. Fedak KM, Bernal A, Capshaw ZA, Gross S. Applying the Bradford Hill criteria in the 21st century: How data integration has changed causal inference in molecular epidemiology. Emerg Themes Epidemiol. 2015; 12:14.

51. Weed DL. Analogy in causal inference: Rethinking Austin Bradford Hill's neglected consideration. Ann Epidemiol. 2018;28(5):343–346.

Abbreviations Used

BP = blood pressure
CVD = cardiovascular disease
Hb = hemoglobin
HCT = hematocrit
ORs = odds ratios
T2DM = type 2 diabetes
TC = total cholesterol
TD = testosterone deficiency
TG = triglyceride
TT = total testosterone
TTh = testosterone therapy
TU = testosterone undecanoate
WC = waist circumference

9

Augmenting Intralesional Collagenase Treatment with Testosterone Therapy Provides Greater Self-Assessed Improvement in Penile Curvature due to Peyronie's Disease

Nadezhda Shlykova[1,2] and Abraham Morgentaler[1,2,*]

Abstract

Introduction: Testosterone (T) deficiency has been reported to be associated with Peyronie's disease (PD). This study investigated response rates to intralesional injections of collagenase clostridium histolyticum (Xiaflex™) (CCx) for penile curvature in men who simultaneously received T therapy (TTh) and in men who received CCx without TTh.

Methods: Search of electronic records identified all men treated with CCx from 2013 to 2018, and whether they also received TTh during that time. Laboratory results for baseline serum T, free T, and luteinizing hormone were available for all men. Response to CCx was categorized as no change, mild change, substantial change, or complete resolution based on subjective reports by patients.

Results: A total of 117 men received treatment with CCx. Of these, 72 received CCx alone (henceforth referred to as XA group) and 45 received CCx plus TTh (referred to as XT group). Mean baseline serum T was 458 ng/dL for the XA group and 384 ng/dL for the XT group ($p = 0.10$). Mean age was 60.4 years for the XT group and 56.5 years for the XA group ($p = 0.028$). Baseline mean curvature was 46° for the XA group and 45° for the XT group. Mean number of treatment cycles (two injections per cycle) was 2.7 for both groups. Overall, 67.5% reported some improvement in curve with CCx. Reports of any improvement were 84.4% for the XT group and 56.9% for the XA group ($p < 0.001$). Conversely, rates of no improvement were 15.6% for the XT group and 43.1% for the XA group. Substantial improvement or complete resolution of curve was noted by 48.8% of the XT group and 20.8% of the XA group ($p = 0.001$).

Conclusions: These pilot observational results suggest that TTh may improve the response to intralesional CCx treatment of PD. A prospective study is warranted to investigate this further.

Keywords: Peyronie's disease; testosterone; testosterone deficiency; hypogonadism; collagenase; Xiaflex

Introduction

Peyronie's disease (PD) is an inflammatory disorder of the tunica albuginea (TA) of the penis that results in collagen deposition and alterations in the elastin framework that lead to creation of fibrous plaques.[1] These inelastic plaques limit expansion of the TA during erection, leading to curvature, reduced length, and girth. Penile trauma or microtrauma is believed to be the inciting event. Significant curvature may result in pain and inability to successfully engage in sexual intercourse. The prevalence of PD is estimated to be 0.5–13%.[2]

[1]Men's Health Boston, Chestnut Hill, Massachusetts, USA.
[2]Beth Israel Deaconess Medical Center, Harvard Medical School, Boston, Massachusetts, USA.

*Address correspondence to: Abraham Morgentaler, MD, Men's Health Boston, 200 Boylston Street, Suite 309, Chestnut Hill, MA 02467, USA, Email: amorgent@bidmc.harvard.edu

Collagenase clostridium histolyticum (CCx) (Xia-flex™) is an FDA-approved intralesional injection used to treat penile curvature due to PD.[3] Treatment consists of up to four cycles, with each cycle comprising two injection procedures on separate days and a penile modeling procedure to stretch the plaque.[3] In combined data from two large double-blind randomized studies, the average improvement in penile curvature with CCx was 34%, or 17°, compared with 18% improvement and 9° in men receiving placebo.[4] A recently published phase 4 study in 204 men reported mean improvement of 20.9° or 39.5% with a further 9.1% improvement with an additional 5 years of follow-up.[5] There is little published information on how various ethnic, biological, or genetic factors may influence response to CCx in men with PD.

In 2009, Moreno and Morgentaler reported in a series of 121 consecutive men presenting with PD that 74% had low baseline concentrations of total or free testosterone (T), and that the severity of T deficiency (TD) was correlated with degree of curvature.[6] Other studies have similarly reported associations between increased plaque size or magnitude of curvature with TD,[7,8] but not all.[9]

This study is a retrospective investigation of subjective self-assessment of change in curvature with CCx in men who simultaneously received TTh during CCx compared with men who received CCx alone. We aimed to test the hypothesis that treatment of TD would improve response to CCx.

Methods
Study population
A search of in-office electronic records identified 117 men who had undergone at least one completed cycle of treatment with CCx at our center during 2013–2018. Chart review was performed for baseline and follow-up information, including number of CCx injections, degree of baseline curvature, laboratory results, and use and type of TTh. There were no cases of ventral curvature treated with CCx. Forty-five men received TTh during CCx treatment (XT group), and 72 men received CCx alone (XA group). Initiation of TTh was within several weeks of first CCx injection in all patients. Forms of TTh included pellets, injections, or topical gels, depending on patient preference and insurance coverage. Chart review was done under Beth Israel Deaconess Medical Center IRB protocol no. 2010P000241.

Hormone testing
All patients underwent routine laboratory testing for total T (TT), free T (FT), estradiol (E), and sex hormone binding globulin (SHBG). Blood tests were obtained during clinic hours between 8 am and 4:30 pm. Although morning determination of T is usually recommended, current evidence indicates that diurnal variation appears to be greatly reduced in men >40 years[10] and absent in men with TD.[11] Immunoassays were used for measurement of all laboratory blood draws (Tosoh Bioscience, San Francisco, Los Angeles, CA) except FT, which was performed through analog assay (Quest Diagnostics Nichols Institute, Valencia, CA). Men were considered candidates for TTh if TT was <300 ng/dL or FT <1.5 ng/dL.

Assessment of change in curvature
The degree of baseline curvature was based on direct measurement after in-office intracavernosal injection of vasoactive medications, photographs brought in by the patient, or patient description. Patients were then placed into one of four categories based on documented self-assessed response to treatment: no change, mild change, substantial change, and complete resolution of the curve.

Statistical analysis
Statistical analysis of the two groups was done with simple t-test focusing on analyzing differences in response to CCx treatment between the two groups. Hypothesis testing was performed with R software 3.3.2 (R Project for Statistical Computing). Demographic data were analyzed to determine baseline differences between treatment groups.

Results
The study population (Table 1) consisted of 117 subjects, with 45 treated with collagenase and T (XT) and 72 who

Table 1. Baseline Patient Characteristics

		Xiaflex+T therapy n=45	Xiaflex n=72	p
Age (years)	Mean (SD)	60.4 (7.80)	56.5 (11.57)	0.03*
Baseline total T	Mean (SD)	384 (247)	458 (198)	0.10
Baseline free T	Mean (SD)	0.74 (0.30)	0.88 (0.37)	0.03*
Baseline angle (°)	Mean (SD)	45 (15)	46 (16)	0.74
SHBG	Mean (SD)	36 (15)	52 (14)	0.43
Estradiol	Mean (SD)	52 (16)	38 (14)	0.83
Diabetes	N (%)	0 (0)	2 (2.90)	0.17
Hypertension	N (%)	16 (7.54)	15 (22.10)	0.04*

*p < 0.05.
SD, standard deviation; SHBG, sex hormone binding globulin.

were treated with collagenase alone (XA). Mean age for the entire population was 58.5 years.

In the XT group, 44.4% had TT of 300 ng/dL or below and 60% had TT of 350 ng/dL or below. In the XA group, 13.9% had TT of 300 ng/dL or below and 25% had TT of 350 ng/dL or below. FT at base line was <1.5 ng/dL in 97.7% of the XT group and 97.2% of the XA group.

The XT group was older than the XA group, at 60.4±7.8 years versus 56.5±11.6 years ($p=0.03$). Baseline curvature was similar for both groups at 45°, and both groups completed 2.7 cycles of CCx. TTh consisted of T undecanoate injections in 7 subjects, T cypionate injections in 3 subjects, T pellets in 31 subjects, and 4 subjects received a mix of T formulations.

Hormones

Baseline concentrations of serum TT were 384 ng/dL ±247 for the XT group and 458 ng/dL ±198 for the XA group ($p=0.1$). FT was slightly lower for the XT group than for the XA group (0.74±0.30 vs. 0.88± 0.37, respectively; $p=0.03$). Differences in SHBG and E were not significantly different between groups. Follow-up TT concentrations rose in the XT group to 616 ng/dL ±299. Follow-up T levels were not obtained in the XA group.

Response to treatment

For the entire study population, 14.5% of subjects reported complete resolution of penile curvature, 35.9% reported mild change, 17.1% reported seeing substantial change, and 32.5% reported no change.

When examined by groups (Table 2), 15.6% of the XT group reported no change in curvature, mild improvement was noted in 35.6%, substantial change was reported by 28.8%, and complete resolution was reported by 20%. In the XA group, no change was reported by 43.1%, mild change was reported by 36.1%, substantial change was reported by 9.7%, and 11.1% claimed complete resolution of curvature. In the XT group, 48.8%

Table 2. Curvature Response to Treatment

Improvement in curvature	Xiaflex+T therapy $n=45$	Xiaflex $n=72$	p
No change	7 (15.6)	31 (43.1)	0.002
Mild change	16 (35.6)	26 (36.1)	0.95
Substantial change	13 (28.8)	7 (9.7)	<0.01
Complete resolution	9 (20)	8 (11.1)	0.18
Substantial and complete resolution	22 (48.8)	15 (20.8)	<0.001

Table 3. Response to Treatment

Improvement in curvature	Xiaflex+T therapy, $n=45$	Xiaflex, $n=72$	p
Any change	38 (84.4)	41 (56.9)	
No change	7 (15.6)	31 (43.1)	
			0.00085

reported substantial improvement or complete resolution, compared with 20.8% for the XA group ($p=0.001$). Overall (Table 3) 84.4% of the XT group reported at least some improvement in curvature compared with 56.9% of the XA group ($p=0.002$). Conversely, 15.6% of the XT group reported no change compared with 43.1% of the XA group ($p=0.002$).

Adverse events

Bruising and swelling consistent with some degree of subcutaneous bleeding were routinely noted. No patient required drainage, surgery, or hospitalization. There were no penile ruptures.

Discussion

PD is a difficult-to-treat condition that causes considerable distress for affected men. The pathophysiology is believed to be related to mechanical stress and microvascular trauma to the TA of the erect penis that results in bleeding into the subtunical space or tunical delamination. Subsequent fibrin deposition initiates an exaggerated wound healing and inflammatory response, including recruitment of macrophages and neutrophils, which, in turn, release cytokines, vasoactive factors, and growth factors, including transforming growth factor (TGF)-β1.[1] Fibroblasts migrate into the area, proliferate, and under the influence of TGF-β1 synthesize collagen, proteoglycans, and fibronectin, while increasing synthesis of tissue inhibitors of collagenase, thus preventing connective tissue scarring during remodeling.[1] The resulting fibrotic area, or plaque, lacks the normal elasticity of adjacent undamaged TA, and in this way impedes tissue compliance and causes curvature and other deformities when the penis engorges during erection.

The evidence suggests an important role for androgens in regulating the fibrotic process of the penis during injury. Wang et al. showed that castration of adult male Sprague-Dawley rats resulted in greater fibrosis, decreased smooth muscle/collagen ratio, and higher expression of TGF-β1, all of which were partly restored with T administration.[12] A review of cavernosal fibrosis by Cho et al. indicated that a number of TGF-β1–driven mechanisms promote fibrosis in the rat model, including RhoA-ROCK1-LIMK2-cofilin and p42-44.[13] The authors proposed that strategies to minimize the impact of TGF-β1–signaling pathways might, therefore, be beneficial for attenuating fibrotic conditions of the penis, such as PD. The gene for TGF-β1 has been found to be overexpressed in PD.[14] Indeed, injection of microspheres containing TGF-β1 into the corpus cavernosum of the rabbit was sufficient to increase connective tissue and reduce smooth muscle content within 3 days.[15] Another possible mechanism by which TD may predispose to PD comes from the work of Shen et al., who showed that TA thickness is reduced to 25% of normal, from 0.16 to 0.04 mm, and with loss of elastic fibers.[16] This suggests a structural vulnerability to tunical injury in men with TD.

Androgens appear to play a critical role in the health of penile tissue, particularly with regard to fibrosis and PD. Inhibition of conversion of T into 5α-dihydrotestosterone with finasteride has been shown to upregulate TGF-β1 in association with deposition of increased collagen fibers in the prostate of adult Wistar rats.[17] T itself has been shown to inhibit TGF-β1 signaling.[18] Thus, the known anti-inflammatory effects of androgens,[19] particularly the suppression of TGF-β1 and its downstream pathways, provide a plausible biochemical mechanism by which TTh may potentially aid men with PD undergoing treatment with intralesional collagenase.

Mechanistically, androgens are thought to regulate the expression and function of inflammatory cytokines, including tumor necrosis factor-α, interleukin (IL)-1β, IL-6, C-reactive protein, and TGF-β1. TTh in men with TD and chronic inflammatory conditions appears to attenuate the inflammatory process.[19] Furthermore, in experimental model, it was shown that T treatment suppresses TGF-β1 signaling that plays a key role in fibrocalcification of the plaques in PD.[20] Furthermore, there is increasing evidence that TGF-β1 may activate lysyl oxidase, the enzyme that plays a key role in cross-linking of collagen and elastin fibers and facilitates the fibrotic process in the penile tissues.[21–23] It remains to be determined whether T treatment regulates TGF-β1 expression and signaling in a way that translates into attenuation of the expression and activity of lysyl oxidase, and reduced fibrosis.

The introduction of an FDA-approved intralesional injection in the form of CCx in 2013 has provided an important new treatment option for men with PD. In the United States, current recommendations are to perform up to four cycles of treatment at 6-week intervals, with each cycle comprising two injections 1–3 days apart, followed by a third visit for in-office modeling, in which the flaccid penis is stretched by the treating health care provider as a form of manual traction. Published results for curvature improvement with CCx have generally been reported with mean of 31–34%, with either standard four cycles of two injections per cycle,[24] or a shortened protocol of three injections at monthly intervals.[25]

In this study, we compared the curvature response with treatment with CCx in 117 men with PD, of whom 45 also received TTh (XT) and 72 who received CCx alone (XA). Baseline curvature was similar at 45° and 46°, respectively. The number of completed treatment cycles for each group was also similar at 2.7; however, the XT group was slightly older. Overall, 67.5% of men observed some improvement in curvature, and 32.5% reported no change.

The primary results of this study revealed that men who received TTh in combination with CCx treatments reported a substantially greater improvement in curvature than men treated with CCx alone. A response categorized as substantial or complete improvement occurred more than twice as often in men who received TTh with CCx (48.9%) than in men who were treated with CCx alone (20.8%). Conversely, failure to observe any change in curvature was reported by only 15.6% of the TTh group compared with 43.1% in the CCx alone group. Although one must interpret observational data such as this with caution, these results suggest the possibility that correction of TD may enhance the response to CCx treatment in men with PD. It also indirectly supports the hypothesis that serum T has some role in development or progression of PD.

A number of studies support the concept that T may be involved in PD. In the original 2009 series by Moreno and Morgentaler involving 121 U.S. men presenting with PD, 74% had low levels of total and/or FT, and the degree of curvature correlated with severity of TD.[6] Nam et al. investigated the impact of TD in 106 men with PD, reporting that men with TD had larger plaque size, greater curvature, and lower erectile function scores.[7]

In a multicenter single-blind study in 2012, Cavallini et al. investigated 106 men with PD and 99 controls, including intralesional verapamil injections in 43 T-deficient men randomized to concurrent treatment with either buccal T or placebo.[8] At baseline, plaque size was greater in men with low bioavailable or FT, however degree of curvature was similar. Response to verapamil injections for reduction in plaque area and curve was improved for men treated with T, but there was no significant change in these parameters for men who received placebo. Those results with verapamil injections are similar to those observed in this study with CCx.

Not all studies demonstrate a relationship between TD and PD. Tal et al. found no association with serum T levels in a specific population of men who developed PD after radical prostatectomy (RP),[26] and more recently, authors from the same institution found no association between serum T concentrations and magnitude of penile deformity in a more general population of 184 men with PD.[9] However, the latter population still comprised greater than one-third (37%) who had undergone RP. Since the etiology of PD is likely to differ in men after RP, these results do not necessarily argue against TD as a contributing factor in non-RP cases of PD. Kirby et al. reported that 52.9% of men with PD had low T concentrations, compared with 45.9% in men with erectile dysfunction (ED).[27] Although no correlation was noted in that study for T levels and plaque size or degree of curvature, there was clearly a high prevalence of TD in the PD population.

There are several important limitations to this study, including its retrospective nature, limited population size, nonuniform assessment of baseline curvature, and subjective response to treatment. The retrospective nature of this study makes it impossible to draw conclusions regarding causality. In addition, we note that the two groups differed with regard to age and baseline T, which, in turn, may have influenced the results. It is also possible that the self-reported improvement among men who received TTh may relate in some way to improved psychological status from correction of TD. Nonetheless, we believe these results are provocative and merit further investigation through a rigorous prospective clinical trial.

Conclusions

Men who received TTh during treatment with CCx for PD demonstrated greater improvement in curvature than men who did not receive TTh. These results argue for a prospective trial to determine whether TTh may provide an optimized response to CCx treatment in men with PD.

References

1. Moreland RB, Nehra A. Pathophysiology of Peyronie's disease. Int J Impot Res. 2002;14:406–410.
2. Stuntz M, Perlaky A, Franka DV, et al. The prevalence of Peyronie's disease in the United States: A population-based study. PLoS One. 2016;11(2): e0150157.
3. https://www.endo.com/File%20Library/Products/Prescribing% 20Information/Xiaflex_prescribing_information.html (last accessed July 31, 2020).
4. Gelbard M, Goldstein I, Hellstrom WJ. Clinical efficacy, safety and tolerability of collagenase Clostridium histolyticum for the treatment of Peyronie disease in 2 large double-blind, randomized, placebo controlled phase 3 studies. J Urol. 2013;190(1):199–207.
5. Goldstein I, Lipshultz LI, McLane M, et al. Long-term safety and curvature deformity characterization in patients previously treated with collagenase clostridium histolyticum for Peyronie's disease. J Urol. 2020;203(6): 1191–1197.
6. Moreno SA, Morgentaler A. Testosterone deficiency and Peyronie's disease: Pilot data suggesting a significant relationship. J Sex Med. 2009; 6(6):1729–1735.
7. Nam HJ, Park HJ, Park NC. Does testosterone deficiency exaggerate the clinical symptoms of Peyronie's disease? Int J Urol. 2011;18(11): 796–800.
8. Cavallini G, Biagiotti G, Lo Giudice C. Association between Peyronie disease and low serum testosterone levels: Detection and therapeutic considerations. J Androl. 2012;33(3):381–388.
9. Mulhall JP, Matsushita K, Nelson CJ. Testosterone levels are not associated with magnitude of deformity in men with Peyronie's disease. J Sex Med. 2019;16(8):1283–1289.
10. Crawford ED, Barqawi AB, O'Donnell C, Morgentaler A. The association of time of day and serum testosterone concentration in a large screening population. BJU Int. 2007;100(3):509–13.
11. Shlykova N, Davidson E, Krakowsky Y, Bolanos J, Traish A, Morgentaler A. Absent diurnal variation in serum testosterone in young men with testosterone deficiency. J Urol. 2020;203(4):817–820.
12. Wang XJ, Xu TY, Xia LL, et al. Castration impairs erectile organ structure and function by inhibiting autophagy and promoting apoptosis of corpus cavernosum smooth muscle cells in rats. Int Urol Nephrol. 2015;47(7): 1105–1115.
13. Cho MC, Song WH, Paick J-S. Suppression of cavernosal fibrosis in a rat model. Sex Med Rev. 2018;6(4):572–582.
14. Gonzalez-Cadavid NF, Magee TR, Ferrini M, Qian A, Vernet D, Rajfer J. Gene expression in Peyronie's disease. Int J Impot Res. 2002;14(5):361–374.
15. Nehra A, Gettman MT, Nugent M, et al. Transforming growth factor-b1 (TGF-b1) is sufficient to induce fibrosis of rabbit corpus cavernosum in vivo. J Urol. 1999;162(3 Pt 1):910–915.
16. Shen ZJ, Zhou XL, Lu YL, Chen ZD. Effect of androgen deprivation on penile ultrastructure. Asian J Androl. 2003;5(1):33–36.
17. Delella FK, de Almeida FLA, Nunes HC, Rinaldi JC, Felisbino SL. Fibrillar collagen genes are not coordinately upregulated with TGF B1 expression in finasteride-treated prostate. Cell Biol Intl. 2017;41(11):1214–1222.
18. Braga M, Bhasin S, Jasuja R, Pervin S, Singh R. Testosterone inhibits transforming growth factor-b signaling during myogenic differentiation and proliferation of mouse satellite cells: Potential role of follistatin in mediating testosterone action. Mol Cell Endocrinol. 2012;350(1):39–52.
19. Traish A, Bolanos J, Nair S, Saad F, Morgentaler A. Do androgens modulate the pathophysiological pathways of inflammation? Appraising the contemporary evidence. J Clin Med. 2018;7(12):pii:E549.
20. Zhang G, Kang Y, Zhou C, et al. Amelioratory effects of testosterone propionate on age-related renal fibrosis via suppression of TGF-β1/Smad signaling and activation of Nrf2-ARE signaling. Sci Rep. 2018;8(1):10726.
21. Wan Z-H, Li G-H, Guo Y-L, et al. Amelioration of cavernosal fibrosis and erectile function by lysyl oxidase inhibition in a rat model of cavernous nerve injury. J Sex Med. 2018;15(3):304–313.
22. Li T, Fu FD, Wu CJ, Qin F, Wang R, Yuan JH. Anti-lysyl oxidase combined with a vacuum device induces penilelengthening by remodeling the tunica albuginea. Asian J Androl. 2020;22:485–492.
23. Gao L, Wu C, Fu F, et al. Effect of lysyl oxidase (LOX) on corpus cavernous fibrosis caused by ischaemic priapism. J Cell Mol Med. 2018;22(3): 2018–2022.

24. Levine LA, Cuzin B, Mark S. Clinical safety and effectiveness of collagenase clostridium histolyticum injection in patients with Peyronie's disease: A phase 3 open-label study. J Sex Med. 2015;12(1):248–258.

25. Abdel-Raheem A, Capece M, Kalejaiye O, et al. Safety and effectiveness of collagenase clostridium histolyticum in the treatment of Peyronie's disease using a new modified shortened protocol. BJU Int. 2017;120(5): 717–723.

26. Tal R, Heck M, Teloken P, et al. Peyronie's disease following radical prostatectomy: Incidence and predictors. J Sex Med. 2010;7(3):1254–1261.

27. Kirby EW, Verges D, Matthews J, et al. Low testosterone has a similar prevalence among men with sexual dysfunction due to either Peyronie's disease or erectile dysfunction and does not correlate with Peyronie's disease severity. J Sex Med. 2015;12(3):690–696.

Abbreviations Used

E = estradiol
FT = free T
IL = interleukin
PD = Peyronie's disease
RP = radical prostatectomy
SHBG = sex hormone binding globulin
T = testosterone
TA = tunica albuginea
TD = T deficiency
TGF = transforming growth factor
TT = total T

10

Effects of Testosterone Therapy on Erythrocytosis and Prostate Adverse Events in Obese Males with Functional Hypogonadism and Type 2 Diabetes in a 2-Year Clinical Trial

Kristina Groti Antonič,[1,2,*] Blaž Antonič,[3] and Marija Pfeifer[2]

Abstract

Aims: Testosterone therapy (TTh) has been postulated to increase the risk of prostate adverse events (PAEs) and erythrocytosis, risk further exacerbated in high-risk obese patients with type 2 diabetes (T2D) and functional hypogonadism (FH). We investigated safety aspects of TTh in obese males with FH and T2D by observing the incidence of PAEs and erythrocytosis and determining when statistically significant difference from the baseline manifests in hematocrit (Hct) and prostate-specific antigen (PSA) levels.

Materials and Methods: Fifty-five obese Caucasian men with FH and T2D participated in a two-part prospective observational clinical study (first year: double-blind randomized placebo-controlled trial employing testosterone undecanoate; second year: open-label follow-up with all participants receiving TTh). Outcomes were assessments of Hct and PSA levels at the baseline, and 3, 6, and 12 months into each of 2 years of the study.

Results: No adverse cardiovascular events or PAEs were observed. Hct first increased at statistically significant level from the baseline after 3 months of TTh in group T and after 6 months of TTh in group P. Individual Hct values for all participants remained <0.52 throughout 2-year course of the study. PSA increased from the baseline in both groups within 3–6 months of trial start regardless of intervention applied (placebo or TTh). Fifty-two patients never exceeded PSA level of 4.0 μg/L nor experienced year-on-year PSA increase >1.4 μg/L. No subject ever reached supraphysiological concentration of total testosterone.

Conclusions: Our results show that TTh may be safe in obese males with FH and T2D. ClinicalTrials.gov ID: NCT0379232.

Keywords: testosterone; prostate-specific antigen; erythrocytosis; hematocrit; functional hypogonadism; prostate adverse events

Introduction

Male hypogonadism is a clinical syndrome resulting from failure of testes to produce physiological concentrations of testosterone and/or normal amounts of spermatozoa due to pathology of hypothalamic-pituitary-testicular axis.[1] Functional hypogonadism (FH) or late-onset hypogonadism is associated with aging and its related comorbidities, including obesity, metabolic syndrome, and type 2 diabetes (T2D).[2–4] Approximately 50% of males with T2D, aged >40 years, exhibit decreased total testosterone (TT) levels.[3,5] Obesity is considered to be the most frequent cause of FH.[6–9] Obesity and T2D are high risk factors for cardiovascular disease (CVD),[2,10–12] and are also

[1]Department of Endocrinology, Diabetes and Metabolic Diseases, University Medical Center Ljubljana, Ljubljana, Slovenia.
[2]Faculty of Medicine, University of Ljubljana, Ljubljana, Slovenia.
[3]Blaž Antonič s.p., Ljubljana, Slovenia.

*Address correspondence to: Kristina Groti Antonič, MD, PhD, Department of Endocrinology, Diabetes and Metabolic Diseases, University Medical Center Ljubljana, Ljubljana SI-1000, Slovenia, E-mail: kristina.groti@kclj.si

risk factors for benign prostatic hyperplasia (BPH); men with T2D are twice as likely to have an enlarged prostate as men without T2D.[13] Pathophysiological mechanisms explaining the correlation between obesity, T2D, risk of BPH, and prostate carcinoma (PCa) are hyperinsulinemic state, increased estrogen-to-androgen ratio, increased sympathetic nervous activity, promotion of inflammation processes, which in turn contribute to ischemia, oxidative stress, and an intraprostatic environment favorable to BPH and PCa.[14]

FH has recently come under greater scrutiny with the widespread use of testosterone therapy (TTh), and concerns regarding the efficacy and safety of TTh have been raised.[15] TTh may exert several benefits with regard to metabolic profile, body composition, psychological, and sexual parameters. Multiple studies have shown that TTh applied to obese men with FH and T2D improves glycemic control; reduces insulin resistance (IR), inflammation, and symptoms of hypogonadism; increases bone mineral density; and improves vascular function and morphology along with improvements in cognitive function.[10,16–21]

TTh has been postulated to potentially increase the risk of prostate adverse events (PAEs) and erythrocytosis.[11] This increased risk for both types of adverse events stems from physiological effects of testosterone. The normal function of the prostate gland is dependent on testosterone, and it has been well documented that administration of testosterone to men with hypogonadism results in a small increase in serum prostate-specific antigen (PSA) level.[22] Meta-analyses of testosterone trials did not show that testosterone increases the risk of PCa.[9,11,23] "Saturation model" hypothesis postulates that once testosterone concentrations have stabilized as a result of TTh, further effects of testosterone on prostate will diminish.[24]

Evidence supports obesity as a risk factor for both BPH and PCa.[14] Increased waist circumference is positively associated with prostate volume, PSA level, and worsened lower urinary tract symptoms (LUTS).[25] Adiposity is associated with increased erythrocyte aggregation; abdominal fat increases blood viscosity due to a rise in hematocrit (Hct), and increased body mass index (BMI) is associated with increased plasma viscosity.[26]

Several challenges exist whenever TTh is being considered. Contraindications must be excluded according to the clinical guidelines.[4,27,28] TTh is not recommended to patients with a history of, or at a high level of risk of PCa, severe BPH, or with high CVD risk.[4,27,28] It is recommended that TTh be applied with caution in men diagnosed with BPH and mild or moderate LUTS, whereas men with severe LUTS should undergo urological evaluation before commencing treatment. Maintaining physiological serum levels of testosterone and monitoring PSA and Hct in patients on TTh is mandatory so that appropriate measures (such as dosage reduction, the withholding of testosterone, and therapeutic phlebotomy) can be performed if erythrocytosis develops. A PSA value >4.0 μg/L or year-on-year increase of 1.4 μg/L or more are the standard indications for prostate biopsy.[4,27,28]

It is the combination of effects of testosterone and the way both obesity and T2D affect prostate and erythropoiesis that makes administering TTh to obese patients with FH and T2D more challenging than to nondiabetic nonobese men. This article attempts to clarify whether TTh can be safely applied to such a high-risk population and to analyze the effect of TTh on Hct and PSA levels.

Objectives

The goal of this report is to evaluate safety aspects of TTh in high-risk population of obese males with T2D and FH by (1) observing the incidence of PAEs and erythrocytosis and by (2) determining the time point where statistically significant difference (increase) from the baseline manifests in Hct and PSA. Three individual cases of significantly elevated PSA in study participants are also detailed.

Materials and Methods

Study design

SETH2 study (Study on Effects of Testosterone Replacement Therapy in Hypogonadal Type 2 Diabetic Patients) was a two-part single-center prospective observational clinical study (first year double-blind randomized placebo-controlled trial; second year open-label follow-up), conducted from January 2014 to March 2018 at General Hospital Celje (Slovenia). Study was approved by the National Medical Ethic Committee (54/04/12) and was conducted in accordance with the Declaration of Helsinki and with all applicable local laws and regulations. Written informed consent was obtained from all study subjects before their participation in the study. The study has been registered at ClinicalTrials.gov (identifier: NCT03792321).

Study population

Fifty-five obese Caucasian male patients with confirmed symptomatic FH, aged 40–70 years, with T2D, participated in SETH2 trial. FH was diagnosed as a biochemical deficiency of circulating testosterone levels (TT <11 nmol/L and free testosterone <220 pmol/L) on at least two separate morning measurements after an overnight fast in addition to exhibiting at least two symptoms of sexual dysfunction (less frequent morning erections, erectile dysfunction, and decreased libido).[4,5,27]

Inclusion criteria were male, confirmed FH, age >35 years, BMI ≥30 kg/m², and T2D treated exclusively with noninsulin antidiabetic medications (metformin and sulfonylureas). Participants did not use concomitant medications that can reduce weight, BMI, and waist circumference.

Exclusion criteria were previously treated FH, history of current prostate or breast cancer, severe BPH or PSA >4.0 μg/L, severe heart failure, acute coronary event or procedure during the 6 months before the study, chronic obstructive lung disease, severe obstructive sleep apnea, and active infection.

Study protocol

Participants were randomized into groups T and P before the first part of the study, and received either intramuscular testosterone undecanoate (TU; Nebido 1000 mg; Bayer AG) or matching placebo for 1 year. Participants and trial investigators were blinded to treatment allocation. Use of placebo was limited to 1 year due to ethical concerns over withholding TTh from hypogonadal patients, so group P subjects were switched to TU for the second part. Group T subjects continued receiving TU for a total of 2 years. First injection of TU/placebo was administered at the first visit (baseline), second injection 6 weeks later (second visit), and each subsequent injection 10 weeks after the previous injection. All participants received TU starting with week 56.

Methods

All patients underwent clinical, biochemical and hormonal assessment at the beginning, after 12 months and after 24 months of the study. Fasting blood samples were taken between 07:00 a.m. and 11:00 a.m. to measure serum TT, estradiol, sex hormone binding globulin (SHBG), albumin, luteinizing hormone, follicle-stimulating hormone, fasting plasma glucose, glycated hemoglobin (HbA$_{1c}$), lipids (total cholesterol, LDL cholesterol, HDL cholesterol, and triglycerides), PSA, routine blood tests (complete blood count, electrolytes, urea, creatinine, and liver tests). TT was

assessed using IMMULITE 2000 chemiluminescent enzyme immunoassay (Siemens Healthcare GmbH). Intra-assay coefficients of variation (CVs) in the relevant result range are 11.7% (at 2.99 nmol/L), 10.0% (5.27 nmol/L), 8.3% (9.70 nmol/L), 7.2% (14.35 nmol/L), and 5.1% (34.36 nmol/L). Interassay CVs at those same respective means are 13.0%, 10.3%, 9.1%, 8.2%, and 7.2%. Safety parameters (complete blood count, PSA, and markers of hepatic and renal functions) were performed at 0, 3, 6, 12, 15, 18, and 24 months.

We calculated free testosterone (cFT) and bioavailable testosterone (BT) from TT, SHBG, and albumin values using online calculator, which employs formulae of Vermuelen.[29]

Outcomes

Assessments of Hct and PSA levels were performed in accordance with the clinical guidelines.[4,27,28] We performed one additional check each year of the study during the first 6 months to get more detailed insight into how Hct and PSA levels respond to introduction of TTh, resulting in three safety tests per each year of the study (at baseline, approximately at 3, 6, and 12 months into each year).

Statistical methods

Results were compared within groups to determine the time point when Hct and PSA changed from their respective baseline values at statistically significant level ($\alpha = 0.05$). Shapiro–Wilk test was used to assess normality of data. Repeated measures analysis of variance (RM-ANOVA) was used to examine normally distributed results and Friedman's nonparametric test was used to examine non-normally distributed results. Adjusted p-values are reported for *post hoc* tests with Bonferroni correction. SPSS Statistics 22.0 (IBM Corporation, New York) was used for statistical analysis.

Results

Study subjects

Baseline demographic, anthropometrical, and laboratory parameters of the study population are provided in Table 1.

Changes in outcome measures

Results for groups P and T are presented separately due to slight differences in TTh administration protocol at the point of introduction of TTh in each study group (lack of initial 6-week loading period for group P upon switch from placebo to TTh).

Table 1. Baseline Study Population Characteristics: Key Anthropometrical, Biochemical, and Clinical Parameters

Parameter	Group T ($n = 28$)	Group P ($n = 27$)	Total ($n = 55$)
Age (years)	58.18 ± 7.93	62.19 ± 5.90	60.15 ± 7.23
BMI (kg/m^2)	34.03 ± 4.37	32.63 ± 3.67	33.34 ± 4.07
HbA$_{1c}$ (%)	8.12 ± 1.04	7.89 ± 0.77	8.00 ± 0.91
HOMA-IR index	11.45 ± 7.34	10.70 ± 6.52	11.08 ± 6.90
Total serum testosterone (nmol/L)	7.24 ± 1.97	7.96 ± 1.34	7.59 ± 1.71
Bioavailable testosterone (nmol/L)	3.74 ± 0.97	4.61 ± 0.95	4.17 ± 1.05
Calculated free testosterone (pmol/L)	155.54 ± 41.11	192.07 ± 44.13	173.47 ± 46.07
Hct level	0.428 ± 0.020	0.436 ± 0.024	0.432 ± 0.022
PSA level (μg/L)	0.645 (0.503 to 1.235)	0.670 (0.390 to 1.190)	0.650 (0.440 to 1.220)
Arterial hypertension, n (%)	25 (89.3)	26 (96.3)	51 (92.7)
Dyslipidemia, n (%)	28 (100.0)	27 (100.0)	55 (100.0)
Current smoker, n (%)	8 (28.6)	13 (48.1)	21 (38.2)

Values are reported as mean ± standard deviation when normally distributed, as median (interquartile range) in the case of PSA and as count (percentage of n) for clinical parameters.

BMI, body mass index; HbA$_{1c}$, glycated hemoglobin; Hct, hematocrit; HOMA-IR, homeostatic model of insulin resistance index; PSA, prostate-specific antigen.

Hct and testosterone levels are reported as mean ± standard deviation. PSA is reported as median (interquartile range).

Changes in Hct are shown in Figure 1 and Table 2. With assumption of sphericity not met for either group P ($p = 0.001$) or T ($p = 0.027$), Greenhouse–Geisser correction was applied to RM-ANOVA, showing that mean

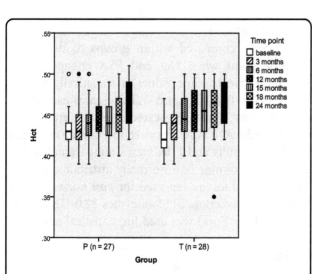

FIG. 1. Hct levels in obese males with FH and T2D on TTh over the 2-year course of the study. Group P received placebo during first year of the study and was switched to testosterone undecanoate afterward. Group T received testosterone undecanoate throughout entire course of the study. FH, functional hypogonadism; Hct, hematocrit; T2D, type 2 diabetes; TTh, testosterone therapy.

Hct level differed significantly between time points in both group P [$F(4.106, 106.757) = 10.708$, $p < 0.001$] and T [$F(4.303, 116.188) = 12.903$, $p < 0.001$]. *Post hoc* pairwise test with Bonferroni correction revealed that mean Hct level changed from 0.444 ± 0.024 at the introduction of TTh in group P to 0.465 ± 0.027 after 12 months of TTh, and from 0.427 ± 0.020 to 0.449 ± 0.028 after 6 months of TTh in group T. Hct increased by 0.021 ± 0.025 in group P and by 0.025 ± 0.026 in group T after first year of TTh in each respective group, whereas no additional increase was observed after extended TTh in group T during second year of the trial ($p = 1.000$ for all pairwise observations). Individual Hct values never exceeded the upper safety limit of 0.52 in either study group at any point of the study.

Changes in PSA level are outlined in Figure 2 and Table 3. Friedman's test confirmed that PSA levels differed at statistically significant level between the time points in both groups P [$\chi^2(6) = 70.529$, $p < 0.001$] and T [$\chi^2(6) = 87.274$, $p < 0.001$]. Dunn–Bonferroni pairwise *post hoc* test showed that PSA increased at statistically significant level from the baseline after 3 months of TTh in group P and after 6 months of TTh in group T. This was reaffirmed by performing RM-ANOVA with Greenhouse–Geisser correction on log-transformed PSA data [$F(2.559, 66.524) = 20.086$, $p < 0.001$ for group P and $F(3.315, 89.496) = 20.791$, $p < 0.001$ for group T], with pairwise Bonferroni-corrected *post hoc* test detecting mean change in log(PSA) after 3 months of TTh in both groups. Median PSA increased from the baseline of 0.645 (0.503–1.235) μg/L to 0.825 (0.610–1.368) μg/L after 12 months of TTh to 1.175 (0.803–1.580) μg/L after 24 months of TTh in group T. Similarly, PSA in group P went from the

Table 2. Changes in Hematocrit in Obese Males with Functional Hypogonadism and Type 2 Diabetes on Testosterone Therapy over the 2-Year Course of the Study

Parameter	Time point	Group T (n = 28)	Change from baseline	Group P (n = 27)	Change from baseline	Change from introduction of TTh
Hct	Baseline	0.427 ± 0.020		0.436 ± 0.024		
	3 Months	0.438 ± 0.026	0.010 ± 0.018 (p = 0.097)	0.434 ± 0.026	−0.001 ± 0.013 (p = 1.000)	
	6 Months	0.449 ± 0.028	**0.021 ± 0.020 (p < 0.001)**	0.442 ± 0.024	0.007 ± 0.018 (p = 1.000)	
	12 Months	0.453 ± 0.031	**0.025 ± 0.026 (p < 0.001)**	0.444 ± 0.024	0.009 ± 0.027 (p = 1.000)	
	15 Months	0.456 ± 0.027	**0.028 ± 0.027 (p < 0.001)**	0.443 ± 0.024	0.007 ± 0.021 (p = 1.000)	−0.002 ± 0.021 (p = 1.000)
	18 Months	0.458 ± 0.033	**0.030 ± 0.028 (p < 0.001)**	0.450 ± 0.029	0.015 ± 0.023 (p = 0.051)	0.006 ± 0.027 (p = 1.000)
	24 Months	0.460 ± 0.027	**0.033 ± 0.027 (p < 0.001)**	0.465 ± 0.027	0.030 ± 0.026 (p < 0.001)	**0.021 ± 0.025 (p = 0.005)**

Group P participants were receiving placebo during first year of the study and was switched to testosterone undecanoate afterward. Group T participants were receiving testosterone undecanoate throughout the entire course of the study. Values are reported as mean ± standard deviation. Statistically significant changes from the point where TTh was introduced in each respective group are marked in bold.

TTh, testosterone therapy.

baseline of 0.670 (0.390–1.190) μg/L to 0.890 (0.500–1.220) μg/L after receiving placebo for 12 months, and then to 0.950 (0.700–1.560) μg/L after 12 months of TTh.

Of 55 patients, 52 never exhibited PSA >4 μg/L or a year-on-year increase >1.4 μg/L; PSA levels for the three exceptions are outlined in Table 4. Study participant number 30 (group T) has been enrolled with pre-existing (diagnosed) BPH, confirmed by prostate biopsy, and was under regular supervision of a urologist; BPH was not severe enough to warrant exclusion

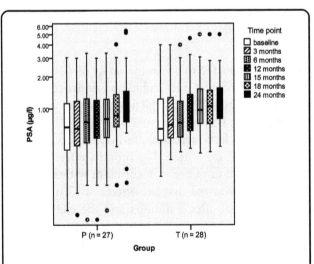

FIG. 2. PSA levels in obese males with FH and T2D on TTh over the 2-year course of the study, displayed on a logarithmic scale due to log-normal distribution of values. Group P received placebo during first year of the study and was switched to testosterone undecanoate afterward. Group T received testosterone undecanoate throughout entire course of the study. PSA, prostate-specific antigen.

from the study. His baseline serum PSA was 4.0 μg/L, and did not change during the first year of TTh. PSA increased to 5.00 μg/L after the second year of TTh, resulting in TTh termination.

Participants numbers 15 and 36 (both group P) were diagnosed with BPH during the second year of the trial, after a marked increase in their PSA after commencing TTh. Patient number 15 PSA increased from 1.17 μg/L at 12 months (the point of introduction of TTh) to 2.67 μg/L 3 months later, and again from 2.70 μg/L at the 18-month mark to 5.20 μg/L after 24 months of the study. Baseline PSA for patient number 36 was 3.03 μg/L and remained steady until the 18-month mark when it first rose >4.00 μg/L (to 4.04 μg/L), and then to 5.40 μg/L at 24 months. Both patients stopped TTh and underwent prostate biopsy; PCa was excluded and BPH was diagnosed in both.

Changes in testosterone levels are detailed in Table 5. Group T mean TT increased from 7.24 ± 1.97 to 17.04 ± 3.07 nmol/L after 12 months of TTh and to 23.50 ± 4.91 nmol/L after 24 months. All group T participants but one reached serum TT concentration above the 11 nmol/L reference value after 12 months of TTh, whereas the sole exception went from baseline TT of 7.5 to 10.6 nmol/L. Statistically significant increase of mean TT in group P after 12 months (from 7.96 ± 1.34 to 9.83 ± 2.21 nmol/L) is of little clinical significance. Mean TT increased considerably more (to 17.92 ± 2.21 nmol/L) after 12 months of TTh (24 months into the study). All group P participants reached TT >11 nmol/L at this point. The calculated values of BT and cFT correlated highly with values of the TT, with clinically relevant increase manifesting in both groups after the first year of TTh (12 months into the study for group T and at 24 months for group P).

Table 3. Changes in Prostate-Specific Antigen in Obese Males with Functional Hypogonadism and Type 2 Diabetes on Testosterone Therapy Over the 2-Year Course of the Study

Parameter	Time point	Group T (n=28)	Change from baseline	Group P (n=27)	Change from baseline	Change from introduction of TTh
PSA (μg/L)	Baseline	**0.645 (0.503 to 1.235)**		**0.670 (0.390 to 1.190)**		
	3 Months	0.700 (0.525 to 1.280)	0.065 (0.020 to 0.120; p=1.000)	0.650 (0.440 to 1.190)	0.020 (−0.010 to 0.070; p=1.000)	
	6 Months	0.735 (0.520 to 1.180)	**0.085 (0.025 to 0.203; p=0.030)**	0.750 (0.460 to 1.280)	0.070 (0.010 to 0.130; p=1.000)	
	12 Months	0.825 (0.610 to 1.368)	**0.180 (0.093 to 0.325; p < 0.001)**	0.890 (0.500 to 1.220)	0.090 (−0.030 to 0.220; p=0.087)	
	15 Months	0.970 (0.713 to 1.595)	**0.245 (0.105 to 0.515; p < 0.001)**	0.800 (0.520 to 1.250)	0.120 (0.010 to 0.250; p=0.031)	0.030 (−0.070 to 0.100; p=1.000)
	18 Months	1.050 (0.720 to 1.488)	**0.255 (0.158 to 0.643; p < 0.001)**	0.860 (0.660 to 1.490)	0.230 (0.090 to 0.420; p < 0.001)	0.100 (0.000 to 0.290; p=0.071)
	24 Months	1.175 (0.803 to 1.580)	**0.370 (0.205 to 0.920; p < 0.001)**	0.950 (0.700 to 1.560)	0.290 (0.160 to 0.520; p < 0.001)	**0.180 (0.010 to 0.350; p = 0.004)**

Group P participants were receiving placebo during first year of the study and was switched to testosterone undecanoate afterward. Group T participants were receiving testosterone undecanoate throughout the entire course of the study. Values are reported as median (interquartile range). Statistically significant changes from the point where TTh was introduced in each respective group are marked in bold.

Table 4. Prostate-Specific Antigen Levels for Three Individuals Who Required Urological Examination at Some Point During the Study due to Elevated Prostate-Specific Antigen

Parameter	Time point	Patient no. 30 (group T)	Patient no. 15 (group P)	Patient no. 36 (group P)
PSA (μg/L)	Baseline	**4.00[a]**	1.22	3.03
	3 Months	4.00	1.16	3.00
	6 Months	4.00	1.30	3.33
	12 Months	4.61	1.17	2.99
	15 Months	5.00	**2.67[b]**	3.35
	18 Months	5.00	2.70	**4.04[c]**
	24 Months	5.00	5.20	5.40

Points where each individual was referred to a urologist are marked in bold.

[a]Patient no. 30 was enrolled into study with known (previously diagnosed) BPH and was under regular supervision of a urologist throughout entire course of the study. Patient was receiving testosterone undecanoate during both years of the study.

[b]Patient no. 15 was referred to a urologist after an increase in PSA (by 1.50 μg/L between two successive tests) 3 months after having been switched from placebo to testosterone undecanoate. Patient was diagnosed with BPH; PCa was excluded.

[c]Patient no. 36 was referred to a urologist after an increase in PSA >4.00 μg/L 6 months after having been switched from placebo to testosterone undecanoate. Patient was diagnosed with BPH; PCa was excluded.

BPH, benign prostatic hyperplasia; PCa, prostate carcinoma.

Harms

No adverse events (PCa, erythrocytosis, and CVD events) or other side effects of TTh have been observed.

Discussion

This study was conducted to assess the safety of TTh in obese men with T2D and FH. Published evidence of TTh safety in this population, which is at higher risk for CVD and PAEs, is scarce.

We showed that Hct increased gradually from the baseline in both groups within 3–6 months after the start of TTh. Our findings are in accordance with several studies, which showed that the effects of TTh on Hct become apparent after 3 months and the plateau is reached within 9–12 months.[30,31] No trial participant ever exceeded the upper Hct limit of 0.52 at any point over the 2-year course of this study.

Increased red blood cell mass (erythrocytosis) is the most common adverse event associated with TTh in clinical practice and in testosterone trials.[4,32] TTh-induced erythrocytosis is associated with stimulation of erythropoietin and reduced ferritin and hepcidin concentrations.[33,34] Large epidemiological studies show that increased Hct levels are associated with increased risk of adverse CVD, because of increase in blood viscosity.[35,36] Guidelines on TTh recommend measuring Hct at baseline, at 3–6 months and annually

Table 5. Changes in Serum Testosterone Levels in Obese Males with Functional Hypogonadism and Type 2 Diabetes on Testosterone Therapy over the 2-Year Course of the Study for Both Study Groups

Parameter	Time point	Group T (n = 28)	Change from baseline	Group P (n = 27)	Change from baseline	Change from introduction of TTh
Total testosterone (nmol/L)	Baseline	7.24 ± 1.97		7.96 ± 1.34		
	12 Months	17.04 ± 3.07	9.80 ± 3.59 ($p < 0.001$)	9.83 ± 1.51	1.87 ± 1.54 ($p < 0.001$)	
	24 Months	23.50 ± 4.91	16.26 ± 4.89 ($p < 0.001$)	17.92 ± 2.21	9.96 ± 2.92 ($p < 0.001$)	8.09 ± 2.08 ($p < 0.001$)
Calculated bioavailable testosterone (nmol/L)	Baseline	3.74 ± 0.97		4.61 ± 0.95		
	12 Months	9.50 ± 1.89	5.76 ± 2.16 ($p < 0.001$)	5.73 ± 0.89	1.12 ± 0.93 ($p < 0.001$)	
	24 Months	13.93 ± 3.39	10.19 ± 3.42 ($p < 0.001$)	10.72 ± 1.84	6.11 ± 1.93 ($p < 0.001$)	4.99 ± 1.91 ($p < 0.001$)
Calculated free testosterone (pmol/L)	Baseline	155.54 ± 41.11		192.07 ± 44.13		
	12 Months	403.84 ± 90.34	248.29 ± 99.45 ($p < 0.001$)	242.00 ± 42.23	49.93 ± 40.67 ($p < 0.001$)	
	24 Months	594.04 ± 147.09	438.50 ± 146.87 ($p < 0.001$)	454.56 ± 87.78	262.49 ± 90.11 ($p < 0.001$)	212.56 ± 84.06 ($p < 0.001$)

Group P participants were receiving placebo during first year of the study and was switched to testosterone undecanoate afterward. Group T participants were receiving testosterone undecanoate throughout the entire course of the study. Values are reported as mean ± standard deviation.

after initiating TTh.[4,27] It is recommended that individuals with baseline (before initiation of TTh) Hct >0.50 undergo a workup before TTh because they have an increased chance of developing Hct level >0.54.

Prostate safety remains one of the most important controversial issues of TTh. We observed a sporadic increase of PSA in both study groups within 3–6 months after the start of the study regardless of intervention (testosterone or placebo), although the rate of increase was higher in group T. The small increase PSA in P group without prostatic symptoms was statistically significant but of questionable clinical relevance. We also observed small but statistically significant increase of testosterone levels in group P, which was attributed to loss of weight and improved glucose control, which we also in this group.[37] In addition to increased testosterone concentrations, decreased BMI, IR, and HbA$_{1c}$[38,39] some other factors can also influence PSA changes: older age, recent ejaculation, certain medications (statin and betamethasone).[40–42] We observed no cases of PCa.

PSA increase after TTh is a response of the physiological stimulation of the prostate by testosterone and its metabolites.[43] Rhoden and Morgentaler[44] showed that even in men with a predisposition to PCa (high-grade intraepithelial neoplasia), 1 year of TTh did not increase PCa incidence. TTh causes a mild increase in serum PSA in most patients without resulting in prostatic changes.[45] According to "saturation hypothesis," although testosterone acts as a critical factor to prostatic tissue growth, there is a saturation point for androgen receptors (AR) at which the human prostate AR are "saturated" by the circulating androgens and, therefore, rather insensitive to further testosterone in-

crease, such as that derived from TTh in cases of mild hypogonadism, so any further increase in testosterone will have no detrimental effects.[24] Studies on the administration of supraphysiological doses of testosterone in healthy volunteers have not demonstrated an increase in PSA or prostate volume for up to 9 months, supporting the central hypothesis of the prostate saturation model that testosterone stimulates prostate tissue, but only up to the point of AR saturation.[46]

In our study TT, cFT, and calculated BT concentrations have increased significantly after initiating TTh in both groups. Crucially, not a single subject in either P or T group ever reached supraphysiological concentrations of testosterone.

Strengths and limitations
Strengths of this study include its prospective randomized placebo-controlled trial design. TTh safety data from placebo-controlled RCTs, especially pertaining to high-risk populations such as obese males with T2D, are invaluable in assessing potential risks of TTh. The fact that no adverse CVD or PAEs have been observed over the 2-year course of our study is potentially attributable to limited study population size and does not constitute conclusive evidence that TTh exerts no negative effects on CVD and prostate health. Our findings have clinical implication for obese male patients with T2D considering TTh and for those receiving treatment.

Conclusions
The results of safety investigations performed throughout the course of our study suggest that 2 years of TTh can be safe even in high-risk population of obese men

with FH and T2D when appropriate safety practices outlined by the clinical guidelines are diligently followed; men on long-term TTh should be monitored with PSA, Hct, and digital rectal examination.[4,27,28,47]

TTh has been associated with modest increases in serum PSA, within safe clinical parameters, but without substantial evidence to support an increased risk of PCa. TTh has been associated with increase in Hct; however, data on the significance of this trend related to patient outcomes is lacking.

Future research should require a dedicated focus on the evaluation of large multicentric cohorts of obese males with T2D to better elucidate risks of TTh related to PCa and erythrocytosis.

Authors' Contributions

K.G.A. and M.P. designed the study. K.G.A. supervised the study, collected study data, and prepared initial article draft. B.A. performed data analysis and prepared figures and tables. K.G.A. and B.A. wrote the article with input from M.P.

References

1. Matsumoto A, Bremner WJ. Testicular disorders. In: Melmed S, Polonsky KS, Larsen PR, and Kronenberg HM (eds.). Williams Textbook of Endocrinology, 13th ed. New York, NY: Elsevier, 2016, pp. 695–784.
2. Corona G, Rastrelli G, Vignozzi L, Mannucci E, Maggi M. Testosterone, cardiovascular disease and the metabolic syndrome. Best Pract Res Clin Endocrinol Metab. 2011;25(2):337–353.
3. Grossmann M. Low testosterone in men with type 2 diabetes: Significance and treatment. J Clin Endocrinol Metab. 2011;96(8):2341–2353.
4. Bhasin S, Brito JP, Cunningham GR, et al. Testosterone therapy in men with hypogonadism: An Endocrine society clinical practice guideline. J Clin Endocrinol Metab. 2018;103(5):1715–1744.
5. Wu FCW, Tajar A, Beynon JM, et al. Identification of late-onset hypogonadism in middle-aged and elderly men. N Engl J Med. 2010;363(2):123–135.
6. Corona G, Rastrelli G, Monami M, et al. Body weight loss reverts obesity-associated hypogonadotropic hypogonadism: A systematic review and meta-analysis. Eur J Endocrinol. 2013;168(6):829–843.
7. Grossmann M, Ng Tang Fui M, Cheung AS. Late-onset hypogonadism: metabolic impact. Andrology. [Epub ahead of print]; DOI: 10.1111/andr.12705.
8. Carrageta DF, Oliveira PF, Alves MG, Monteiro MP. Obesity and male hypogonadism: Tales of a vicious cycle. Obes Rev Off J Int Assoc Study Obes. 2019;20(8):1148–1158.
9. Fernandez CJ, Chacko EC, Pappachan JM. Male obesity-related secondary hypogonadism—pathophysiology, clinical implications and management. Eur Endocrinol. 2019;15(2):83–90.
10. Kapoor D, Goodwin E, Channer KS, Jones TH. Testosterone replacement therapy improves insulin resistance, glycaemic control, visceral adiposity and hypercholesterolaemia in hypogonadal men with type 2 diabetes. Eur J Endocrinol. 2006;154(6):899–906.
11. Snyder PJ, Peachey H, Berlin JA, et al. Effects of testosterone replacement in hypogonadal men. J Clin Endocrinol Metab. 2000;85(8):2670–2677.
12. Wang C, Jackson G, Jones TH, et al. Low testosterone associated with obesity and the metabolic syndrome contributes to sexual dysfunction and cardiovascular disease risk in men with type 2 diabetes. Diabetes Care. 2011;34(7):1669–1675.
13. Parsons JK, Carter HB, Partin AW, et al. Metabolic factors associated with benign prostatic hyperplasia. J Clin Endocrinol Metab. 2006;91(7):2562–2568.
14. Parikesit D, Mochtar CA, Umbas R, Hamid ARAH. The impact of obesity towards prostate diseases. Prostate Int. 2016;4(1):1–6.
15. Tharakan T, Miah S, Jayasena C, Minhas S. Investigating the basis of sexual dysfunction during late-onset hypogonadism. F1000Research. 2019;8: F1000 Faculty Rev-331.
16. Haider A, Saad F, Doros G, Gooren L. Hypogonadal obese men with and without diabetes mellitus type 2 lose weight and show improvement in cardiovascular risk factors when treated with testosterone: An observational study. Obes Res Clin Pract. 2014;8(4):e339–e349.
17. Yassin D-J, Yassin A, Hammerer PG, Traish A, Doros G. 705 Long-term testosterone treatment over 5 years leads to progressive weight loss and waist size reduction as well as improvement of metabolic syndrome parameters in elderly men with hypogonadism. Eur Urol Suppl. 2014; 13(1):e705.
18. Yassin A, Haider A, Haider KS, et al. Testosterone therapy in men with hypogonadism prevents progression from prediabetes to type 2 diabetes: Eight-year data from a registry study. Diabetes Care. 2019;42(6): 1104–1111.
19. Zitzmann M, Vorona E, Wenk M, Saad F, Nieschlag E. Testosterone administration decreases carotid artery intima media thickness as a marker of impaired vascular integrity in middle-aged overweight men. J Mens Health. 2009;6(3):243.
20. Traish AM, Haider A, Doros G, Saad F. Long-term testosterone therapy in hypogonadal men ameliorates elements of the metabolic syndrome: An observational, long-term registry study. Int J Clin Pract. 2014;68(3): 314–329.
21. Saad F, Caliber M, Doros G, Haider KS, Haider A. Long-term treatment with testosterone undecanoate injections in men with hypogonadism alleviates erectile dysfunction and reduces risk of major adverse cardiovascular events, prostate cancer, and mortality. Aging Male. 2020;23(1):81–92.
22. Gerstenbluth RE, Maniam PN, Corty EW, Seftel AD. Prostate-specific antigen changes in hypogonadal men treated with testosterone replacement. J Androl. 2002;23(6):922–926.
23. Cui Y, Zong H, Yan H, Zhang Y. The effect of testosterone replacement therapy on prostate cancer: A systematic review and meta-analysis. Prostate Cancer Prostatic Dis. 2014;17(2):132–143.
24. Morgentaler A, Traish AM. Shifting the paradigm of testosterone and prostate cancer: The saturation model and the limits of androgen-dependent growth. Eur Urol. 2009;55(2):310–320.
25. Lee RK, Chung D, Chughtai B, Te AE, Kaplan SA. Central obesity as measured by waist circumference is predictive of severity of lower urinary tract symptoms. BJU Int. 2012;110(4):540–545.
26. Guiraudou M, Varlet-Marie E, Raynaud de Mauverger E, Brun J-F. Obesity-related increase in whole blood viscosity includes different profiles according to fat localization. Clin Hemorheol Microcirc. 2013; 55(1):63–73.
27. Corona G, Goulis DG, Huhtaniemi I, et al. European Academy of Andrology (EAA) guidelines on investigation, treatment and monitoring of functional hypogonadism in males. Andrology. 2020;8(5):970–987.
28. Barbonetti A, D'Andrea S, Francavilla S. Testosterone replacement therapy. Andrology. [Epub ahead of print]; DOI: 10.1111/andr.12774.
29. Free and Bioavailable Testosterone calculator. www.issam.ch/freetesto.htm Accessed July 1, 2020.
30. Saad F, Gooren L, Haider A, Yassin A. An exploratory study of the effects of 12 month administration of the novel long-acting testosterone undecanoate on measures of sexual function and the metabolic syndrome. Arch Androl. 2007;53(6):353–357.
31. Saad F, Aversa A, Isidori AM, Zafalon L, Zitzmann M, Gooren L. Onset of effects of testosterone treatment and time span until maximum effects are achieved. Eur J Endocrinol. 2011;165(5):675–685.
32. Calof OM, Singh AB, Lee ML, et al. Adverse events associated with testosterone replacement in middle-aged and older men: A meta-analysis of randomized, placebo-controlled trials. J Gerontol Ser A. 2005;60(11): 1451–1457.

33. Bachman E, Travison TG, Basaria S, et al. Testosterone induces erythrocytosis via increased erythropoietin and suppressed hepcidin: Evidence for a new erythropoietin/hemoglobin set point. J Gerontol A Biol Sci Med Sci. 2014;69(6):725–735.

34. Dhindsa S, Ghanim H, Batra M, et al. Effect of testosterone on hepcidin, ferroportin, ferritin and iron binding capacity in patients with hypogonadotropic hypogonadism and type 2 diabetes. Clin Endocrinol (Oxf). 2016;85(5):772–780.

35. Spitzer M, Huang G, Basaria S, Travison TG, Bhasin S. Risks and benefits of testosterone therapy in older men. Nat Rev Endocrinol. 2013;9(7): 414–424.

36. Danesh J, Collins R, Peto R, Lowe GD. Haematocrit, viscosity, erythrocyte sedimentation rate: Meta-analyses of prospective studies of coronary heart disease. Eur Heart J. 2000;21(7):515–520.

37. Groti K, Žuran I, Antonič B, Foršnarič L, Pfeifer M. The impact of testosterone replacement therapy on glycemic control, vascular function, and components of the metabolic syndrome in obese hypogonadal men with type 2 diabetes. Aging Male. 2018;21(3):1–12.

38. Elrifai A, Kotb AF, Sharaki O, Abdelhady M. Correlation of body mass index with serum total PSA, total testosterone and prostatic volume in a sample of men. Pol Ann Med. 2016;23(1):1–5.

39. Parekh N, Lin Y, Marcella S, Kant AK, Lu-Yao G. Associations of lifestyle and physiologic factors with prostate-specific antigen concentrations: Evidence from the National Health and Nutrition Examination Survey (2001–2004). Cancer Epidemiol Biomark Amp Prev. 2008;17(9): 2467.

40. Boudreau DM, Yu O, Buist DSM, Miglioretti DL. Statin use and prostate cancer risk in a large population-based setting. Cancer Causes Control. 2008;19(7):767–774.

41. Iguchi K, Hashimoto M, Kubota M, et al. Effects of 14 frequently used drugs on prostate-specific antigen expression in prostate cancer LNCaP cells. Oncol Lett. 2014;7(5):1665–1668.

42. Morgentaler A, Benesh JA, Denes BS, Kan-Dobrosky N, Harb D, Miller MG. Factors influencing prostate-specific antigen response among men treated with testosterone therapy for 6 months. J Sex Med. 2014;11(11): 2818–2825.

43. Meikle AW, Arver S, Dobs AS, et al. Prostate size in hypogonadal men treated with a nonscrotal permeation-enhanced testosterone transdermal system. Urology. 1997;49(2):191–196.

44. Rhoden EL, Morgentaler A. Testosterone replacement therapy in hypogonadal men at high risk for prostate cancer: Results of 1 year of treatment in men with prostatic intraepithelial neoplasia. J Urol. 2003;170(6): 2348–2351.

45. Rhoden EL, Morgentaler A. Risks of testosterone-replacement therapy and recommendations for monitoring. N Engl J Med. 2004;350(5): 482–492.

46. Cooper CS, Perry PJ, Sparks AE, MacIndoe JH, Yates WR, Williams RD. Effect of exogenous testosterone on prostate volume, serum and semen prostate specific antigen levels in healthy young men. J Urol. 1998;159(2): 441–443.

47. Wang C, Nieschlag E, Swerdloff R, et al. Investigation, treatment and monitoring of late-onset hypogonadism in males: ISA, ISSAM, EAU, EAA and ASA recommendations. Eur J Endocrinol. 2008;159(5):507–514.

Abbreviations Used

AR = androgen receptors
BMI = body mass index
BPH = benign prostatic hyperplasia
BT = bioavailable testosterone
cFT = calculated free testosterone
CVD = cardiovascular disease
CVs = coefficients of variation
FH = functional hypogonadism
HbA_{1c} = glycated hemoglobin
Hct = hematocrit
IR = insulin resistance
LUTS = lower urinary tract symptoms
PAEs = prostate adverse events
PCa = prostate carcinoma
PSA = prostate-specific antigen
RM-ANOVA = repeated measures analysis of variance
SHBG = sex hormone binding globulin
T2D = type 2 diabetes
TT = total testosterone
TTh = testosterone therapy

11

Strategies for Testosterone Therapy in Men with Metastatic Prostate Cancer in Clinical Practice: Introducing Modified Bipolar Androgen Therapy

Abraham Morgentaler[*]

Abstract

Purpose: To investigate prostate-specific antigen (PSA) and clinical responses to a variety of treatment strategies involving testosterone therapy (TTh) in men with metastatic prostate cancer (mPCa).

Materials and Methods: Case records were reviewed for three men with advanced PCa treated with TTh for improved quality of life. Two had bone metastases and nephrostomies at baseline. The third had biochemical recurrence, and continued TTh after developing bone metastases. All rejected androgen deprivation therapy, desired improved quality of life with TTh, and accepted the risk of rapid PCa progression and death.

Results: All men experienced substantial symptomatic and health benefits during TTh, including improved strength, vigor, and sexuality. Two reversed substantial weight loss. A 94-year-old man with baseline PSA of 546 ng/mL survived 11 months with continuous TTh, with last PSA of 2493 ng/mL. Two men in their 60s received some form of TTh for 3.5 and 8 years, respectively, and are still alive. None experienced sudden major adverse events. Continuous TTh resulted in progressive rise in PSA to high values. The combination of TTh and enzalutamide provided moderate protection against weakness and fatigue with PSA <10ng/mL for 6 months. PSA values fluctuated from <1.0 to >100 ng/mL within 1–2 months depending on recent androgen status. The most promising strategy appears to be a modified bipolar androgen therapy consisting of repeating cycles of 8 weeks of high-dose TTh followed by 4 weeks of enzalutamide, allowing for prolonged periods of vigor while maintaining PSA control.

Conclusions: These pilot results support explorations of new hormonal strategies involving TTh for men with mPCa.

Keywords: metastatic; modified bipolar androgen therapy; prostate cancer; testosterone; testosterone therapy; androgens

Introduction

Over the last two decades there has been a major re-evaluation of the biology of androgens and prostate cancer (PCa).[1] Whereas it has been long believed that offering testosterone therapy (TTh) to a man with PCa was like "pouring gasoline on a fire,"[2] numerous case series and observational studies have failed to demonstrate increased risk of disease recurrence or progression with TTh after radical prostatectomy,[3] radiation therapy,[4] and even in men on active surveillance.[5,6] This lack of progression may be attributed to saturation, namely, the finite ability of androgens to stimulate PCa growth, with a maximum achieved at a relatively low serum testosterone concentration of ~250 ng/mL.[7] It is now commonplace for health care providers to offer TTh to men after definitive treatment for localized PCa at low risk for recurrence. In 2016, Ory et al. reported low recurrence and progression rates in men with PCa

Men's Health Boston, Division of Urology, Department of Surgery, Beth Israel Deaconess Medical Center, Harvard Medical School, Chestnut Hill, Massachusetts, USA.

*Address correspondence to: Abraham Morgentaler, MD, Men's Health Boston, 200 Boylston Street, Suite A309, Chestnut Hill, MA 02467, USA, Email: amorgent@bidmc.harvard.edu

who received TTh after surgery, radiation, or on active surveillance, concluding, "…our study supports the hypothesis that testosterone therapy may be oncologically safe in hypogonadal men after definitive treatment or in those on active surveillance for prostate cancer."[8]

However, there is extremely limited clinical experience with TTh among men with metastatic PCa (mPCa), due to the concern that any rise in serum T, even transiently as seen with testosterone flare with luteinizing hormone-releasing hormone agonists, may cause rapid disease progression, with associated morbidity and mortality.[9] Standard treatment for many decades for men with metastatic PCa is androgen deprivation therapy (ADT),[10] with the addition of newer agents as needed that are even more effective at lowering serum T or blocking its actions.[11]

Yet there is evidence to suggest TTh may not be as dangerous as previously believed. *In vitro* and animal experiments have shown growth suppression of androgen-sensitive PCa tumors with high androgen concentrations,[12,13] and androgens have been shown to induce reversion of androgen-sensitive phenotypes in PCa cell lines that have developed androgen insensitivity.[14] Of greatest clinical relevance, landmark studies involving serial cycling of supraphysiological and castrate levels of T within a 4-week period, called bipolar androgen therapy (BAT) in men with castrate-resistant PCa, have shown strong evidence of clinical response.[15,16] These studies suggest a possible role for TTh in men with mPCa.

Presented here are clinical and prostate-specific antigen (PSA) responses to a variety of TTh strategies in three men with mPCa. The most promising of these strategies appears to be a modified BAT (mBAT) protocol to maximize duration of TTh and its associated benefits followed by a shorter period of androgen blockade.

Materials and Methods
Medical records were reviewed for three men with mPCa treated with TTh. Two had previously undergone ADT and found it intolerable. The third repeatedly declined ADT while seeking a more natural form of treatment. All three men had extensively researched their options and understood that TTh was considered an absolute contraindication that could cause rapid morbidity and death. Extensive detailed informed consent was obtained, and all patients provided written consent. Review of these data was performed with approval by the institutional review board for Beth Israel Deaconess Medical Center.

Case 1
This 94-year-old scientist underwent prostate biopsy 2 years earlier for PSA 320 ng/mL, revealing Gleason 9. Bone scan showed diffuse metastases. He was treated with leuprolide for 6 months but discontinued treatment due to severe weakness and fatigue. At time of consultation in July 2015, he had suffered 30 lb (13.6 kg) weight loss and had bilateral nephrostomy tubes for obstruction. Bilateral small pleural effusions were present.

The patient requested TTh so that he could regain enough energy to resume exercise and correspondence with his colleagues. PSA was 546 ng/mL and testosterone was 259 ng/dL. Treatment began with injections of testosterone cypionate 200 mg IM every 2 weeks, with dosage increased to 400 mg every 2 weeks after 5 months of treatment. Results of PSA during TTh are shown in Figure 1. By 1 month, he felt improved and was exercising vigorously three times weekly, fatigue resolved, and he had resumed his correspondence. He no longer required a daily nap, and resumed his scientific work. At 3 months he had gained 10 lbs from initial weight of 108 lbs. He died 11 months after beginning TTh, after developing shortness of breath with prominent pleural effusions. Cytology of aspirated pleural effusion revealed PCa. At no time did he experience bone pain. His last documented PSA was 2493 ng/mL.

Case 2
This 65-year-old businessman was first diagnosed with Gleason 8 PCa in 2011 and had undergone treatment with two courses high-intensity focused ultrasound, external beam radiation, and sipuleucel-T. He had been treated with TTh for >10 years before this. Baseline testosterone without TTh was 134 ng/dL. PSA rose to 31 ng/mL with resumption of T injections in 2012 and became undetectable after treatment with degarelix and enzalutamide. When first seen by me in 2014, his bone scan and CT were negative. He complained of severe fatigue, lack of energy, and absent libido that caused him substantial distress. A number of strategies to improve his quality of life involving androgens were undertaken. PSA results are shown in Figure 2 for several planned strategies involving TTh. In addition, he had experimented with several short-term androgenic strategies to improve his strength, which are as follows.

Oxandrolone.   The oral androgen, oxandrolone, was taken for 3 months during degarelix treatment. Workouts improved, but libido did not. Testosterone

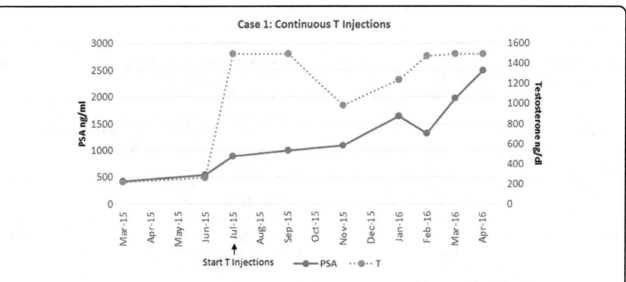

FIG. 1. PSA response to continuous T cypionate injections in a 94-year-old man with diffuse bony metastases and bilateral nephrostomy tubes. Baseline PSA was 546 ng/mL. Testosterone cypionate was administered in doses of 200 mg intramuscularly every 2 weeks. In early February 2016, dose was increased to 400 mg every 2 weeks. He died in late May 2016. Testosterone levels reported as >1500 ng/dL are represented here as 1500 ng/dL. PSA, prostate-specific antigen.

levels were 25–30 ng/dL. PSA rose from 0.03 to 0.64 ng/mL, and dropped to 0.05 ng/mL with discontinuation of oxandrolone.

Selective androgen receptor modulator. A 2-week trial of a noncommercial selective androgen receptor modulator (SARM) resulted in a PSA rise from 21 to 31 ng/mL after 2 weeks, despite a testosterone concentration of only 88 ng/dL.

Short-acting T treatments. Nasal testosterone gel (Natesto™) was applied 30–60 min before exercise. Blood tests obtained immediately before and 1 h after application revealed testosterone concentrations of 182 and 615 ng/dL, respectively. PSA was 0.66 ng/mL at baseline and 0.70 ng/mL at 1 h. No exercise benefit was noted.

Injections of short-acting testosterone propionate 25 mg three times per week provided no symptomatic benefit; however, 75 mg every 4–7 days provided transient improvement in energy and exercise tolerance for 2–3 days. After 3 months, PSA rose from 0.64 to 0.78 ng/mL.

Planned strategies. Bone scan first revealed bone metastases in April 2016. The PSA and clinical response to

a number of planned TTh strategies before and after this date are shown in Figure 2, including continuous T injections, combination of TTh with enzalutamide, intermittent use of TTh during enzalutamide treatment, and BAT. Throughout, the goal of adding TTh was to diminish fatigue and weakness and allow for improved quality of life. Additional treatments since development of metastatic disease have included pembrolizumab, and a repurposed drug protocol (doxycycline, metformin). Peak PSA with TTh was 397 ng/mL. Bone marrow biopsy for evaluation of anemia in October 2019 revealed replacement of bone marrow with PCa. At last contact in April 2020, his PSA was slowly declining, with a last value of 51 ng/mL on apalutamide, abiraterone, and prednisone.

Case 3

A 61-year-old consultant was seen in December 2015, 5 years after radical prostatectomy for Gleason 9 PCa with positive lymph nodes. A right nephrostomy was in place for ureteral obstruction from adenopathy. PSA was 31 ng/mL and bone scan revealed metastatic disease in the pelvis. Total testosterone was 181 ng/dL. Symptoms included weight loss, decreased libido, poor erections, weakness, and decreased strength. He was

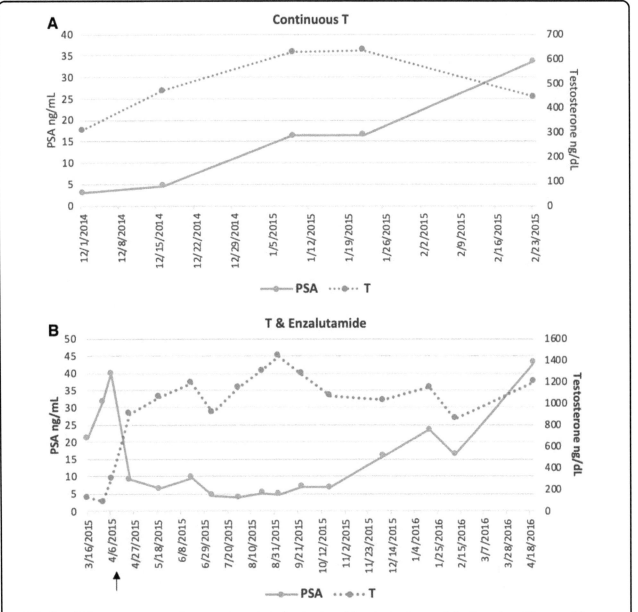

FIG. 2. PSA response to various treatment strategies involving testosterone injections in a 65-year-old man at presentation in December 2014 with biochemical recurrence after high-intensity focused ultrasound, external beam radiation, and sipuleucel-T. Initial PSA was 2.9 ng/mL. Bone metastases were first identified on April 2016. Bone marrow replacement with prostate cancer noted in October 2019. **(A)** Continuous weekly injections of T cypionate 80–120 mg intramuscularly. **(B)** Combination treatment with enzalutamide and testosterone injections. Enzalutamide was taken at 40–160 mg po daily. Testosterone cypionate was administered weekly at 120–200 mg intramuscularly. Arrow indicates beginning of combination treatment. Enzalutamide holidays and reduced doses began on October 2015, accompanied by rising PSA.
(C) Enzalutamide with infrequent testosterone treatments. Enzalutamide 160 mg taken daily with occasional injections of testosterone cypionate, short-acting testosterone propionate, and nasal testosterone gel. Blood tests taken 2 weeks or longer after injections. **(D)** BAT. Eleven monthly injections of testosterone cypionate 400 mg intramuscularly (arrows) during treatment with leuprolide. Enzalutamide 160 mg added for final 10–14 days of each cycle beginning on May 2017, as indicated. Enzalutamide discontinued after completion of BAT cycle on October 2017, associated with rise in PSA from 12 to 59 ng/mL. BAT, bipolar androgen therapy.

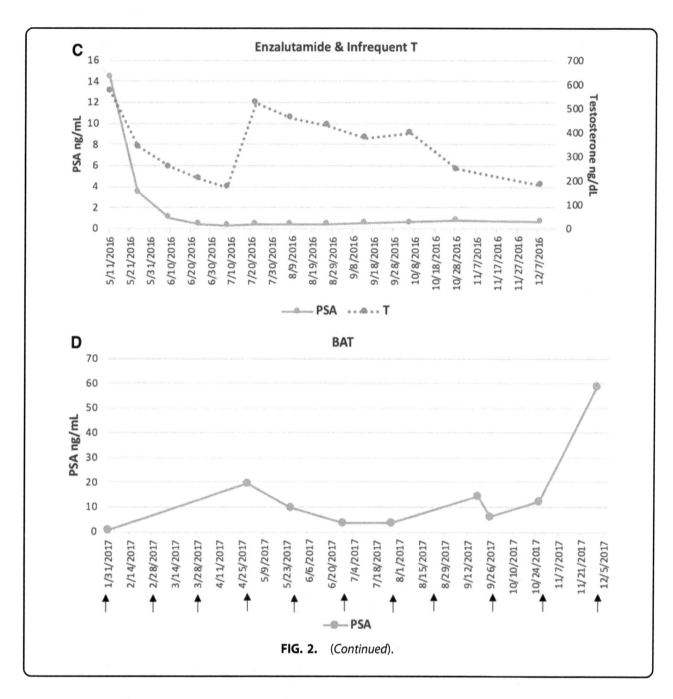

FIG. 2. *(Continued).*

5′8″ and weighed 135 lbs. He had refused ADT, and specifically requested TTh.

Treatment was initiated with injections of T cypionate 400 mg every 2 weeks. Energy, mood, and libido improved. He gained weight, strength, and resumed sexual activity. The PSA response is shown in Figure 3A. He discontinued TTh when PSA reached 185 ng/mL and bone scan revealed extension of bony disease in the pelvis. He denied bone pain. Interestingly, CT 2 months later revealed decreased size of para-aortic adenopathy from 16.7 to 9.8 mm.

In December 2016, bone scan showed a new metastatic focus at the base of the skull, and he agreed to treatment with enzalutamide 160 mg po daily. Although PSA declined to 1.0 ng/mL, he complained of severe weakness and weight loss, and again requested TTh. A mBAT program was developed in response to the patient's request to maximize the time on TTh and minimize the time on antiandrogen therapy. This consisted of testosterone cypionate injections 400 mg every 2 weeks for 8 weeks, followed by 4 weeks of enzalutamide. PSA response is shown in Figure 2B. He rapidly gained

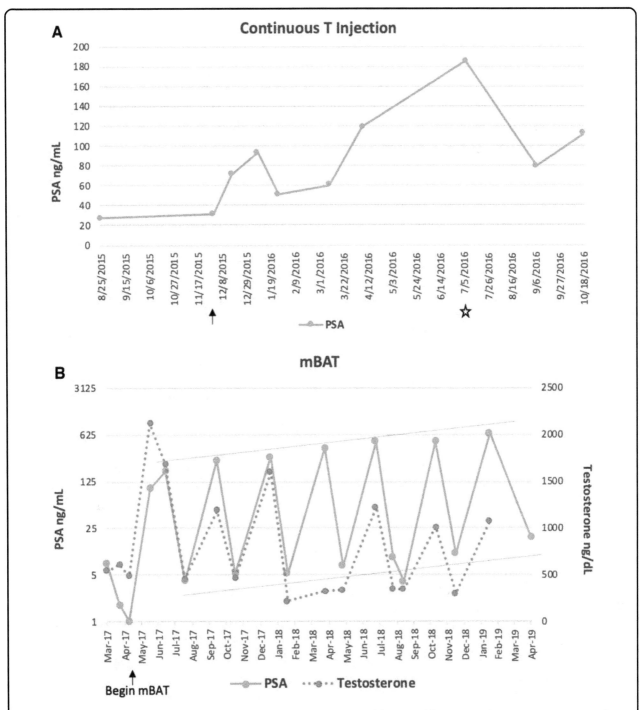

FIG. 3. PSA response to testosterone injections in a 61-year-old man with metastatic prostate cancer and nephrostomy tube, 5 years after radical prostatectomy with positive lymph nodes. PSA at presentation was 31 ng/mL. **(A)** Continuous T injections. Testosterone cypionate injections 400 mg intramuscularly were administered every 2 weeks. Note initial rise to 93 ng/mL with subsequent decline to 51–60 ng/mL for 3–4 months before rising steadily to 185 ng/mL at 7 months. Arrow indicates start of testosterone injections. Star indicates discontinuation of testosterone injections. **(B)** mBAT. Twelve-week cycles were initiated, consisting of 8 weeks of testosterone cypionate 400 mg intramuscularly every 2 weeks, followed by 4 weeks of daily enzalutamide 160 mg orally. Blood tests obtained at end of testosterone and enzalutamide periods. Arrow indicates start of mBAT. PSA shown in log scale to preserve details of PSA values at nadirs. Note upward slope of peaks and nadirs. Imaging studies showed no progression for ~2 years, until April 2019 when new lesions appeared on bone scan and mBAT was discontinued. mBAT, modified BAT.

energy, strength, muscle mass, and resumed sexual activity. PSA levels rose and fell during TTh and enzalutamide periods, respectively, reaching a highest peak of 645 ng/mL after ~2 years. Nadirs were consistently 5–10 ng/mL, gradually increasing with each cycle. Once, when the nadir PSA was 9.2 ng/mL, an additional 2 weeks of enzalutamide reduced PSA to 4.0 ng/mL, after which T injections resumed.

After 2.5 years of stable imaging studies on mBAT, progression was noted on bone scan in May 2019. He discontinued T injections. At last contact, PSA was 4.6 ng/mL in March 2020 after intermittent treatment with enzalutamide alone.

Discussion

After two decades of accumulating evidence of lack of harm with TTh in a variety of circumstances of men with nonmetastatic PCa,[1] it is longer reasonable to assume TTh is universally harmful in men with mPCa. Indeed, several reports suggest that TTh may even be associated with favorable cancer outcomes. Mathew reported stable PSA of ~1 ng/mL during 27 months of TTh in a 78-year-old man with adenopathy after radical prostatectomy.[17] In a study of 850 men who underwent radical prostatectomy, Ahlering et al. recently reported a lower biochemical recurrence rate (7.2%) among 152 men who received postoperative TTh compared with 419 proportionately matched controls who did not receive TTh (12.6%).[18]

The most intriguing evidence for a possible role for TTh in men with mPCa comes from the BAT trials involving rapidly cycling supraphysiological and castrate levels of serum T. These landmark trials demonstrated 50% or greater declines in PSA in 7 of 14 evaluable men with castrate-resistant mPCa and radiographic responses in 5 of 10 evaluable cases.[15] A subsequent trial also re-established androgen sensitivity in men with CRPC. Importantly, BAT was well tolerated despite regular excursions of serum T into the supraphysiological range.

Several immediate observations can be made from this study. First, there are men with mPCa who value quality of life over duration of life, and are willing to accept substantial risk to achieve this. Second, all experienced major benefits from TTh, including increased sense of well-being and physical activity level. Two men reversed substantial weight loss, and two experienced return of sexual desire and ability. Third, none experienced precipitous or unexpected adverse events, such as pathological fracture, spinal cord compression,

pulmonary embolus, or disabling bone pain, despite TTh use for 11 months, 3.5 years, and 8 years, respectively. Fourth, there is no indication TTh shortened the lives of these men. One died at 95 years nearly a year after presenting with extensive metastatic disease, and two are still alive and active 4 and 8 years after diagnosis of metastatic disease.

Continuous TTh was associated with an immediate rise in PSA in all men, followed by a plateau period that lasted 2 weeks in one, and 3–4 months in the others, before rising again. Since PSA production is itself androgen dependent, the initial rise was consistent with the saturation model,[7] and it is proposed that the subsequent plateau reflected tumor volume at the time of initiation of TTh, with the subsequent PSA rise representing progressively greater tumor volume over time. The improved health and vigor experienced by these men during continuous TTh argues that such treatment merits formal investigation as a possible treatment option for men for whom quality of life is paramount, and particularly for end of life.

It is noteworthy that PSA rose with all versions of androgen-type therapy, including oxandrolone, and a noncommercial SARM. However, intermittent, short-term, or short-acting TTh failed to cause a rise in PSA, as long as enough time was allowed for T to decline before blood was drawn for PSA testing. Although PSA remained low throughout the period of treatment with enzalutamide combined with infrequent administration of TTh, the patient experienced the chronic bothersome fatigue and absent libido seen with standard ADT or antiandrogen therapy, except for brief periods after testosterone administration. This strategy does demonstrate that in this particular patient, there did not appear to be any lasting adverse PSA effect from occasional testosterone use; however, it was not a successful strategy for improvement in quality of life. The absence of precipitous events in this small group, coupled with eventual return of PSA to low levels here, and with BAT and mBAT, raises the possibility that episodic periods of normal or even elevated testosterone may not cause irreparable harm.

We are unaccustomed to PSA values in advanced PCa with robust T concentrations and without ADT or antiandrogens. The high PSA values seen with continuous T injections were startling and caused two men to discontinue treatment. Any similar studies in the future would require mental recalibration for PSA levels. To illustrate, in one BAT study,[16] median baseline PSA was 39.8 ng/mL, whereas in a 1989 study of men with mPCa, median PSA in two groups was >10-fold higher at 546 and 678 ng/mL.[19] In the BAT study, all men were already on ADT, and in the 1989 study they were not.

The combination of TTh and enzalutamide was investigated to determine whether this may allay the weakness routinely experienced with ADT. Enzalutamide blocks androgen binding to AR and its subsequent translocation to the nucleus,[11] whereas skeletal muscle contains a second androgenic pathway independent of AR through a G protein-coupled membrane receptor.[20] Patient 2 took this regimen for 11 months, self-adjusting T and enzalutamide doses to optimize energy and minimize fatigue, with moderate subjective benefit. PSA dropped from 40 to 5–10 ng/mL for ∼7 months, before rising with reduced dosage of enzalutamide. It appears nearly any PSA within a very wide range can be achieved by manipulating the relative amounts of androgen and antiandrogens, until hormone-insensitivity occurs.

This same patient underwent 11 monthly cycles of BAT once bone metastases were identified.

Enzalutamide was added after the fourth cycle for the last 10–14 days of each cycle to lower the PSA nadir without interfering with the benefits experienced during intervals of high testosterone concentrations. He looked forward to those periods but was frustrated by their short duration.

The most promising of the strategies presented here is mBAT, which provided extended predictable periods of TTh benefits while maintaining PSA control. Whereas BAT proved that repeating cycles of high serum T followed by low serum T could offer therapeutic benefits to men with advanced PCa,[15] the rapid cycles within a 4-week period may not provide an optimal patient experience since the period of normal or even elevated serum T is relatively short. mBAT was developed specifically for clinical use, to improve quality of life due to the prolonged TTh period of 8 weeks, while hopefully providing similar benefits as BAT with regard to cancer control through the bipolar mechanism. A similar peak-and-valley PSA response was seen as with BAT,[15] but in this case occurring for a 3-month interval rather than monthly. Subjectively, patient 3 felt extremely well during his 8 weeks of TTh, and found 4 weeks of enzalutamide tolerable. Enzalutamide was selected for its ability to immediately "quench" the effects of high testosterone; however, other agents could be used to achieve the antiandrogenic effect. Interestingly, both PSA peaks and nadirs gradually rose over time. We surmise the rise in peak values represented increased tumor volume. The rise in the nadir values, in contrast, appears due to the prolonged half-life of PSA, since additional time on enzalutamide at one point resulted in a further drop in PSA. Additional patients have now been treated with mBAT, with promising results. Those cases will be presented when the data are more mature.

It bears comment that an apparent reduction in tumor burden was noted in Case 3, with reduction of para-aortic adenopathy from 16.7 to 9.8 mm after 2 months of continuous high-dose testosterone injections. This is reminiscent of the decreased tumor burden noted in several cases of men treated with BAT,[15] and consistent with in vitro studies showing that high androgen concentrations inhibit growth of androgen-sensitive PCa cell lines.[12–14] Clearly, the relationship of testosterone with PCa growth is more complex than previously believed.

These various TTh strategies underscore the limitations of PSA as a marker of disease status in men with advanced PCa. Low values with ADT or antiandrogens may be observed in men with either minimal disease or diffuse metastases. To correctly interpret PSA results, it is necessary to not only know the current testosterone concentration but also its recent history, as changes in PSA concentrations lag behind changes in serum testosterone by at least several days. A high PSA may be seen together with a low serum testosterone, or vice versa, as testosterone is administered or withdrawn. A low PSA in the setting of ADT cannot be interpreted to indicate minimal disease, since the value may soon be in the hundreds with relatively short periods of TTh.

In conclusion, these results suggest a potential role for TTh in selected men with advanced or metastatic PCa, especially for those who prioritize quality of life. Further investigation is warranted to identify treatment strategies that provide adequate cancer control without the full negative impact of ADT on quality of life. Since there are no randomized controlled trials adequately powered to address safety for any of the strategies presented here, no clinical recommendations can be made on the basis of these three patients. Nonetheless, in the absence of an effective cure for mPCa, these results support a personalized approach to hormonal treatment in men with advanced PCa, particularly at end of life.

References

1. Kaplan, AL, Hu JC, Morgentaler A, Mulhall JP, Schulman CC, Montorsi F. Testosterone therapy in men with prostate cancer. Eurol Urol. 2015;69: 894–903.
2. Morgentaler A. Testosterone and prostate cancer: An historical perspective on a modern myth. Eur Urol. 2006;50:935–939.
3. Pastuszak AW, Pearlman AM, Lai WS, et al. Testosterone replacement therapy in patients with prostate cancer after radical prostatectomy. J Urol. 2013;190:639–644.
4. Pastuszak AW, Khanna A, Badhiwala N, et al. Testosterone therapy after radiation therapy for low, intermediate and high risk prostate cancer. J Urol. 2015;194:1271–1276.
5. Morgentaler A, Lipshultz LI, Avila D, Jr, Bennett R, Sweeney M, Khera M. Testosterone therapy in men with untreated prostate cancer. J Urol. 2011; 185:1256–1261.
6. Kacker R, Mariam H, San Francisco IF, et al. Can testosterone therapy be offered to men on active surveillance for prostate cancer? Preliminary results. Asian J Androl. 2016;18:16–20.
7. Morgentaler A, Traish A. Shifting the paradigm of testosterone and prostate cancer: The saturation model and the limits of androgen-dependent growth. Eur Urol. 2009;55:310–320.
8. Ory J, Flannigan R, Lundeen C, Huang JG, Pommerville P, Goldenberg SL. Testosterone therapy in patients with treated and untreated prostate cancer: Impact on oncologic outcomes. J Urol. 2016;196:1082–1089.
9. Krakowsky Y, Morgentaler A. risk of testosterone flare in the era of the saturation model: One more historical myth. Eur Urol Focus. 2019;5:81–89.
10. Mottet N, Cornford P, van den Bergh EB, De Santis M, Fanti S, Gillessen S. Prostate cancer. https://uroweb.org/guideline/prostate-cancer/#note_616 (last accessed September 2, 2020).
11. Zheng X, Zhao X, Xu H, et al. Efficacy and safety of abiraterone and enzalutamide for castration-resistant prostate cancer: A systematic review and meta-analysis of randomized controlled trials. Medicine (Baltimore). 2019;98:e17748.
12. Song W, Khera M. Physiological normal levels of androgen inhibit proliferation of prostate cancer cells *in vitro*. Asian J Androl. 2014;16(6):864–868.
13. Song W, Soni V, Soni S, Khera M. Testosterone inhibits the growth of prostate cancer xenografts in nude mice. BMC Cancer. 2017;17:635.
14. Chuu C, Hipakka RA, Fukuchi J, et al. Androgen causes growth suppression and reversion of androgen-independent prostate cancer xenografts to an androgen-stimulated phenotype in athymic mice. Cancer Res. 2005; 65:2082–2084.
15. Schweizer MT, Antonarakis ES, Wang H, et al. Effect of bipolar androgen therapy for asymptomatic men with castration-resistant prostate cancer: Results from a pilot clinical study. Sci Transl Med. 2015;7(269):269ra2.
16. Teply BA, Wang H, Luber B, et al. Bipolar androgen therapy in men with metastatic castration-resistant prostate cancer after progression on enzalutamide: An open-label, phase 2, multicohort study. Lancet Oncol. 2018;19:76–86.
17. Mathew P. Prolonged control of progressive castration-resistant metastatic prostate cancer with testosterone replacement therapy: The case for a prospective trial. Ann Oncol. 2008;19:395–403.
18. Ahlering TE, Huynh LM, Towe M, et al. Testosterone replacement therapy reduces biochemical recurrence after radical prostatectomy. BJUI. 2020; 126:91–96.
19. Kuhn JM, Billebaud T, Navratil H, et al. Prevention of the transient adverse effects of a gonadotropin-releasing hormone analogue (buserelin) in metastatic prostatic carcinoma hy administration of an antiandrogen (nilutamide). NEJM. 1989;321:413–418.
20. Estrada M, Espinosa A, Muller M, Jaimovich E. Testosterone stimulates intracellular calcium release and mitogen-activated protein kinases via a G protein-coupled receptor in skeletal muscle cells. Endocrinology. 2003; 144:3586–3597.

Abbreviations Used

ADT = androgen deprivation therapy
BAT = bipolar androgen therapy
CT = computed tomography
mBAT = modified bipolar androgen therapy
mPCa = metastatic prostate cancer
PSA = prostate-specific antigen
SARM = selective androgen receptor modulator
TTh = testosterone therapy

12

Testosterone Therapy for Prevention and Treatment of Obesity in Men

Monica Caliber[1-3] and Farid Saad[4-6],*

Abstract

Testosterone deficiency (TD) is common in men with obesity. The association between TD and obesity is bidirectional; low testosterone (T) is a contributing cause to obesity, and obesity is a contributing cause to low T, creating a vicious circle. Most guidelines recommend weight loss by diet/exercise as the first point of intervention to stop this vicious cycle. However, it requires a large amount of weight loss that is maintained over time. In clinical practice, this is rarely achieved by lifestyle interventions. Bariatric surgery is currently the main obesity treatment modality that results in a large amount of weight loss with decent weight loss maintenance. However, bariatric surgery is an invasive and expensive procedure, with risk for complications. Considering the high prevalence of TD in men with obesity, a more practical and sustainable obesity treatment for men is testosterone therapy (TTh). Thanks to the metabolic effects of T, TTh results in more fat loss and preservation of fat-free mass, compared with diet/exercise interventions alone. In contrast to weight loss achieved by diet/exercise and bariatric surgery, TTh significantly preserves both muscle and bone mass. Further, TTh has psychological effects that may increase the motivation and ability of men to adhere to diet/exercise programs. Real-world evidence studies of long-term TTh for up to 11 years provide compelling evidence that TTh holds tremendous potential as a new treatment modality for obesity in men, with long-term weight loss maintenance and health benefits far exceeding those achieved by lifestyle interventions, approved obesity drugs, as well as bariatric surgery.

Keywords: obesity; testosterone deficiency; testosterone therapy; weight loss; body fat; fat loss; lean mass; muscle; body composition; type 2 diabetes; myocardial infarction; stroke; mortality

Introduction

The prevalence and disease burden of obesity continues to rise worldwide.[1-4] Among men, 40% have obesity.[5] Importantly, waist circumference (WC) in men is increasing more rapidly than body weight and body mass index (BMI).[6] Although both general and abdominal obesity are associated with an increased risk of premature mortality,[7] it has been shown that abdominal obesity may be a stronger risk factor for mortality than BMI.[8-11]

Cardiovascular disease (CVD), diabetes, and kidney disease are among the leading causes of obesity-related death and disability-adjusted life years (DALYs, a measure of overall disease burden, expressed as the number of years lost due to ill health or disability).[2] Developed countries are facing a public health crisis related to

[1]Medical Writer, Fort Lauderdale, Florida, USA.
[2]American Medical Writers Association (AMWA), Rockville, Maryland, USA.
[3]International Society for Medical Publication Professionals (ISMPP), Tarrytown, New York, USA.
[4]Medical Affairs Consultant, Hamburg, Germany.
[5]Research Department, Gulf Medical University, Ajman, United Arab Emirates.
[6]Dresden International University, Center of Medicine and Health Sciences, Dresden, Germany.

*Address correspondence to: Farid Saad, DVM, PhD, Medical Affairs Consultant, Hinsbleek 1, 22391 Hamburg, Germany, Email: farid.saad@bayer.com

overweight and obesity, which has likely been a key driver of the reversal of the decline in CVD mortality rates in these countries.[12] In particular, the finding that overweight and obesity are affecting CVD mortality in younger age cohorts where lifetime exposure to obesity has been much shorter than in older cohorts are very concerning and are likely to adversely impact CVD mortality trends and hence life expectancy in future.[12]

A large meta-analysis of prospective studies in four continents showed that men with obesity had three times the death rate than women with obesity.[1] This is consistent with previous observations that, at equivalent BMI levels, men have greater insulin resistance, ectopic (e.g., liver) fat mass, and prevalence of type 2 diabetes mellitus (T2DM).[13] The greater obesity-related disease burden in men was confirmed in a recent analysis of the Global Burden of Disease Study, which showed that global deaths and DALYs attributable to obesity are significantly higher in men than women (aged <70 years old).[14]

The aim of this review is to summarize evidence regarding the need for sex-specific interventions to treat obesity in men, focusing on the link between obesity and testosterone deficiency (TD) and the clinical utility of long-term testosterone therapy (TTh) as a treatment for obesity in men.

The Need for Sex-Specific Interventions to Treat Obesity in Men

The influence of sex hormones on metabolism and regulation of energy balance, body composition, body fat distribution, and appetite is well established.[15] Sex has emerged as a significant predictive factor in the development of CVD associated with metabolic dysregulation, such as obesity.[16] Even though the prevalence of obesity (BMI $\geq 30 \, kg/m^2$) is slightly higher in women than men, men suffer from more obesity-related comorbidities and are at a higher risk of obesity-related premature death.[1,17–19]

A study that investigated patterns of weight regain among men and women during a long-term follow-up found that men have poorer weight loss maintenance than women.[20] The Look Action for Health in Diabetes (AHEAD) trial likewise found sex differences in response to an intensive lifestyle intervention (ILI); although both men and women lost body fat and lean mass compared with the control group at year 1, by year 8, men in the ILI group had regained all body fat but not the lost lean mass, so that there was no dif-

ference in body fat but a significantly reduced lean mass compared with the control group at study end. In contrast, women in the ILI group had a significantly reduced amount of body fat but no difference in lean body mass compared with the control group at year 8.[21]

Sex-specific activation of the androgen receptor in the hypothalamus, skeletal muscle, liver, adipose tissue, and pancreatic islet β cells accounts for maintenance or disruption (in the case of TD) in energy metabolism and glucose homeostasis in men.[22] Therefore, the androgen receptor is a logical target for obesity interventions in men. However, there is a paucity of clinical trials examining sex-specific interventions and outcomes of obesity treatments (lifestyle-based or pharmacological).[15] The study of sex differences in obesity and regulation of energy expenditure, appetite, and body composition is an area rich with clinical research opportunities. As countries around the world struggle to deal with increasing population obesity, it will be important to focus on sex differences when designing obesity interventions to achieve improved health and economic outcomes.[15]

There are also psychological differences between men and women, which have implications for obesity treatments. For instance, it seems that men have more difficulty perceiving they have obesity, because of the desire to be muscular and have the masculinity of a large body size.[23] Unsurprisingly, a key motivator for men to start a weight loss treatment is an actual diagnosis of obesity, as opposed to simply being overweight.[23] Men from various cultures reported that being overweight did not concern them, and in some cases represented an ideal weight, as they did not want to be "too thin."[23] Further, men are more reluctant than women to undergo strict diets, and prefer to attend "men-only" treatments.[23] Effective obesity interventions for men, therefore, need to frame messages that are suited to the male mindset and appeal to the masculinity ideal. One male-specific benefit of weight loss is reduction in erectile dysfunction (ED).[24] The ability to perform sexually can, in turn, boost men's self-confidence and motivation to adhere to weight loss programs. Therefore, obesity interventions in men should not only focus on weight loss; they should also place greater emphasis on boosting sexual function/performance, and pleasure will likely provide far better adherence and sustained health outcomes.

As explained in the remaining sections of this review, long-term TTh qualifies as a highly effective treatment for obesity, resulting in marked weight loss/body fat reduction even without dietary restriction, and preservation of lean (muscle) mass. Being well known as the "male sex hormone," TTh is obviously a "men only" treatment. With its well-documented effects on muscle gain and sex drive/function, TTh is uniquely positioned to appeal to the masculine desires of men, while curbing an epidemic public health threat.

Obesity (BMI ≥30 kg/m^2) Versus Abdominal Obesity (WC ≥94 cm)

Clinical guidelines diagnose obesity as BMI ≥30 kg/m^2.[25–27] This is problematic for several reasons. BMI does not distinguish between body fat mass and muscle mass, which have an opposite impact on health outcomes. In addition, BMI does not provide information about abdominal obesity, which is a greater risk factor for premature atherosclerosis, heart disease, and mortality than overall obesity.[28] It is, therefore, alarming that the prevalence of abdominal obesity in the NHANES III survey is exceeding that of BMI-defined obesity (≥30 kg/m^2).[29]

The WC is the most common measure of abdominal obesity. For Caucasian/Europid populations, medical organizations recommend the WC thresholds of ≥94 cm (37 inches) in men and ≥80 cm (31 inches) in women for diagnosing abdominal obesity.[30] Waist size typically increases with increasing body weight, whereas abdominal obesity can occur even in normal weight (BMI 18.5 to 24.9) people.[31] In fact, the prevalence of normal weight abdominal obesity is increasing, now affecting at least one in three adults.[32]

The WC is more strongly associated with all-cause[7,9,11,33] and heart disease mortality[33,34] than BMI. Importantly, abdominal obesity is associated with higher mortality risk, independent of BMI.[8–11] For any given BMI category, apparently healthy individuals with a larger WC have an increased risk of premature mortality compared with those with a smaller WC.[8–11] Even among individuals with normal weight, abdominal obesity is associated with higher mortality than BMI-defined obesity.[31] Therefore, when interpreting outcomes of TTh studies, changes in WC are more clinically meaningful than changes in body weight (BMI).

Bidirectional Link Between Obesity and TD

It is well documented that the association between obesity and TD is bidirectional.[35,36] Obesity is the most common and strongest risk factor for TD, more so than aging itself (as explained below).[37–40]

Meta-analysis evidence that obesity is a cause of TD comes from studies of weight loss (induced by either low-calorie dieting or bariatric surgery) that show that increases in T levels are proportional to the amount of weight lost.[41] However, it should be pointed out that a large degree of sustained weight loss is required to elevate T levels that are enough to be of clinical significance. In men with TD, diet-associated weight loss leads to modest increases in T, 2.87 nmol/L (83 mg/dL) with 10% loss of body weight.[41] Bariatric surgery (30% loss of body weight) is associated with a more marked increase in total T of 8.73 nmol/L (252 mg/dL),[42] and it has been suggested that this may contribute to the health benefits seen in men after bariatric surgery.[41]

A Mendelian randomization analysis confirmed the causal effect of BMI on serum T in men; weight loss resulting in a reduction of BMI from 30 to 25 kg/m^2 was estimated to correspond to a 13% increase in serum T.[43] Similar results were found in the prospective Massachusetts Male Aging Study (MMAS).[37] Although normalization of T levels is a possible mechanism contributing to the beneficial health effect of bariatric surgery in excessive obesity, the increase in endogenous T levels with nonsurgical weight loss interventions is minor and of questionable clinical significance. Support for this comes from a randomized controlled trial (RCT) of TTh plus diet in men with obesity; a rigorous diet program leading to 11 kg (24 lb) weight loss in the placebo group increased serum T by only 2.9 nmol/L (84 mg/dL).[44] Not surprisingly, there was no improvement of hypogonadal symptoms,[45] and this effect was not sustained 18 months after the trial.[46]

These data suggest that although obesity is a strong cause of TD, efforts to treat TD by typical diet/exercise weight loss interventions are futile.

There is also solid evidence supporting the reverse direction that low T is a causal contributor to development of obesity. Experimental induction of hypogonadism in healthy men aged 20–50 years significantly increases body fat mass already after 12 weeks[47] and 16 weeks,[48] and men with prostate cancer (PCa) receiving androgen deprivation therapy show marked increases in total body fat mass and abdominal visceral fat within 6 months.[49] A prospective study of 3351 community-dwelling men showed that men with low T had higher BMI, WC, and risk of metabolic syndrome (MetS) after a 10-year follow-up.[50] Interestingly, men with higher baseline T levels not only had the lowest BMI, WC, and risk of MetS, but they also had the lowest risk of incident CVD events—irrespective of physical activity level—and had the lowest risk of dying from CVD.[50] Low T is a particularly strong predictor of the development of central adiposity[51] with visceral fat accumulation.[52] Another prospective study specifically examined the association between baseline T levels and visceral fat accumulation (measured by computed tomography) after a follow-up of 7.5 years.[52] Men with low T at baseline had a significantly greater increase in visceral fat, even after adjustment for baseline visceral and subcutaneous fat mass, BMI, age, T2DM status (oral glucose tolerance test by the World Health Organization diagnostic criteria), and fasting C-peptide.[52] A real-world evidence (RWE) study of men with TD and various body weight categories investigated the effect of long-term TTh for up to 11 years.[42] All men in the control group, regardless of baseline weight status, experienced a marked increase in body weight and WC.[42] Importantly, the greatest increases in body weight and WC occurred after 6 years in men with normal weight and overweight at baseline. As expected, T levels significantly declined over time, from 9.5 to 8.5 nmol/L in the normal weight, from 9.6 to 8.2 nmol/L in the overweight, and from 9.8 to 7.7 in the obese groups, respectively.[42] This suggests that the causal role of TD in the development of obesity takes multiple years to fully manifest.

Further proof of the causal role of TD in the pathogenesis of obesity comes from a growing number of studies showing that TTh significantly reduces markers of obesity (including body weight, WC, waist-to-height ratio, and BMI),[42,53–55] total body fat mass,[47,48,56–61] and intra-abdominal fat mass.[61–64] The remaining sections in this review will summarize important studies regarding the potential use of TTh as a treatment for obesity in men with TD.

Obesity Is More Strongly Linked to Low Testosterone than Age

A common misperception is that advancing age is the main cause of TD. Although the prevalence of TD increases with advancing age, this is mainly due to comorbidities—particularly obesity and T2DM—rather than aging *per se*.[37,65–72] As a consequence of the growing obesity epidemic among all age groups, the prevalence of TD in young men is increasing.[73] A meta-analysis of 18 studies (comprising a total of 4546 men with obesity, age ranging from 27.9 to 61.9 years, and BMI ranging from 24.8 to 50.3 kg/m²) found a TD prevalence as high as 50–80%.[74] Studies

using total T and free T showed the same trend of increasing prevalence of TD with increasing BMI.[74]

The Coronary Artery Risk Development in Young Adults (CARDIA) study showed that increasing obesity, particularly abdominal obesity, is associated with decreasing T levels in young men aged 18–30 years.[75,76]

A report from the Centers for Disease Control showed that among men, the prevalence of obesity was 40.3% in those aged 20–39, 46.4% among those aged 40–59, and 42.2% among those aged 60 and older.[73] In other words, obesity is nearly as common in younger men as in older men. Not surprisingly, up to 33–58% of young men (age 35 years or younger) with obesity have TD.[77–79] Another study found that among young men (aged 33–45 years) with obesity attending primary care, the prevalence of TD was as high as up to 75%.[80] This is similar to the TD prevalence seen in older men with obesity.[81–84]

The MMAS showed that an increase in BMI of 4–5 kg/m² was associated with a reduction in T levels comparable to that seen during ~10 years of aging in men whose body weight remained unchanged.[37] In the European Male Aging Study (EMAS), obese men (BMI ≥30 kg/m²) had a 30% lower T level—equivalent to almost three decades of aging—and a 13-fold increase in TD prevalence compared with men with a BMI of <25 kg/m².[38,39] Prospective data from EMAS showed that a 10% weight gain (+12.3 kg) and 10% weight loss (−13.7 kg) was associated with a proportional decrease (−2.4 nmol/L) and increase (+2.9 nmol/L) in T levels during a 4-year follow-up, respectively.[40] Obesity is associated with low T levels even in young men aged 24–41 years, a finding that supports the notion that obesity is a stronger risk factor for TD than age itself.[75]

Facing the current epidemic of obesity, it is critical for health care professionals to know that body fatness is more strongly associated with low T levels than age.[29,72,85] Therefore, T levels should be measured in men with excess body fat and/or large waist size, regardless of age, and TTh should be offered to all men who have no contraindications.[26]

Clinical Utility of TTh as a Treatment for Obesity: Long-Term RWE

The RWE from long-term observational studies have provided compelling support for the use of TTh as a sustainable and feasible treatment for obesity.[42,53–55,86–93] These observational studies comprise men with TD and various degrees of obesity and weight classes, ranging from normal weight to obesity class III, who are receiving long-term treatment with T undecanoate injections in real-life urology practices.

Because the health benefits of TTh are time dependent, these RWE studies provide valuable data about the true clinical significance of TTh, which cannot be derived from RCTs due to their short-term nature. The longest duration TTh RCTs are 3 years. In contrast, RWE data on metabolic/sexual, skeletal, and prostate outcomes have been continuously collected for 12 years,[93] 6 years,[94] and 17 years,[95] respectively.

One RWE study examined the effects of long-term TTh on anthropometric and metabolic parameters in 411 men with TD (mean age 60 years) and different degrees of obesity: class I (BMI 30–34.9 kg/m^2; $n=214$), class II (BMI 35–39.9 kg/m^2; $n=150$), and class III (BMI $\geq$40 kg/m^2; $n=47$). TTh was given as T undecanoate injections in 12 weeks intervals for up to 8 years.[55] In all three classes of obesity, TTh resulted in significant weight loss and a decrease in WC and BMI (Table 1). In men with class I and class II obesity, BMI dropped to below 30 kg/m^2, hence moving men from the obese state to the overweight state (Table 1).[55]

In a 10-year follow-up of 115 patients who had been continuously treated with T undecanoate injections, BMI decreased from 31 to 27 kg/m^2. The decrease was significant versus baseline ($p<0.0001$) and significant versus previous year for the first 8 years.[87] Body weight decreased from 97.3 to 84.6 kg. The weight loss was progressive and reached 18.5% (range 6.19% to 31.97%) after 10 years. At baseline, nearly all men (97.4%) had an elevated WC ($\geq$94 cm), out of which 67% had a substantially elevated WC ($\geq$102 cm). Mean WC decreased progressively from 106.5 to 92.3 cm (12%). The decrease was significant versus baseline ($p<0.0001$) and significant versus previous year for the first 7 years.[87]

Interestingly, men with moderate-to-severe ED or lower urinary tract symptoms have a more severe cardiovascular (CV) risk profile and benefit more from TTh than men with mild symptoms.[91,93] In men with obesity and various degrees of ED, treatment with T undecanoate injections for up to 12 years reduced body weight by ~18 kg (−16%), WC by 10 cm, and BMI by 6 kg/m^2 (from 33 to 27 kg/m^2).[93] Considering the high prevalence of ED in men with obesity, it is remarkable that erectile function continued to significantly improve for each successive year for 9 years.[93]

A more recent analysis of RWE data examined the effect of TTh for up to 11 years in men ($n=823$) with various weight classes.[42] Of these men, 474 (57.6%) had obesity, 286 (34.8%) overweight, and 63 (7.7%) normal weight. In 428 men (281 with obesity, 121 with overweight, and 26 with normal weight), T undecanoate 1000 mg injections were administered every 12 weeks after an initial 6-week interval, for up to 11 years. The remaining 395 men served as a control group. Anthropometric and metabolic parameters were measured at least twice yearly, and changes were adjusted for confounding factors to account for baseline differences between groups. In the normal weight group, T treated men had a weight loss of −3.4 kg (−4.8%), whereas untreated men had a weight gain of 6.1 kg (+8%). In the overweight group, T-treated men had a weight loss of −8.5 kg (−9.6%), whereas untreated men had a weight gain of 6.0 kg (+6.9%). In the obese group, T-treated men had a weight loss of −23.2 kg (−20.6%), whereas untreated men had a weight gain of 4.2 kg (+5.1%). Corresponding changes were seen in WC and BMI. The WC decreased in T-treated men (increased in untreated men) by −3.4 cm (+5.6 cm), −4.7 cm (+5.5 cm), and −12.9 cm (+5.6 cm) in the normal weight, overweight, and

Table 1. Changes in Obesity Parameters After Testosterone Therapy for up to 8 Years

	Class I obesity BMI 30–34.9	Class II obesity 35–39.9	Class III obesity BMI ≥40
Total testosterone	+8.16 nmol/L (from 8.74 to 17.02[a] nmol/L)	+7.29 nmol/L (from 9.3 to 16.86[a] nmol/L)	+6.41 nmol/L (from 9.34 to 15.99[a] nmol/L)
Free testosterone	+235 ng/dL (from 252 to 491[a] ng/dL)	+210 ng/dL (from 268 to 486[a] ng/dL)	+185 ng/dL (from 269 to 461[a] ng/dL)
Body weight	−17.4 kg or −16.8% (from 102.6 kg to 84.1 kg)	−25.3 kg or −21.5% (from 116.8 to 91.3 kg)	−30.5 kg or −23.6% (from 129.0 to 98.9 kg)
Waist circumference	−10.6 cm (from 106.8 to 95.1 cm)	−13.9 cm (from 113.5 to 100.0 cm)	−14.3 cm (from 118.5 to 103.8 cm)
BMI	−5.52 (from 32.69 to 27.07)	−8.15 (from 37.32 to 29.49)	−9.96 (from 41.93 to 32.46)

Data from: Saad et al.[55]

[a]When interpreting elevations in T levels (total and free), one has to keep in mind that these reported levels are trough levels, i.e. the lowest level measured immediately before the next injection. Trough levels can serve as an indicator of whether therapeutic T levels have been achieved..

BMI, body mass index.

obese groups, respectively. The differences in percent body weight change between groups, after adjustments for confounding factors, became significant in the normal weight group after year 1, and in the overweight and obese groups after year 2 (Fig. 1A). The differences in WC change between groups, after adjustments for confounding factors, became significant in the normal weight group after year 5, in the overweight group after year 2, and in the obese group after year 1 (Fig. 1B). The changes in body weight and WC were accompanied by corresponding changes in lipids and glucose control (improvement in T-treated men and worsening in untreated men).

In another RWE analysis, 316 men with prediabetes (defined as hemoglobin A1c [HbA_{1c}] 5.7–6.4%) and TD (defined as total T levels ≤12.1 nmol/L combined with symptoms) were included.[54] Of these, 229 men received T undecanoate injections for 8 years, and 87 men served as untreated control subjects. Metabolic and anthropometric parameters were measured twice yearly. At baseline, in both groups, BMI, HbA_{1c}, and International Index of Erectile Function, Erectile Function Domain (IIEF-EF) were 30 kg/m^2, 5.9%, and 11, respectively. TTh led to substantial improvement in glycemic parameters, with significant reductions in fasting blood glucose and HbA_{1c}. In contrast, in the untreated group, glycemic parameters worsened over time. At the last observation, all 229 patients (100%) in the TTh group had an HbA_{1c} of <6.5% (48 mmol/mol), and 205 of these 229 patients (90%) achieved normal glucose regulation with an HbA_{1c} <5.7% (39 mmol/mol). In the untreated group, only 1 patient (of 87, i.e., 1%) had HbA_{1c} <5.7% (39 mmol/mol) whereas 35 men (40.2%) had progressed to frank T2DM with HbA_{1c} >6.5% (48 mmol/mol).[54] Men in the TTh group achieved a weight loss of 8% at 8 years, whereas untreated men experienced a weight gain of 9%. This corresponded to a weight loss of 9.2 kg in T-treated patients and a weight gain of 8 kg in the untreated group. The WC decreased by 6.8 cm in the TTh group whereas it increased by 7.4 cm in the untreated group.[54] This is the first study to show that long-term TTh not only completely prevents progression of prediabetes to frank T2DM but also restores normal glucose regulation in most men.

Another RWE analysis of 356 men with T2DM and TD examined whether long-term TTh can result in remission of T2DM.[92] Remission of T2DM was defined as HbA_{1c} <6.5% and discontinuation of all diabetes drugs, including metformin. All patients received standard T2DM treatment. One hundred seventy-eight men additionally received treatment with T undecanoate injections 1000 mg every 12 weeks after an initial 6-week interval. The remaining 178 men did not receive TTh and served as a control group.[92] The T-treated men had a progressive and sustained reduction in body weight of −22.1 kg (−19.3%) and WC of −13.3 cm. In contrast, the control group had an increase in body weight and WC of +6.8 kg (+7.4%) and +7.1 cm, respectively. In parallel with the reduction in body weight and WC, T-treated men had significant progressive and sustained reductions in fasting glucose, HbA_{1c}, and fasting insulin throughout the entire treatment period. In contrast, the control group had progressive elevations in fasting glucose, HbA_{1c}, and fasting insulin. The T-treated men who had been on insulin at baseline had a reduction in insulin dose requirement compared with the control group, suggesting improved β cell function. In contrast, 20 patients in the control group were started on insulin treatment during the observation time, suggesting deteriorated β cell function. Remarkably, among T-treated men, 34.3% (61 out of 178 patients) achieved remission of T2DM (22 of these patients had been on insulin at baseline). The average time to discontinuation of diabetes medications was 8.6 years; the average time in remission was 2.5 years. There were no relapses. Overall, 46.6% of patients achieved normal glucose regulation (these patients, if not yet in remission, are eligible for discontinuation of diabetes drugs, which will be explored in an upcoming update of this ongoing study), 83.1% reached the HbA_{1c} target of 6.5%, and 90% reached the HbA_{1c} target of 7.0%. In contrast, no remission of T2DM or reduction in glucose or HbA_{1c} levels was noted in the control group.[92]

Importance of Uninterrupted TTh and Achievement of Therapeutic Testosterone Levels

A prerequisite for achievement of maximal metabolic and body composition benefits (loss of excess body fat with preserved or increased fat-free mass [FFM]) of TTh is long-term uninterrupted treatment. Multiple studies have shown that the beneficial effects of TTh are not maintained if treatment is discontinued.[46,53,96–100] This applies not only to improvements in body composition but also to improvements in muscle strength, erectile function, HbA_{1c}, total cholesterol, low-density lipoprotein cholesterol (LDL), high-density lipoprotein cholesterol (HDL), triglycerides, AMS, IPSS, IIEF-EF, residual voiding volume and bladder wall thickness, quality of life, and likely

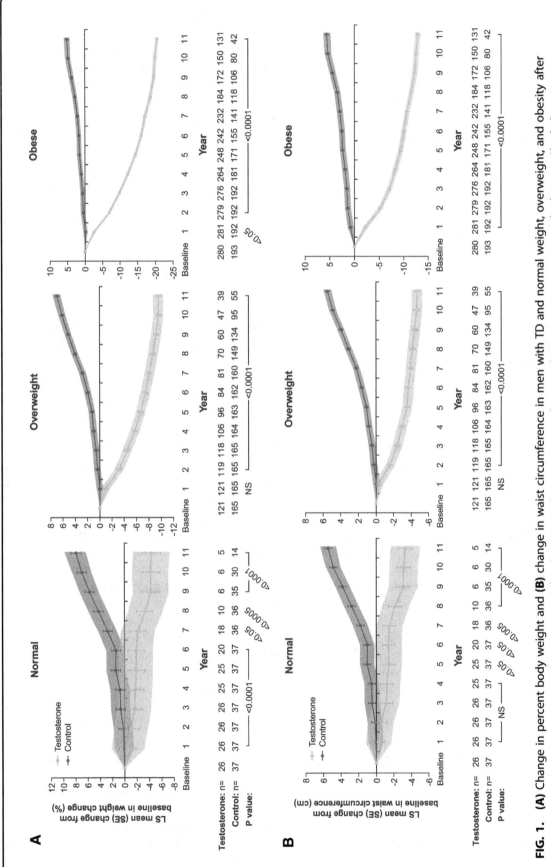

FIG. 1. **(A)** Change in percent body weight and **(B)** change in waist circumference in men with TD and normal weight, overweight, and obesity after treatment with T undecanoate injections, compared with untreated men. Data are shown as least squares means ± standard errors. Shaded areas represent 95% confidence intervals. *p*-Values indicate statistical significance between groups for each year. TD, testosterone deficiency. From: Saad et al.[42]

most—if not all—other T-related outcomes.[46,53,96–100] Nevertheless, beneficial effects return when TTh is resumed.[98] As pointed out in the British Society for Sexual Medicine guidelines on Adult Testosterone Deficiency, cessation of TTh results in progressive reappearance of symptoms and reversal of benefits (commonly within 6 months), so TTh is likely to be required lifelong for persistent symptom resolution and maintenance of health benefits.[65]

A related issue occurs when TTh is not properly dosed to achieve a high enough elevation of T levels (within the physiological range) for therapeutic efficacy. There are different T threshold levels for different responses to TTh; hence, TTh needs to achieve sustained therapeutic T levels to be effective.[101]

The Hormonal Regulators of Muscle and Metabolism in Aging (HORMA) Trial found that increases in total T of 1046 ng/dL (95% confidence interval [CI] = 1040–1051) and 898 ng/dL (95% CI = 892–904) were necessary to achieve median increases in lean body mass of 1.5 kg and appendicular skeletal muscle mass of 0.8 kg, respectively, which, in turn, were required to significantly enhance one-repetition maximum strength.[102] Therefore, for maximal benefits the dose of TTh should be titrated to achieve target T blood levels.[102]

The correlation between declining T levels during TTh and suboptimal response can be seen in several studies. For instance, in a long-term TTh study, body fat % dropped from 31.5% at baseline to 26.5% at month 24.[103] This was accompanied by an increase in total and free T levels from 9.1 to 19.1 nmol/L (263 to 551 ng/dL) and from 6.2 to 14.3 ng/dL, respectively. However, at month 96, total and free T levels had dropped to 372 and 8.68 ng/dL respectively, with body fat % no longer being significantly different from baseline,[103] suggesting inadequate dosing/adherence to TTh. Similarly, other studies have found that men who receive TTh that fails to normalize (restore) T levels (due to inadequate dose or adherence) do not experience a reduction in myocardial infarction (MI), stroke, atrial fibrillation or all-cause mortality, which is seen in men who receive TTh that does normalize (restore) T levels.[104–106] Suboptimal TTh also occurs in randomized controlled trials. In the Testosterone's Effects on Atherosclerosis Progression in Aging Men (TEAAM) trial, 156 men were randomized to receive TTh and 152 were randomized to receive placebo for 3 years. Despite aiming at achieving T levels between 500 and 900 ng/dL, at 6, 18, and 36 months total T levels were ~640, 600, and 460 ng/dL, respectively, and free T levels were 12, 11, and 8.5 ng/dL, respectively.

Because target T blood levels (T thresholds) likely vary between individuals, it is important to regularly monitor T levels during TTh, and in cases of suboptimal or lack of response, increase the TTh dose for a sufficient length of time and then re-evaluate.[107,108] In a secondary analysis of the BLAST study, examining T levels associated with clinical and biochemical improvements, it was pointed out that men with severe obesity may need shorter dosing intervals of T undecanoate—around 10 weeks between injections as opposed to 12 weeks—to achieve ideal therapeutic T levels, especially if the target levels of >15 nmol/L recommended in clinical guidelines are to be reached within 3–6 months.[101]

TTh in Comparison to Traditional Obesity Treatments

To fully appreciate the potential of TTh as an obesity treatment modality, it is informative to compare the weight loss and changes in body composition achieved with TTh with those achieved in traditional obesity interventions. A meta-analysis of weight loss trials reported a mean weight loss of 5 to 8.5 kg (5% to 9%) during the first 6 months from interventions with reduced-energy diets and/or weight-loss medications, with weight loss plateaus commonly occurring at ~6 months.[109] A systematic review of long-term weight loss studies found that diet/lifestyle interventions result in <5 kg weight loss after 2–4 years and obesity drugs result in 5–10 kg weight loss after 1–2 years.[110] After completing structured weight-loss programs, subjects regained half of the lost weight after 1 year and nearly three quarter during the first three years; less than 3% of subjects maintained their weight loss at all annual visits for 4–5 years after completion of a weight-loss program.[20,111,112] Meta-analysis shows that people on average maintain a weight loss of 3 kg and a reduced weight of 3% of initial body weight after 5 years.[113] Obesity medications approved for long-term use, when prescribed with lifestyle interventions, produce additional weight loss relative to placebo ranging from ~3% to 9% of initial weight at 1 year.[114] However, a major limitation of diet/exercise and obesity drug interventions is high dropout and a large proportion of subjects lost to follow-up.[110,115]

The Look AHEAD trial showed that an ILI resulted in a weight loss of −6% after 4 years.[116] In the RWE study of TTh in men with various severity of obesity (summarized above), weight loss at year 4 ranged from −10% to −15%, depending on obesity grade.[55]

An 8-year analysis of The Look AHEAD trial (baseline BMI of 35 kg/m^2) reported a weight loss of 7.9, 3.7, and 4.0 kg for year 1, 4, and 8, respectively.[21] The corresponding weight loss in men on long-term TTh was 3, 10.7, and 17.4 kg in class I obese men, 3.8, 16.6, and 25.3 kg in class II obese men, and 3.5, 18.5, and 30.5 kg in class III obese men (Table 2).[55]

As shown in Table 2, there was a marked weight regain after the first year in the ILI. In contrast, long-term TTh resulted in a sustained and progressive weight loss, with no plateau or weight regain. After 8 years, weight loss was four- to eight-fold greater with TTh than ILI.

The Look AHEAD trial, which is the longest duration ILI with body composition data, clearly shows a marked loss of FFM.[21] In a sex-specific analysis, differences in fat mass among men in the intervention and control groups were not significant at year 8; however, men in the intervention group had a significantly greater loss of FFM at all time points.[21] From baseline to year 1, fat mass and FFM did not change in men in the control group, whereas men in the intervention group had a weight loss of 9.4 kg, of which nearly 3 kg (30%) was FFM. From year 1–8, there was little change in the fat mass and FFM in the control group, and FFM in the intervention group. However, the year 1–8 weight gain in men (as well as women) in the intervention group was ~100% fat mass.[21]

As of this writing, there is no long-term TTh trial with body composition data that included a control group. Nevertheless, body composition trials of TTh (summarized below) show that TTh results in a greater reduction in fat mass per unit weight loss (in other words, preservation of FFM) compared with diet/exercise interventions. The large reduction in WC seen in the RWE studies outlined earlier confirms the beneficial effect of TTh on body composition and body fat distribution.

Weight loss is only one aspect of obesity treatment. Perhaps more important is the issue of weight loss maintenance. Weight-loss programs based on diet, exercise, and obesity drugs can help people lose weight, whereas maintaining weight loss seems to be the greatest challenge.[117–119] Even when obesity drugs are used during the maintenance phase, the vast majority regain most of the lost weight.[120] Considering that long-term TTh results in a progressive sustained reduction in obesity markers, combined with data showing that men may be more likely to regain weight after weight loss programs,[20,121] TTh holds tremendous potential as a unique obesity treatment for men.

TTh in Comparison to Bariatric Surgery

Among approved obesity treatments, bariatric surgery results in the greatest long-term weight loss maintenance,[122,123] with an average reduction in body weight after 2, 10, 15, and 20 years in the magnitude of −23%, −17%, −16%, and −18%, respectively.[122] A meta-analysis showed a weight-loss maintenance of 22.2% (30.1 kg) 20 years after bariatric surgery.[123] In a multicenter longitudinal study of 2348 bariatric surgery patients, after roux-en-Y gastric bypass (RYGB) and laparoscopic adjustable gastric banding (LAGB) the 7-year mean weight loss was 28.4% (−38.2 kg) and 14.9% (−18.8 kg), respectively.[124] Between years 3 and 7, there was a mean weight regain of 3.9% (RYGB) and 1.4% (LAGB). Among RYGB patients, 75% maintained at least 20% weight loss, and 50% of LAGB patients maintained at least 16% weight loss through 7 years. The remission of T2DM at year 7 was 60% for RYGB and 20.3% for LABG.[124]

Compared with usual care, bariatric surgery is associated with a long-term reduction in overall mortality [adjusted hazard ratio (HR) = 0.71, 95% CI 0.54–0.92; $p = 0.01$] and decreased incidence of T2DM (adjusted HR = 0.17; $p < 0.001$), MI (adjusted HR = 0.71; $p = 0.02$), and stroke (adjusted HR = 0.66; $p = 0.008$).[122] One study found that remission of T2DM after bariatric surgery was achieved in 58.2% ($n = 2090$) of patients at 2 years, and in 46.6% of patients at 5 years.[125] Although T2DM remission can be as high as 74% at 1 year postsurgery, T2DM relapse increased over time with a longer follow-up duration.[125,126]

As summarized earlier, TTh for 8 years results in weight loss corresponding to 16.8% to 23.6%, depending on baseline obesity grade (Table 1).[55] An 11-year

Table 2. Long-Term Weight Loss with Testosterone Therapy Compared with Intensive Lifestyle Intervention[a]

	Year 1 weight loss (kg)	Year 4 weight loss (kg)	Year 8 weight loss (kg)
Look AHEAD trial BMI 35	9.4	5.0	3.0
Class I obesity BMI 30–34.9	3.0	10.7	17.4
Class II obesity 35–39.9	3.8	16.6	25.3
Class III obesity BMI ≥40	3.5	18.5	30.5

[a]References.[21,55,116]
Data from: Saad et al.,[55] and the Look AHEAD (Action for Health in Diabetes) study.[21,116]
AHEAD, Action for Health in Diabetes.

analysis of RWE data showed that men who had been receiving TTh had a weight loss of −23.2 kg (−20.6%), whereas untreated men had a weight gain of 4.2 kg (+5.1%).[127] The marked weight loss seen during long-term TTh is accompanied by a reduced incidence of T2DM[54] and remission of T2DM in 34.3% of patients.[92] In an RWE analysis, the average time to discontinuation of diabetes medications (i.e., achievement of T2DM remission) was 8.6 years.[92] During a follow-up time of 2.5 years, there were no relapses.[92] Longer-term follow-up of this RWE cohort will tell whether T2DM relapse will occur. Currently, data suggest that with increasing the duration of TTh, the greater the rate of T2DM remission, that is, opposite to that seen with bariatric surgery.

As outlined later, TTh also compares favorably regarding long-term reduction in overall mortality, MI, and stroke. Although bariatric surgery results in greater short-term (<2 years) weight loss and T2DM, it is an invasive and very expensive procedure. Due to its risk for complications and high cost, it is only an option for a small minority of men with obesity and will hence not help curb the global obesity epidemic.

Effect of Traditional Obesity Treatments and Bariatric Surgery on Bone Mineral Density and Fractures

In addition to loss of FFM (discussed in the next section), another negative effect of diet-based obesity intervention[128,129] and bariatric surgery is significant loss of bone mineral density (BMD). Studies of both diet-induced weight loss and bariatric surgery show changes in bone markers, reflecting an increased bone turnover, evidenced by increased urinary excretion of deoxypyridinoline and serum levels of osteocalcin.[130] A 30-month follow-up study of a 1-year lifestyle intervention trial found a significant progressive reduction in total hip BMD despite lack of change in FFM or appendicular lean mass.[131] Weight loss of 10% or more beginning at age 50 years increases the risk of hip fracture in older men.[132] Among patients with T2DM, a weight loss of ≥20% is a significant risk factor for fractures, especially for men.[133] The Osteoporotic Fractures in Men (MrOS) study demonstrated that the impact of weight loss in older men on rates of bone loss is increased in the presence of low T levels.[134] Support for this comes from another MrOS analysis showing that low free T is an independent predictor of low BMD and increased prevalence of fractures.[135]

Bariatric surgery appears to be a particularly strong risk factor for BMD loss[136,137] and fractures.[138–140] A 7-year prospective study after RYGB (baseline mean age 43 ± 8 years, BMI 42 ± 6 kg/m^2) found continuous decline in BMD and deterioration of bone microarchitecture, as well as reduced estimated bone strength compared with baseline and 2 years postsurgery.[137] A meta-analysis concluded that bariatric surgery significantly increases fracture risk.[138]

In contrast, long-term TTh for 6 years results in a significant progressive improvement of BMD and T-scores, while simultaneously reducing obesity markers (body weight and WC).[94] Another long-term study found that TTh for 8 years significantly increased vertebral and femoral BMD, despite sub-optimal TTh dosing.[103] The anabolic effect of TTh on the bone was unequivocally demonstrated in the Testosterone Trials (T-Trials).[141] These findings underscore that full realization of the osteoanabolic effects of TTh can only be realized in the long term.

When given in conjunction with a diet program, TTh modulates bone remodeling markers in a way indicative of a favorable long-term effect on BMD.[142] TTh is the only available treatment that results in long-term sustained weight loss combined with increased BMD. Further study is needed to find out whether this translates into a reduced incidence of fractures.

Weight Loss Versus Fat Loss

Obesity treatment interventions commonly target weight loss alone,[26,115,143] without attention to effects on body composition and health outcomes.[144–148] In fact, regulatory agencies require that obesity drug trials have change in body weight as the primary efficacy end-point.[149] This is a problem, as a myopic focus on weight loss alone can mask important body composition improvements, such as reduction in total and/or visceral fat mass accompanied by preservation,[44] or even gain in FFM.[150] Further, it can lead to frustration and dropout among patients with obesity who think that weight loss is the only desirable result.

The goal of obesity treatment is to lose excess body fat mass while preserving FFM, which consists of 40–68% muscle mass.[127,151,152] The preservation of FFM is critical, because loss of FFM may increase risk for weight regain and increased fatness, by lowering maintenance energy requirement and triggering increased hunger/appetite.[153] Further, FFM is important for maintenance of metabolic health,[151] bone mass/skeletal integrity,[154] and quality of life.[155] Higher FFM (muscle mass) is associated with a significantly reduced risk of the MetS,[156] nonalcoholic fatty liver disease,[157] T2DM,[158] as well as lower mortality risk, independently of body fat mass, CV, and metabolic risk factors.[159–162] In older age, ≥65 years, loss of FFM is a particularly strong risk factor for mortality, independently of body fat.[163] Hence, the preservation of FFM during weight loss is important for both successful weight loss maintenance as well as reduction of comorbidities and mortality risk.

A concern with traditional obesity treatment modalities is that they cause a significant loss of FFM.[127] Currently, no guidelines are available that define how much FFM loss is excessive during or after weight loss interventions. According to the "Quarter FFM Rule," in healthy weight loss, the fraction of weight loss that can be attributed to FFM should not exceed 25%.[164] Although the percentage of weight loss that constitutes FFM is influenced by variables such as physical activity, diet composition, degree of caloric restriction, etc., 25% is a reasonable reference point for examination of the degree to which different weight loss interventions achieve preservation of FFM and a healthy weight loss.

A meta-analysis of lifestyle interventions for weight loss (minimum intervention period including follow-up of ≥12 months) found that 25% of weight loss comprises FFM.[165] A systematic review found that the mean FFM loss as a percentage of weight loss after dietary and drug-based weight-loss interventions resulting in a weight loss of >10 kg is 27% and 31%, respectively.[166] In a sex-specific body composition analysis at 1, 2, and 5 years after bariatric surgery, baseline body weight and FFM in men was 137.4 kg and 77.8 kg, respectively.[167] At 1, 2, and 5 years postsurgery, body weight (weight loss) was 94.4 kg (−43 kg), 98.1 kg (−39.3 kg), and 105.4 kg (−32 kg), and FFM (FFM loss) was 69.1 kg (−8.7 kg), 70.2 (−7.6 kg), and 69.9 kg (−8.7 kg). The percentage of weight lost as FFM was, hence, 20% at year 1, 19% at year 2, and 25% at year 5.[167] However, bariatric surgery can cause FFM loss as high as 53% of weight loss 2 years postsurgery.[168] A head-to-head comparison showed that bariatric surgery results in a significantly greater reduction in muscle mass than diet/exercise programs after 1 year.[169]

Effect of TTh on Body Composition During Diet-Induced Weight Loss

Currently, there are only a few RCTs with body composition data that specifically investigated the effect of TTh in the context of weight loss in men with obesity.

A notable diet RCT by Ng Tang Fui et al. investigated whether TTh has beneficial effects on weight loss and body composition over and above caloric restriction alone.[44] Men with obesity (BMI ≥30 kg/m²) and low T ≤ 12 nmol/L (346 ng/dL) were randomized to receive TTh with T undecanoate injections every 10 weeks (n = 49, baseline weight 118.3 kg) or matching placebo (n = 51, baseline weight 120.7 kg) for 56 weeks. Both groups underwent a very-low calorie diet during week 1 to 10, which was followed by a weight maintenance period of 46 weeks. Subjects were advised to perform at least 30 min of moderate-intensity exercise each day and completed exercise questionnaires and accelerometer testing (at weeks 0, 10, and 56) to reinforce and encourage participation in exercise. After the very-low calorie diet (phase 1, week 0 to 10), subjects were put on a less stringent calorie-restricted diet for the remaining 46 weeks (phase 2, week 11 to 56). At the end of the 10-week diet phase, weight loss was 12 kg and 13.5 kg in the T-group and placebo group, respectively (difference between groups not significant). There was a trend toward a 0.4 kg greater reduction in body fat mass and a 0.9 kg smaller reduction in lean mass in the T-group. At the end of phase 2 (week 56), weight loss remained largely stable in the T-group (+0.6 kg, p = 0.62), whereas there was weight regain in the placebo group (+2.6 kg, p = 0.06). At study end, men on TTh had, compared with placebo, lost significantly more body fat mass (−2.9 kg vs. −0.4 kg, p = 0.04) and visceral fat (−2678 mm² vs. −1099 mm², p = 0.04), and regained the diet-induced loss of lean mass (+3.4 kg vs. +0.9 kg, p = 0.002). As the combined loss of body fat and lean mass in men on placebo was similar to the amount of fat mass lost in men on TTh, there was no difference in body weight at study end. It is remarkable that men who had received TTh had a 7.3-fold greater reduction in total body fat and a 2.4-fold greater reduction in visceral fat mass than men on placebo.

A unique benefit of TTh in the context of weight loss is preservation of FFM (muscle mass). At the end of phase 1 (after 10 weeks on a very-low calorie diet), the fraction of weight loss comprising FFM was 32.5% and 35.5% in men on TTh and placebo, respectively. At study end (week 56), the fraction of weight loss comprising FFM was 5.3% in men on TTh and 36.7% in men on placebo. To the best of our knowledge, 5.3% is the smallest reduction in FFM ever reported in weight-loss trials. Support for the conclusion that TTh preserves muscle mass comes from the finding that men on TTh had a significantly higher appendicular lean mass and increased handgrip strength than men on placebo.

At the end of phase 1 (week 10), both groups had increased daily step count ($p < 0.01$) and activity levels ($p < 0.05$). However, at study end (week 56), daily step count was increased only in men on TTh, as was percentage of daily nonsedentary time (due to spending less time in sedentary activities and more time in light activities. Notably, the dropout rate was higher among men assigned to placebo compared with TTh. This suggests that TTh may make it easier for men with obesity to adhere to diet/exercise programs.

A likely explanation for the lack of preservation of lean mass during the initial diet phase may be the short duration of 10 weeks, as T-induced changes in lean mass or FFM typically require several months to manifest.[170] It should be pointed out that the greater reduction in body fat and preservation of lean mass in the T-group occurred despite a modest increase in endogenous total and free T levels (+2.9 nmol/L [+84 ng/dL] and +30.3 pmol/L [+10.5 pg/mL], respectively) in the placebo group.[44] This diet-induced elevation in T levels is similar to what has been seen in previous weight-loss studies,[41,171] and it suggests that the endogenous rise in T subsequent to dieting is not sufficient to prevent diet-related loss of lean mass.

The results from Ng Tang Fui et al. confirm findings from previous smaller studies showing that TTh combined with lifestyle modification results in better outcomes than lifestyle modification alone. In 2009, a small RCT with 16 subjects who were newly diagnosed with T2DM and MetS showed for the first time that the combination of TTh and lifestyle intervention leads to greater therapeutic improvement in glycemic control, and reverses the MetS, after 52 weeks of treatment.[172] An 18-week (4.5 months) RCT in men with obesity and obstructive sleep apnea showed that the combination of TTh and lifestyle modification improved insulin sensitivity, ameliorated fatty liver, and increased muscle mass, in comparison to placebo and lifestyle modification alone.[173] In elderly men (age 65–85 years), TTh for 12 weeks combined with a resistance exercise program did not have any effect on body composition compared with placebo.[174] This is likely due to the short 3-month duration.

An RCT of 167 generally healthy community-dwelling older men (age 66 years) found that TTh for 12 months combined with resistance exercise training resulted in a greater reduction in fat mass by 1.2 kg, a greater increase in FFM by 1.7 kg, and a 0.3 kg greater increase in arm FFM than resistance exercise training alone.[175]

An observational, parallel-arm, open-label 54-week study investigated the effect of hypocaloric diet plus exercise (DPE; $n = 12$) or DPE plus treatment with T undecanoate injections (DPE + T; $n = 12$), followed by 24 weeks of DPE alone in 24 men with obesity (BMI 42 kg/kg^2; age 54 years).[97] After 54 weeks, the DPE + T group had improvement in epicardial fat thickness, ejection fraction, diastolic function, carotid intima-media thickness (CIMT), and endothelial function ($p < 0.01$ vs. controls). Also, hormonal (T, $p < 0.0001$; GH, $p < 0.01$), metabolic (Homeostatic Model Assessment of Insulin Resistance [HOMA-IR], $p < 0.01$; microalbuminuria, $p < 0.01$), lipid (total cholesterol, $p < 0.05$), and inflammatory (fibrinogen, $p < 0.05$) parameters improved. After 24 weeks from T withdrawal, most parameters returned to baseline. A 33% dropout rate was reported in the DPE group, whereas there was no dropout among men receiving TTh.[97]

Effect of TTh on Body Composition Without Dieting

Studies with body composition outcomes highlight the importance of looking beyond weight change when evaluating the potential clinical utility of TTh for prevention of obesity. It should be pointed out that shorter-term studies of TTh in the absence of dieting may show lack of change in body weight or even an increased body weight, but they still have beneficial effects on body composition by reducing body fat and increasing FFM.

For example, in men with normal weight and low T (13.6 nmol/L or 392 ng/dL), TTh for 1 year selectively reduced visceral fat accumulation without change in total body FM and increased total body FFM and total body and thigh skeletal muscle mass.[64] In another study of men with obesity (BMI 40 kg/m^2) and hypogonadism (231 ng/dL), TTh for 24 weeks reduced subcutaneous fat mass by −3.3 kg and increased lean mass by 3.4 kg.[150] Despite a lack of change in body weight, there was a significant improvement in insulin sensitivity.[150] In men with overweight, TTh for 6 months increased lean body mass by 3.6 kg while simultaneously decreasing total fat mass by −1.2 kg, resulting in a net gain in body weight despite a significant reduction in percent body fat.[176]

One RCT aimed at investigating the effect of TTh with T undecanoate injections versus placebo on CV risk factors, atherosclerosis progression, and body composition in a population of men with hypogonadism and MetS and T2DM.[177] After 12 months, men in the T-group had a reduction in body fat percent and WC by −18.5% and −8.5 cm, and an increase in FFM by 4.8 kg, despite no change in body weight. This was accompanied by a marked improvement in insulin sensitivity (HOMA-IR, $p < 0.001$) and reduction in HbA_{1c} ($p < 0.01$), high-sensitivity C-reactive protein ($p < 0.001$), as well as CIMT ($p < 0.0001$). In contrast, no changes were seen in the placebo group.[177]

In 161 men with TD and baseline BMI of 26 kg/m², TTh for 52 weeks reduced body fat from 28.8% to 24.5%.[178] In a long-term follow-up of this study, body fat declined from 31.5% to 26.5% at month 24, whereas T levels increased from 263 to 551 ng/dL. Thereafter, there was a reduction in T levels, so that at month 96 the mean T level was 372 ng/dL. As the T level declined, body fat increased, so that at the end of the study there was no difference in body fat compared with baseline.[103] This underscores the importance of maintaining high enough elevations of T levels throughout the entire treatment period.

In contrast to RCTs of TTh in men with normal weight and overweight, which show improvement in body composition with no change or increase in body weight,[179] RCTs that included mostly men with obesity show significant reduction in body weight and WC.[53,180,181] The first double-blind, placebo-controlled study conducted exclusively in men with T2DM and obesity was published in 2014. Patients ($n = 211$) were recruited from general practices for a 30-week RCT of TTh with T undecanoate injections, followed by 52 weeks of open-label treatment.[180] After 30 weeks, there was a significant reduction in WC by −2.5 cm and a small nonsignificant reduction in body weight. After 82 weeks, there was a significant weight loss of −2.7 kg and reduction in WC by −4.2 cm. At both time points, there were significant improvements in HbA_{1c} and total cholesterol. Hypogonadism symptoms had significantly improved at week 82, but not week 30.[180] This suggests that 30 weeks (7.5 months) is not enough for weight loss and symptomatic improvement. Further support for the importance of long-term TTh comes from a long-term follow-up of this study, which found that WC and erectile function continued to improve for 4 years with ongoing uninterrupted TTh.[53] Remarkably, the progressive improvement in erectile function for nearly 4 years was independent of PDE5i use.[53]

Another RCT of TTh in 55 men with obesity and T2DM showed that treatment with T undecanoate injections versus placebo injections for 1 year significantly reduced HOMA-IR by −4.64 versus −0.52, HbA_{1c} (%) by −0.94 versus −0.24, fasting glucose (mmol/L) by −1.23 versus −0.13, fasting insulin (mE/L) by −8.52 versus −0.51 and CIMT (mm), a surrogate measure of atherosclerosis, by −0.10 versus −0.05.[182] Endothelial function, measured by flow mediated dilatation (FMD, %), improved by 2.40 versus −0.08. Although the between-group difference in body weight and WC was not significant after 1 year, in a follow-up of this study, where the placebo group was switched over to treatment with T undecanoate injections and the T group continued receiving T undecanoate injections for a second year, there was a significant reduction in body weight and.[181] In men who had been receiving T undecanoate injections for 2 years (which increased total T to 23.5 nmol/L and free T (calculated) to 594 pmol/L), there was a significant reduction in WC by 3.51 cm and BMI by −1.6 kg/m².[181] This was accompanied by further improvement in insulin resistance/glucose control, lipids, atherosclerosis, and endothelial function; HOMA-IR (−5.94, final reading 5.51), fasting glucose (−1.83 mmol/L, final reading 8.23 mmol/L), HbA_{1c} (−1.51%, final reading 6.6%), total cholesterol (−0.97 nmol/L, final reading 4.34 nmol/L), LDL (−0.40 nmol/L, final reading 2.39 nmol/L), HDL (+0.15 nmol/L, final reading 1.15 nmol/L), triglycerides (−0.99 nmol/L, final reading 1.86 nmol/L), non-HDL (1.12 nmol/L, final reading 3.19 nmol/L), FMD (+2.46%, final reading 7.14), and CIMT (−0.14 mm, final reading 0.73). It should be pointed out that these beneficial effects of TTh were achieved without any diet or exercise intervention. This RCT with follow-up shows that TTh for at least 2 years may be needed in some populations of men to achieve significant improvements in body weight, WC, insulin resistance/glucose control, lipids, atherosclerosis, and endothelial function.

More studies of TTh with long-term body composition data are needed to elucidate how the effects of T treatment on fat loss, FFM gain, and metabolic outcomes are influenced by TTh dose, treatment duration, as well as diet and exercise (or lack thereof), in men with obesity, the MetS and/or T2DM.

Reduction in CV Events and Mortality with Long-Term TTh in Daily Clinical Practice

Considering that obesity is a strong CV risk factor, and the widespread misperception about TTh and CV risk, it is important to examine long-term RWE data of TTh in men with obesity. In one RWE study, 77 men with obesity, hypogonadism, and a history of CVD were treated with T undecanoate injections for up to 8 years.[88] No patient suffered a major adverse CV event during the entire 8 year-long observation time. It was concluded that TTh in men with a history of CVD may be effective as an add-on treatment for secondary prevention of CV events.[88]

In the first RWE study analysis that included a control group, 360 men with obesity and TD received T undecanoate injections for up to 10 years.[89] This TTh group was compared with a control group of 296 men who had opted to not receive TTh. There were 26 cases of nonfatal MI and 30 cases of nonfatal stroke in the control group and none in the TTh group. In the nontreated control group, there were 21 deaths, 19 of which were due to CV events (5 MI, 4 stroke, 7 heart failure, 2 thromboembolisms, 1 lung embolism). In the TTh group, there were only 2 deaths, and none was related to CV events (one was due to postsurgical thromboembolism and the other due to traffic accident). The estimated reduction in mortality for the TTh compared with the control group was between 66% and 92%.[89] This is the first large RWE study showing a significant reduction in hard clinical end-points with long-term TTh.

In the prediabetes RWE study described earlier, the incidence of nonfatal MI and mortality was 0.4% and 7.4% in the TTh group, and 5.7% and 16.1% in the control group, respectively.[54] Similarly, in the T2DM remission RWE study, there was no MI or stroke in T-treated men. Among untreated men, 31% had MI and 25% stroke. Mortality rate was 7% in T-treated men and 29% in untreated men.[92]

The effect on hard clinical end-points after treatment with T undecanoate injections for up to 11 years in men with different weight classes, compared with untreated men, is illustrated in Figure 2.[42] Remarkably, there were no cases of MI nor stroke in any of the TTh groups.

Adverse events in men with different weight classes during treatment with T undecanoate injections for up to 11 years could be compared with untreated (control) patients.[42]

In men with various degrees of ED, TTh was given to 412 patients for up to 12 years, whereas 393 served as a control group.[93] In the TTh groups, no MI nor stroke occurred during the entire observation period (Fig. 3). In the untreated groups, MI and stroke oc-

curred in 18.9% and 14.9% of patients with moderate/severe ED, respectively, and 16% and 15.3% in patients with no/mild ED. In the TTh groups, death from all causes occurred in 6.5% and 2.3% of men with no/mild ED and moderate/severe ED, respectively. In the untreated groups, death occurred in 14.6% and 21.3% of men with no/mild ED and moderate/severe ED, respectively. In the T-treated groups, PCa occurred in 0% and 2.3% of men with no/mild ED and moderate/severe ED, respectively. In the untreated groups, PCa occurred in 6.9% and 6.8% of men with no/mild ED and moderate/severe ED, respectively.

Discussion and Conclusion

T is a key metabolic hormone with well-documented effects on body fat, muscle mass, and the skeleton.[36,141,170,179,183,184] TD is particularly common in men with obesity. Because T is a key metabolic hormone, achieving and maintaining weight loss in men who have TD is extremely difficult. Numerous studies have shown that adding TTh to lifestyle interventions increases fat loss while preserving or increasing FFM.[97,172,173,175]

Loss of FFM and regain of body fat over time is a major drawback of diet and/or drug-based obesity treatment interventions.[127] Preservation of FFM during weight loss is critical, as reduction in FFM may counteract the beneficial health effects of weight loss,[185] as well as increase risk for weight regain.[153] In studies of diet/exercise interventions, around 25–35% of weight loss comprises FFM. After bariatric surgery, 20–50% of weight loss comprises FFM.[167,168] The RCT data show that dieting men who receive placebo lose both body fat and lean mass, whereas weight loss in dieting men receiving TTh was almost exclusively body fat.[44] After 1 year of reduced caloric intake, the fraction of weight loss comprising FFM was 36.7% in men on placebo but only 5.3% in men on TTh. This suggests that TTh augments diet-induced loss of body fat and prevents loss of FFM. The mechanisms underlying the anabolic effect of TTh on muscle during diet interventions are starting to get elucidated, and it has been concluded that TTh is a viable strategy for preserving muscle mass during caloric restriction.[186]

Although RCTs are considered to provide the highest quality evidence, efficacy of an intervention under controlled conditions is not synonymous with effectiveness, that is, intervention outcomes in "real-world" conditions.[187–189] Because obesity is a chronic condition that is greatly influenced by lifestyle,

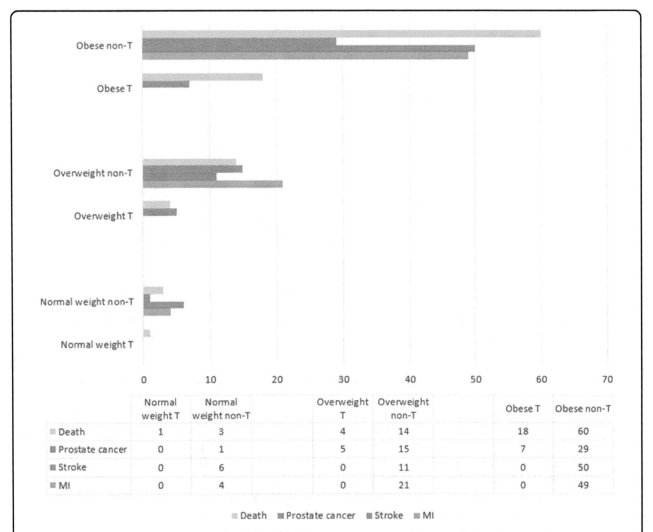

	Normal weight T	Normal weight non-T	Overweight T	Overweight non-T	Obese T	Obese non-T
Death	1	3	4	14	18	60
Prostate cancer	0	1	5	15	7	29
Stroke	0	6	0	11	0	50
MI	0	4	0	21	0	49

Death   Prostate cancer   Stroke   MI

FIG. 2. Incidence of death, nonfatal myocardial infarction, nonfatal stroke, and prostate cancer in men with TD and normal weight, overweight, and obesity after treatment with T undecanoate injections (T), compared with untreated men (non-T). MI, myocardial infarction. Data from: Saad et al.[42]

evidence for how weight loss/maintenance interventions work in daily living conditions in the long term is essential.

Long-term RWE studies of men with TD and obesity who receive TTh in routine clinical practice show large amounts of weight loss that is progressive and sustained over time, with no plateau reported for up to 11 years.[42] This is opposite to the experience with obesity drugs, which have declining drug efficacy/effectiveness over time, often culminating in a weight-loss plateau within ~1 year.[190] Further, because T is a key metabolic hormone, by correcting TD, TTh creates a metabolic environment that facilitates fat loss and long-term maintenance of an improved body composition.

The prevalence of severe obesity (BMI $\geq 35\,\mathrm{kg/m^2}$) is rising at an alarming pace; by 2030, it is projected to affect one in four adults.[191,192] Considering that conventional weight-loss interventions (diet, exercise, drugs) have minimal impact in patients with severe obesity,[193] it is particularly noteworthy that long-term TTh for up to 8 years reduced BMI from 37.3 to 29.5 in men with grade II obesity (BMI 35–39.9) and from 41.9 to 32.4 in men with grade III obesity.[55] This suggests that TTh also offers significant clinical value for men with more severe obesity.

The RWE studies have additionally provided valuable insight about the consequences of untreated TD.[42] Men with TD who do not receive TTh have an

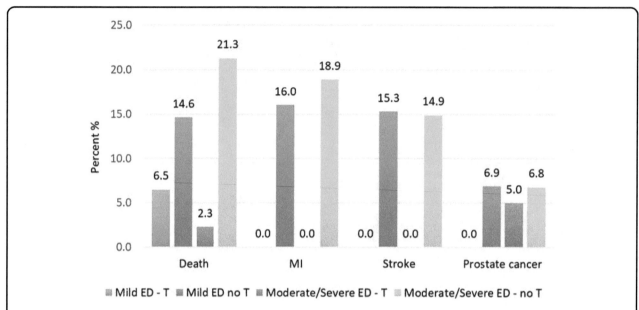

FIG. 3. Adverse events (%) in patients with no/mild and moderate/severe ED during treatment with T undecanoate injections for up to 12 years (T), compared with untreated (control) patients (no T). ED, erectile dysfunction; T, testosterone. Data from: Saad et al.[93]

increase in body weight and WC over time, regardless of baseline bodyweight. It is remarkable that in men with obesity, long-term TTh results in a weight loss of similar magnitude as that achieved with bariatric surgery. Change in body weight and BMI are the most frequently used measures to evaluate bariatric surgery outcomes. However, body weight-based metrics do not provide information about change in body composition (body fat and lean mass), which is what ultimately matters in terms of chronic disease risk, particularly T2DM and CVD. Bariatric surgery results in a large amount of weight loss and better weight loss maintenance compared with diet/exercise interventions; however, this is followed by a disproportional regain of body fat during the second and third year after bariatric surgery.[194,195] A sex-specific analysis showed that men have increases in all adipose tissue depots between 12 and 24 months postsurgery with weight regain.[196] In parallel with the significant post-surgery body fat rebound, there is progressive worsening of lipid parameters, suggesting that the adverse switch in the change in body composition between the first and third year may underlie the observed recurrence of CV risk factors over time.[194,195] In stark contrast, the weight loss and reduction in WC observed in RWE studies of long-term TTh is progressive over time and accompanied by marked improvement in

glycemic control and lipid profile. Support for the beneficial effects of TTh on body composition comes from 36-month RCTs showing progressive reduction in body fat percent with TTh versus placebo.[56,197] However, a prerequisite for achievement of body fat loss with TTh is adequate dosing of TTh and adherence to treatment, so that a sufficient T level elevation is reached and maintained in the long term.[103]

In addition to increased fat loss and preservation of FFM, TTh may make it easier for men to adhere to diet/exercise programs.[44] Support for this comes from experimental studies showing that TTh increases spontaneous physical activity by enhancing CNS sensitivity to dopamine.[198] Previous studies have shown that TTh consistently improves mood and feelings of energy, and it reduces fatigue[199–204]; this, in turn, may bolster motivation and the ability to adhere to diet/exercise programs.[172,205,206]

Effective intervention to curb the rapidly growing obesity epidemic, which is affecting men of all ages, is urgently needed. Long-term "real-life" studies provide compelling evidence that TTh offers significant clinical utility in the treatment of men with obesity, as well as in the prevention of obesity development, in men with TD.[42,55,87,93] This is accompanied by T2DM remission[92] and a significant reduction in T2DM incidence,[54] MI, stroke, PCa, and mortality.[54,88,89,92,93] Because obesity is a gateway to ill health,[207] especially T2DM and CVD, a large-scale initiative for widespread implementation of TTh, as part of medical care for men with obesity, is highly warranted.

References

1. Di Angelantonio E, Bhupathiraju Sh N, Wormser D, et al. Body-mass index and all-cause mortality: Individual-participant-data meta-analysis of 239 prospective studies in four continents. Lancet. 2016;388(10046):776–786.
2. Afshin A, Forouzanfar MH, Reitsma MB, et al. Health effects of overweight and obesity in 195 countries over 25 years. N Engl J Med. 2017;377(1):13–27.
3. Kivimäki M, Kuosma E, Ferrie JE, et al. Overweight, obesity, and risk of cardiometabolic multimorbidity: Pooled analysis of individual-level data for 120 813 adults from 16 cohort studies from the USA and Europe. Lancet Public Health. 2017;2(6):e277–e285.
4. GBD 2017 Causes of Death Collaborators. Global, regional, and national age-sex-specific mortality for 282 causes of death in 195 countries and territories, 1980–2017: A systematic analysis for the Global Burden of Disease Study 2017. Lancet. 2018;392(10159):1736–1788.
5. Hales CM, Fryar CD, Carroll MD, Freedman DS, Ogden CL. Trends in obesity and severe obesity prevalence in US youth and adults by sex and age, 2007–2008 to 2015–2016. JAMA. 2018;319(16):1723–1725.
6. Han TS, Correa E, Lean ME, et al. Changes in prevalence of obesity and high waist circumference over four years across European regions: The European male ageing study (EMAS). Endocrine. 2017;55(2):456–469.
7. Pischon T, Boeing H, Hoffmann K, et al. General and abdominal adiposity and risk of death in Europe. N Engl J Med. 2008;359(20):2105–2120.
8. Després JP. Excess visceral adipose tissue/ectopic fat the missing link in the obesity paradox? J Am Coll Cardiol. 2011;57(19):1887–1889.
9. Cerhan JR, Moore SC, Jacobs EJ, et al. A pooled analysis of waist circumference and mortality in 650,000 adults. Mayo Clin Proc. 2014;89(3):335–345.
10. Song X, Jousilahti P, Stehouwer CD, et al. Cardiovascular and all-cause mortality in relation to various anthropometric measures of obesity in Europeans. Nutr Metab Cardiovasc Dis. 2015;25(3):295–304.
11. Jacobs EJ, Newton CC, Wang Y, et al. Waist circumference and all-cause mortality in a large US cohort. Arch Intern Med. 2010;170(15):1293–1301.
12. Adair T, Lopez AD. The role of overweight and obesity in adverse cardiovascular disease mortality trends: An analysis of multiple cause of death data from Australia and the USA. BMC Med. 2020;18(1):199.
13. Sattar N. Gender aspects in type 2 diabetes mellitus and cardiometabolic risk. Best Pract Res Clin Endocrinol Metab. 2013;27(4):501–507.
14. Dai H, Alsalhe TA, Chalghaf N, Riccò M, Bragazzi NL, Wu J. The global burden of disease attributable to high body mass index in 195 countries and territories, 1990–2017: An analysis of the Global Burden of Disease Study. PLoS Med. 2020;17(7):e1003198.
15. Lovejoy JC, Sainsbury A. Sex differences in obesity and the regulation of energy homeostasis. Obes Rev. 2009;10(2):154–167.
16. Faulkner JL, Belin de Chantemèle EJ. Sex hormones, aging and cardio-metabolic syndrome. Biol Sex Differ. 2019;10(1):30.
17. Bhaskaran K, Dos-Santos-Silva I, Leon DA, Douglas IJ, Smeeth L. Association of BMI with overall and cause-specific mortality: A population-based cohort study of 3·6 million adults in the UK. Lancet Diabetes Endocrinol. 2018;6(12):944–953.
18. Vidra N, Trias-Llimos S, Janssen F. Impact of obesity on life expectancy among different European countries: Secondary analysis of population-level data over the 1975–2012 period. BMJ Open. 2019;9(7):e028086.
19. Seidell JC, Verschuren WMM, van Leer EM, Kromhout D. Overweight, underweight, and mortality: A prospective study of 48287 men and women. Arch Intern Med. 1996;156(9):958–963.
20. Kramer FM, Jeffery RW, Forster JL, Snell MK. Long-term follow-up of behavioral treatment for obesity: Patterns of weight regain among men and women. Int J Obes. 1989;13(2):123–136.
21. Pownall HJ, Bray GA, Wagenknecht LE, et al. Changes in body composition over 8 years in a randomized trial of a lifestyle intervention: The look AHEAD study. Obesity (Silver Spring). 2015;23(3):565–572.
22. Navarro G, Allard C, Xu W, Mauvais-Jarvis F. The role of androgens in metabolism, obesity, and diabetes in males and females. Obesity (Silver Spring). 2015;23(4):713–719.
23. Archibald D, Douglas F, Hoddinott P, et al. A qualitative evidence synthesis on the management of male obesity. BMJ Open. 2015;5(10):e008372.
24. Men's Health Forum (UK). How to make weight loss services work for men. Available at https://www.menshealthforum.org.uk/sites/default/files/pdf/how_to_weight_final_lr_1.pdf. Accessed May 10, 2020.
25. Bray GA, Heisel WE, Afshin A, et al. The science of obesity management: An endocrine society scientific statement. Endocr Rev. 2018;39(2):79–132.
26. Garvey WT, Mechanick JI, Brett EM, et al. American Association of Clinical Endocrinologists and American College of Endocrinology comprehensive clinical practice guidelines for medical care of patients with obesity. Endocr Pract. 2016;22 Suppl 3:1–203.
27. Jensen MD, Ryan DH, Apovian CM, et al. 2013 AHA/ACC/TOS guideline for the management of overweight and obesity in adults: A report of the American College of Cardiology/American Heart Association Task Force on practice guidelines and the obesity society. J Am Coll Cardiol. 2014;63(25 Pt B):2985–3023.
28. Carmienke S, Freitag MH, Pischon T, et al. General and abdominal obesity parameters and their combination in relation to mortality: A systematic review and meta-regression analysis. Eur J Clin Nutr. 2013;67(6):573–585.
29. Rohrmann S, Shiels MS, Lopez DS, et al. Body fatness and sex steroid hormone concentrations in US men: Results from NHANES III. Cancer Causes Control. 2011;22(8):1141–1151.
30. Alberti KG, Eckel RH, Grundy SM, et al. Harmonizing the metabolic syndrome: A joint interim statement of the International Diabetes Federation Task Force on Epidemiology and Prevention; National Heart, Lung, and Blood Institute; American Heart Association; World Heart Federation; International Atherosclerosis Society; and International Association for the Study of Obesity. Circulation. 2009;120(16):1640–1645.
31. Sahakyan KR, Somers VK, Rodriguez-Escudero JP, et al. Normal-weight central obesity: Implications for total and cardiovascular mortality. Ann Intern Med. 2015;163(11):827–835.
32. Mainous AG, 3rd, Tanner RJ, Jo A, Anton SD. Prevalence of prediabetes and abdominal obesity among healthy-weight adults: 18-year trend. Ann Fam Med. 2016;14(4):304–310.
33. Mulligan AA, Lentjes MAH, Luben RN, Wareham NJ, Khaw KT. Changes in waist circumference and risk of all-cause and CVD mortality: Results from the European Prospective Investigation into Cancer in Norfolk (EPIC-Norfolk) cohort study. BMC Cardiovasc Disord. 2019;19(1):238.
34. Song X, Jousilahti P, Stehouwer CD, et al. Comparison of various surrogate obesity indicators as predictors of cardiovascular mortality in four European populations. Eur J Clin Nutr. 2013;67(12):1298–1302.
35. Molina-Vega M, Munoz-Garach A, Damas-Fuentes M, Fernandez-Garcia JC, Tinahones FJ. Secondary male hypogonadism: A prevalent but overlooked comorbidity of obesity. Asian J Androl. 2018;20(6):531–538.
36. Kelly DM, Jones TH. Testosterone and obesity. Obes Rev. 2015;16(7):581–606.
37. Travison TG, Araujo AB, Kupelian V, O'Donnell AB, McKinlay JB. The relative contributions of aging, health, and lifestyle factors to serum testosterone decline in men. J Clin Endocrinol Metab. 2007;92(2):549–555.
38. Wu FC, Tajar A, Pye SR, et al. Hypothalamic-pituitary-testicular axis disruptions in older men are differentially linked to age and modifiable risk factors: The European Male Aging Study. J Clin Endocrinol Metab. 2008;93(7):2737–2745.

39. Wu FC, Tajar A, Beynon JM, et al. Identification of late-onset hypogonadism in middle-aged and elderly men. N Engl J Med. 2010; 363(2):123–135.

40. Camacho EM, Huhtaniemi IT, O'Neill TW, et al. Age-associated changes in hypothalamic-pituitary-testicular function in middle-aged and older men are modified by weight change and lifestyle factors: Longitudinal results from the European Male Ageing Study. Eur J Endocrinol. 2013; 168(3):445–455.

41. Corona G, Rastrelli G, Monami M, et al. Body weight loss reverts obesity-associated hypogonadotropic hypogonadism: A systematic review and meta-analysis. Eur J Endocrinol. 2013;168(6):829–843.

42. Saad F, Doros G, Haider KS, Haider A. Differential effects of 11 years of long-term injectable testosterone undecanoate therapy on anthropometric and metabolic parameters in hypogonadal men with normal weight, overweight and obesity in comparison with untreated controls: Real-world data from a controlled registry study. Int J Obes. 2020;44(6): 1264–1278.

43. Eriksson J, Haring R, Grarup N, et al. Causal relationship between obesity and serum testosterone status in men: A bi-directional mendelian randomization analysis. PLoS One. 2017;12(4):e0176277.

44. Ng Tang Fui M, Prendergast LA, Dupuis P, et al. Effects of testosterone treatment on body fat and lean mass in obese men on a hypocaloric diet: A randomised controlled trial. BMC Med. 2016;14(1):153.

45. Ng Tang Fui M, Hoermann R, Prendergast LA, Zajac JD, Grossmann M. Symptomatic response to testosterone treatment in dieting obese men with low testosterone levels in a randomized, placebo-controlled clinical trial. Int J Obes (Lond). 2017;41(3):420–426.

46. Ng Tang Fui M, Hoermann R, Zajac JD, Grossmann M. The effects of testosterone on body composition in obese men are not sustained after cessation of testosterone treatment. Clin Endocrinol (Oxf). 2017;87(4): 336–343.

47. Thirumalai A, Rubinow KB, Cooper LA, et al. Dose-response effects of sex hormone concentrations on body composition and adipokines in medically castrated healthy men administered graded doses of testosterone gel. Clin Endocrinol (Oxf). 2017;87(1):59–67.

48. Finkelstein JS, Lee H, Burnett-Bowie SA, et al. Gonadal steroids and body composition, strength, and sexual function in men. N Engl J Med. 2013; 369(11):1011–1022.

49. Hamilton EJ, Gianatti E, Strauss BJ, et al. Increase in visceral and subcutaneous abdominal fat in men with prostate cancer treated with androgen deprivation therapy. Clin Endocrinol (Oxf). 2011;74(3): 377–383.

50. Chasland LC, Knuiman MW, Divitini ML, et al. Higher circulating androgens and higher physical activity levels are associated with less central adiposity and lower risk of cardiovascular death in older men. Clin Endocrinol (Oxf). 2019;90(2):375–383.

51. Khaw KT, Barrett-Connor E. Lower endogenous androgens predict central adiposity in men. Ann Epidemiol. 1992;2(5):675–682.

52. Tsai EC, Boyko EJ, Leonetti DL, Fujimoto WY. Low serum testosterone level as a predictor of increased visceral fat in Japanese-American men. Int J Obes Relat Metab Disord. 2000;24(4):485–491.

53. Hackett G, Cole N, Mulay A, Strange RC, Ramachandran S. Long-term testosterone therapy in type 2 diabetes is associated with decreasing waist circumference and improving erectile function. World J Mens Health. 2020;38(1):68–77.

54. Yassin A, Haider A, Haider KS, et al. Testosterone therapy in men with hypogonadism prevents progression from prediabetes to type 2 diabetes: Eight-year data from a registry study. Diabetes Care. 2019;6(42): 1104–1111.

55. Saad F, Yassin A, Doros G, Haider A. Effects of long-term treatment with testosterone on weight and waist size in 411 hypogonadal men with obesity classes I-III: Observational data from two registry studies. Int J Obes (Lond). 2016;40(1):162–170.

56. Page ST, Amory JK, Bowman FD, et al. Exogenous testosterone (T) alone or with finasteride increases physical performance, grip strength, and lean body mass in older men with low serum T. J Clin Endocrinol Metab. 2005;90(3):1502–1510.

57. Snyder PJ, Peachey H, Hannoush P, et al. Effect of testosterone treatment on body composition and muscle strength in men over 65 years of age. J Clin Endocrinol Metab. 1999;84(8):2647–2653.

58. Kenny AM, Prestwood KM, Gruman CA, Marcello KM, Raisz LG. Effects of transdermal testosterone on bone and muscle in older men with low

59. bioavailable testosterone levels. J Gerontol A Biol Sci Med Sci. 2001; 56(5):M266–M272.

59. Wittert GA, Chapman IM, Haren MT, Mackintosh S, Coates P, Morley JE. Oral testosterone supplementation increases muscle and decreases fat mass in healthy elderly males with low-normal gonadal status. J Gerontol A Biol Sci Med Sci. 2003;58(7):618–625.

60. Wang C, Swerdloff RS, Iranmanesh A, et al. Transdermal testosterone gel improves sexual function, mood, muscle strength, and body composition parameters in hypogonadal men. J Clin Endocrinol Metab. 2000; 85(8):2839–2853.

61. Sattler F, He J, Chukwuneke J, et al. Testosterone supplementation improves carbohydrate and lipid metabolism in some older men with abdominal obesity. J Gerontol Geriatr Res. 2014;3(3):1000159.

62. Marin P, Holmang S, Gustafsson C, et al. Androgen treatment of abdominally obese men. Obes Res. 1993;1(4):245–251.

63. Marin P, Holmang S, Jonsson L, et al. The effects of testosterone treatment on body composition and metabolism in middle-aged obese men. Int J Obes Relat Metab Disord. 1992;16(12):991–997.

64. Allan CA, Strauss BJ, Burger HG, Forbes EA, McLachlan RI. Testosterone therapy prevents gain in visceral adipose tissue and loss of skeletal muscle in nonobese aging men. J Clin Endocrinol Metab. 2008;93(1): 139–146.

65. Hackett G, Kirby M, Edwards D, et al. British society for sexual medicine guidelines on adult testosterone deficiency, with statements for UK practice. J Sex Med. 2017;14(12):1504–1523.

66. Harman SM, Metter EJ, Tobin JD, Pearson J, Blackman MR. Longitudinal effects of aging on serum total and free testosterone levels in healthy men. Baltimore Longitudinal Study of Aging. J Clin Endocrinol Metab. 2001;86(2):724–731.

67. Feldman HA, Longcope C, Derby CA, et al. Age trends in the level of serum testosterone and other hormones in middle-aged men: Longitudinal results from the Massachusetts male aging study. J Clin Endocrinol Metab. 2002;87(2):589–598.

68. Lapauw B, Goemaere S, Zmierczak H, et al. The decline of serum testosterone levels in community-dwelling men over 70 years of age: Descriptive data and predictors of longitudinal changes. Eur J Endocrinol. 2008;159(4):459–468.

69. Mohr BA, Guay AT, O'Donnell AB, McKinlay JB. Normal, bound and nonbound testosterone levels in normally ageing men: Results from the Massachusetts Male Ageing Study. Clin Endocrinol (Oxf). 2005;62(1): 64–73.

70. Haring R, Ittermann T, Volzke H, et al. Prevalence, incidence and risk factors of testosterone deficiency in a population-based cohort of men: Results from the study of health in Pomerania. Aging Male. 2010;13(4): 247–257.

71. Liu PY, Beilin J, Meier C, et al. Age-related changes in serum testosterone and sex hormone binding globulin in Australian men: Longitudinal analyses of two geographically separate regional cohorts. J Clin Endocrinol Metab. 2007;92(9):3599–3603.

72. Couillard C, Gagnon J, Bergeron J, et al. Contribution of body fatness and adipose tissue distribution to the age variation in plasma steroid hormone concentrations in men: The HERITAGE Family Study. J Clin Endocrinol Metab. 2000;85(3):1026–1031.

73. Hales CM, Carroll MD, Fryar CD, Ogden CL. Prevalence of obesity among adults and youth: United States, 2015–2016. NCHS Data Brief. 2017(288): 1–8.

74. van Hulsteijn LT, Pasquali R, Casanueva F, et al. Prevalence of endocrine disorders in obese patients: Systematic review and meta-analysis. Eur J Endocrinol. 2020;182(1):11–21.

75. Gapstur SM, Gann PH, Kopp P, Colangelo L, Longcope C, Liu K. Serum androgen concentrations in young men: A longitudinal analysis of associations with age, obesity, and race. The CARDIA male hormone study. Cancer Epidemiol Biomarkers Prev. 2002;11(10 Pt 1):1041–1047.

76. Gapstur SM, Kopp P, Gann PH, Chiu BC, Colangelo LA, Liu K. Changes in BMI modulate age-associated changes in sex hormone binding globulin and total testosterone, but not bioavailable testosterone in young adult men: The CARDIA Male Hormone Study. Int J Obes (Lond). 2007;31(4): 685–691.

77. Dhindsa S, Ghanim H, Batra M, Dandona P. Hypogonadotropic hypogonadism in men with diabesity. Diabetes Care. 2018;41(7):1516–1525.

78. Chandel A, Dhindsa S, Topiwala S, Chaudhuri A, Dandona P. Testosterone concentration in young patients with diabetes. Diabetes Care. 2008;31(10):2013–2017.

79. Mogri M, Dhindsa S, Quattrin T, Ghanim H, Dandona P. Testosterone concentrations in young pubertal and post-pubertal obese males. Clin Endocrinol (Oxf). 2013;78(4):593–599.

80. Molina-Vega M, Asenjo-Plaza M, García-Ruiz MC, et al. Cross-sectional, primary care-based study of the prevalence of hypoandrogenemia in nondiabetic young men with obesity. Obesity (Silver Spring). 2019; 27(10):1584–1590.

81. Pellitero S, Olaizola I, Alastrue A, et al. Hypogonadotropic hypogonadism in morbidly obese males is reversed after bariatric surgery. Obes Surg. 2012;22(12):1835–1842.

82. Mulligan T, Frick MF, Zuraw QC, Stemhagen A, McWhirter C. Prevalence of hypogonadism in males aged at least 45 years: The HIM study. Int J Clin Pract. 2006;60(7):762–769.

83. Calderón B, Gómez-Martín JM, Vega-Piñero B, et al. Prevalence of male secondary hypogonadism in moderate to severe obesity and its relationship with insulin resistance and excess body weight. Andrology. 2016;4(1):62–67.

84. Dhindsa S, Miller MG, McWhirter CL, et al. Testosterone concentrations in diabetic and nondiabetic obese men. Diabetes Care. 2010;33(6): 1186–1192.

85. Trabert B, Graubard BI, Nyante SJ, et al. Relationship of sex steroid hormones with body size and with body composition measured by dual-energy X-ray absorptiometry in US men. Cancer Causes Control. 2012;23(12):1881–1891.

86. Francomano D, Lenzi A, Aversa A. Effects of five-year treatment with testosterone undecanoate on metabolic and hormonal parameters in ageing men with metabolic syndrome. Int J Endocrinol. 2014;2014: 527470.

87. Yassin AA, Nettleship J, Almehmadi Y, Salman M, Saad F. Effects of continuous long-term testosterone therapy (TTh) on anthropometric, endocrine and metabolic parameters for up to 10 years in 115 hypogonadal elderly men: Real-life experience from an observational registry study. Andrologia. 2016;48(7):793–799.

88. Haider A, Yassin A, Haider KS, Doros G, Saad F, Rosano GM. Men with testosterone deficiency and a history of cardiovascular diseases benefit from long-term testosterone therapy: Observational, real-life data from a registry study. Vasc Health Risk Manag. 2016;12:251–261.

89. Traish AM, Haider A, Haider KS, Doros G, Saad F. Long-term testosterone therapy improves cardiometabolic function and reduces risk of cardiovascular disease in men with hypogonadism: A real-life observational registry study setting comparing treated and untreated (control) groups. J Cardiovasc Pharmacol Ther. 2017;22(5):414–433.

90. Zitzmann M, Traish A, Kliesch S. Long-term treatment of hypogonadal men: Results from a 9-year-registry J Urol. 2017;197:e1220–e1221.

91. Saad F, Doros G, Haider KS, Haider A. Hypogonadal men with moderate-to-severe lower urinary tract symptoms have a more severe cardiometabolic risk profile and benefit more from testosterone therapy than men with mild lower urinary tract symptoms. Investig Clin Urol. 2018;59(6):399–409.

92. Haider KS, Haider A, Saad F, et al. Remission of type 2 diabetes following long-term treatment with injectable testosterone undecanoate in patients with hypogonadism and type 2 diabetes: 11-year data from a real-world registry study. Diabetes Obes Metab. 2020 [Epub ahead of print]; DOI: 10.1111/dom.14122.

93. Saad F, Caliber M, Doros G, Haider KS, Haider A. Long-term treatment with testosterone undecanoate injections in men with hypogonadism alleviates erectile dysfunction and reduces risk of major adverse cardiovascular events, prostate cancer, and mortality. Aging Male. 2020; 23(1):81–92.

94. Haider A, Meergans U, Traish A, et al. Progressive improvement of T-scores in men with osteoporosis and subnormal serum testosterone levels upon treatment with testosterone over six years. Int J Endocrinol. 2014;2014:496948.

95. Haider A, Zitzmann M, Doros G, Isbarn H, Hammerer P, Yassin A. Incidence of prostate cancer in hypogonadal men receiving testosterone therapy: Observations from five year-median follow-up of three registries. J Urol. 2015;193(1):80–86.

96. O'Connell MD, Roberts SA, Srinivas-Shankar U, et al. Do the effects of testosterone on muscle strength, physical function, body composition, and quality of life persist six months after treatment in intermediate-frail and frail elderly men? J Clin Endocrinol Metab. 2011;96(2):454–458.

97. Francomano D, Bruzziches R, Barbaro G, Lenzi A, Aversa A. Effects of testosterone undecanoate replacement and withdrawal on cardio-metabolic, hormonal and body composition outcomes in severely obese hypogonadal men: A pilot study. J Endocrinol Invest. 2014;37(4):401–411.

98. Yassin A, Almehmadi Y, Saad F, Doros G, Gooren L. Effects of intermission and resumption of long-term testosterone replacement therapy on body weight and metabolic parameters in hypogonadal in middle-aged and elderly men. Clin Endocrinol (Oxf). 2016;84(1):107–114.

99. Yassin A, Nettleship JE, Talib RA, Almehmadi Y, Doros G. Effects of testosterone replacement therapy withdrawal and re-treatment in hypogonadal elderly men upon urinary, voiding function and prostate safety parameters. Aging Male. 2016;19(1):64–69.

100. Morgunov LY, Denisova IA, Rozhkova TI, Stakhovskaya LV, Skvortsova VI. Hypogonadism and its treatment following ischaemic stroke in men with type 2 diabetes mellitus. Aging Male. 2020;23(1):71–80.

101. Hackett G, Cole N, Bhartia M, et al. The response to testosterone undecanoate in men with type 2 diabetes is dependent on achieving threshold serum levels (the BLAST study). Int J Clin Pract. 2014;68(2): 203–215.

102. Sattler F, Bhasin S, He J, et al. Testosterone threshold levels and lean tissue mass targets needed to enhance skeletal muscle strength and function: The HORMA trial. J Gerontol A Biol Sci Med Sci. 2011; 66(1):122–129.

103. Permpongkosol S, Khupulsup K, Leelaphiwat S, Pavavattananusorn S, Thongpradit S, Petchthong T. Effects of 8-year treatment of long-acting testosterone undecanoate on metabolic parameters, urinary symptoms, bone mineral density, and sexual function in men with late-onset hypogonadism. J Sex Med. 2016;13(8):1199–1211.

104. Sharma R, Oni OA, Gupta K, et al. Normalization of testosterone level is associated with reduced incidence of myocardial infarction and mortality in men. Eur Heart J. 2015;36(40):2706–2715.

105. Sharma R, Oni OA, Gupta K, et al. Normalization of testosterone levels after testosterone replacement therapy is associated with decreased incidence of atrial fibrillation. J Am Heart Assoc. 2017;6(5): e004880.

106. Oni OA, Dehkordi SHH, Jazayeri MA, et al. Relation of testosterone normalization to mortality and myocardial infarction in men with previous myocardial infarction. Am J Cardiol. 2019;124(8):1171–1178.

107. Saad F, Aversa A, Isidori AM, Zafalon L, Zitzmann M, Gooren L. Onset of effects of testosterone treatment and time span until maximum effects are achieved. Eur J Endocrinol. 2011;165(5):675–685.

108. Caliber M, Hackett G. Important lessons about testosterone therapy-weight loss vs. testosterone therapy for symptom resolution, classical vs. functional hypogonadism, and shortterm vs. lifelong testosterone therapy. Aging Male. 2019 [Epub ahead of print]; DOI: 10.1080/13685538.2018.1549211.

109. Franz MJ, VanWormer JJ, Crain AL, et al. Weight-loss outcomes: A systematic review and meta-analysis of weight-loss clinical trials with a minimum 1-year follow-up. J Am Diet Assoc. 2007;107(10): 1755–1767.

110. Douketis JD, Macie C, Thabane L, Williamson DF. Systematic review of long-term weight loss studies in obese adults: Clinical significance and applicability to clinical practice. Int J Obes (Lond). 2005;29(10): 1153–1167.

111. Anderson JW, Vichitbandra S, Qian W, Kryscio RJ. Long-term weight maintenance after an intensive weight-loss program. J Am Coll Nutr. 1999;18(6):620–627.

112. Curioni CC, Lourenço PM. Long-term weight loss after diet and exercise: A systematic review. Int J Obes (Lond). 2005;29(10):1168–1174.

113. Anderson JW, Konz EC, Frederich RC, Wood CL. Long-term weight-loss maintenance: A meta-analysis of US studies. Am J Clin Nutr. 2001;74(5): 579–584.

114. Yanovski SZ, Yanovski JA. Long-term drug treatment for obesity: A systematic and clinical review. JAMA. 2014;311(1):74–86.

115. Khera R, Murad MH, Chandar AK, et al. Association of pharmacological treatments for obesity with weight loss and adverse events: A systematic review and meta-analysis. JAMA. 2016;315(22):2424–2434.

116. Look Ahead Research Group. Long-term effects of a lifestyle intervention on weight and cardiovascular risk factors in individuals with type 2

diabetes mellitus: Four-year results of the Look AHEAD trial. Arch Intern Med. 2010;170(17):1566–1575.

117. MacLean PS, Wing RR, Davidson T, et al. NIH working group report: Innovative research to improve maintenance of weight loss. Obesity (Silver Spring). 2015;23(1):7–15.

118. Fischer M, Oberänder N, Weimann A. Four main barriers to weight loss maintenance? A quantitative analysis of difficulties experienced by obese patients after successful weight reduction. Eur J Clin Nutr. 2020; 74(8):1192–1200.

119. Nordmo M, Danielsen YS, Nordmo M. The challenge of keeping it off, a descriptive systematic review of high-quality, follow-up studies of obesity treatments. Obes Rev. 2020;21(1):e12949.

120. Mathus-Vliegen EM. Long-term maintenance of weight loss with sibutramine in a GP setting following a specialist guided very-low-calorie diet: A double-blind, placebo-controlled, parallel group study. Eur J Clin Nutr. 2005;59 Suppl 1:S31–S38; discussion S39.

121. Funk MD, Lee M, Vidoni ML, Reininger BM. Weight loss and weight gain among participants in a community-based weight loss challenge. BMC Obes. 2019;6:2.

122. Sjöström L. Review of the key results from the Swedish Obese Subjects (SOS) trial—A prospective controlled intervention study of bariatric surgery. J Intern Med. 2013;273(3):219–234.

123. O'Brien PE, Hindle A, Brennan L, et al. Long-term outcomes after bariatric surgery: A systematic review and meta-analysis of weight loss at 10 or more years for all bariatric procedures and a single-centre review of 20-year outcomes after adjustable gastric banding. Obes Surg. 2019; 29(1):3–14.

124. Courcoulas AP, King WC, Belle SH, et al. Seven-year weight trajectories and health outcomes in the longitudinal assessment of bariatric surgery (LABS) study. JAMA Surg. 2018;153(5):427–434.

125. Jans A, Näslund I, Ottosson J, Szabo E, Näslund E, Stenberg E. Duration of type 2 diabetes and remission rates after bariatric surgery in Sweden 2007–2015: A registry-based cohort study. PLoS Med. 2019;16(11): e1002985.

126. Pessoa BM, Browning MG, Mazzini GS, et al. Factors mediating type 2 diabetes remission and relapse after gastric bypass surgery. J Am Coll Surg. 2020;230(1):7–16.

127. Marks BL, Rippe JM. The importance of fat free mass maintenance in weight loss programmes. Sports Med. 1996;22(5):273–281.

128. Soltani S, Hunter GR, Kazemi A, Shab-Bidar S. The effects of weight loss approaches on bone mineral density in adults: A systematic review and meta-analysis of randomized controlled trials. Osteoporos Int. 2016; 27(9):2655–2671.

129. Ensrud KE, Fullman RL, Barrett-Connor E, et al. Voluntary weight reduction in older men increases hip bone loss: The osteoporotic fractures in men study. J Clin Endocrinol Metab. 2005;90(4):1998–2004.

130. Guney E, Kisakol G, Ozgen G, Yilmaz C, Yilmaz R, Kabalak T. Effect of weight loss on bone metabolism: Comparison of vertical banded gastroplasty and medical intervention. Obes Surg. 2003;13(3):383–388.

131. Waters DL, Vawter R, Qualls C, Chode S, Armamento-Villareal R, Villareal DT. Long-term maintenance of weight loss after lifestyle intervention in frail, obese older adults. J Nutr Health Aging. 2013;17(1):3–7.

132. Langlois JA, Visser M, Davidovic LS, Maggi S, Li G, Harris TB. Hip fracture risk in older white men is associated with change in body weight from age 50 years to old age. Arch Intern Med. 1998;158(9): 990–996.

133. Komorita Y, Iwase M, Fujii H, et al. Impact of body weight loss from maximum weight on fragility bone fractures in Japanese patients with type 2 diabetes: The Fukuoka Diabetes Registry. Diabetes Care. 2018; 41(5):1061.

134. Ensrud KE, Lewis CE, Lambert LC, et al. Endogenous sex steroids, weight change and rates of hip bone loss in older men: The MrOS study. Osteoporos Int. 2006;17(9):1329–1336.

135. Mellström D, Johnell O, Ljunggren O, et al. Free testosterone is an independent predictor of BMD and prevalent fractures in elderly men: MrOS Sweden. J Bone Miner Res. 2006;21(4):529–535.

136. Maghrabi AH, Wolski K, Abood B, et al. Two-year outcomes on bone density and fracture incidence in patients with T2DM randomized to bariatric surgery versus intensive medical therapy. Obesity (Silver Spring). 2015;23(12):2344–2348.

137. Hansen S, Jørgensen NR, Hermann AP, Støving RK. Continuous decline in bone mineral density and deterioration of bone microarchitecture 7 years after Roux-en-Y gastric bypass surgery. Eur J Endocrinol. 2020; 182(3):303–311.

138. Ablett AD, Boyle BR, Avenell A. Fractures in adults after weight loss from bariatric surgery and weight management programs for obesity: Systematic review and meta-analysis. Obes Surg. 2019;29(4):1327–1342.

139. Zhang Q, Chen Y, Li J, et al. A meta-analysis of the effects of bariatric surgery on fracture risk. Obes Rev. 2018;19(5):728–736.

140. Khalid SI, Omotosho PA, Spagnoli A, Torquati A. Association of bariatric surgery with risk of fracture in patients with severe obesity. JAMA Netw Open. 2020;3(6):e207419.

141. Snyder PJ, Kopperdahl DL, Stephens-Shields AJ, et al. Effect of testosterone treatment on volumetric bone density and strength in older men with low testosterone: A controlled clinical trial. JAMA Intern Med. 2017;177(4):471–479.

142. Ng Tang Fui M, Hoermann R, Nolan B, Clarke M, Zajac JD, Grossmann M. Effect of testosterone treatment on bone remodelling markers and mineral density in obese dieting men in a randomized clinical trial. Sci Rep. 2018;8(1):9099.

143. Jensen MD, Ryan DH, Apovian CM, et al. 2013 AHA/ACC/TOS guideline for the management of overweight and obesity in adults: A report of the American College of Cardiology/American Heart Association Task Force on Practice Guidelines and The Obesity Society. Circulation. 2014; 129(25 Suppl 2):S102–S138.

144. Gadde KM, Allison DB, Ryan DH, et al. Effects of low-dose, controlled-release, phentermine plus topiramate combination on weight and associated comorbidities in overweight and obese adults (CONQUER): A randomised, placebo-controlled, phase 3 trial. Lancet. 2011;377(9774): 1341–1352.

145. Pi-Sunyer X, Astrup A, Fujioka K, et al. A randomized, controlled trial of 3.0 mg of liraglutide in weight management. N Engl J Med. 2015; 373(1):11–22.

146. Smith SR, Weissman NJ, Anderson CM, et al. Multicenter, placebo-controlled trial of lorcaserin for weight management. N Engl J Med. 2010;363(3):245–256.

147. Greenway FL, Fujioka K, Plodkowski RA, et al. Effect of naltrexone plus bupropion on weight loss in overweight and obese adults (COR-I): A multicentre, randomised, double-blind, placebo-controlled, phase 3 trial. Lancet. 2010;376(9741):595–605.

148. Stubbs RJ, Morris L, Pallister C, Horgan G, Lavin JH. Weight outcomes audit in 1.3 million adults during their first 3 months' attendance in a commercial weight management programme. BMC Public Health. 2015; 15:882.

149. Colman E. Food and Drug Administration's obesity drug guidance document: A short history. Circulation. 2012;125(17):2156–2164.

150. Dhindsa S, Ghanim H, Batra M, et al. Insulin resistance and inflammation in hypogonadotropic hypogonadism and their reduction after testosterone replacement in men with type 2 diabetes. Diabetes Care. 2016; 39(1):82–91.

151. Wolfe RR. The underappreciated role of muscle in health and disease. Am J Clin Nutr. 2006;84(3):475–482.

152. Prior BM, Modlesky CM, Evans EM, et al. Muscularity and the density of the fat-free mass in athletes. J Appl Physiol (1985). 2001;90(4): 1523–1531.

153. Dulloo AG, Jacquet J, Miles-Chan JL, Schutz Y. Passive and active roles of fat-free mass in the control of energy intake and body composition regulation. Eur J Clin Nutr. 2017;71(3):353–357.

154. Bano G, Pigozzo S, Piovesan F, et al. Influence of serum 25-hydroxyvitamin D levels, fat-free mass, and fat mass on bone density, geometry and strength, in healthy young and elderly adults. Exp Gerontol. 2018;113:193–198.

155. Trombetti A, Reid KF, Hars M, et al. Age-associated declines in muscle mass, strength, power, and physical performance: Impact on fear of falling and quality of life. Osteoporos Int. 2016;27(2): 463–471.

156. Park BS, Yoon JS. Relative skeletal muscle mass is associated with development of metabolic syndrome. Diabetes Metab J. 2013;37(6): 458–464.

157. Kim G, Lee SE, Lee YB, et al. Relationship between relative skeletal muscle mass and nonalcoholic fatty liver disease: A 7-year longitudinal study. Hepatology. 2018;68(5):1755–1768.

158. Kalyani RR, Metter EJ, Xue QL, et al. The relationship of lean body mass with aging to the development of diabetes. J Endocr Soc. 2020;4(7):bvaa043.

159. Srikanthan P, Karlamangla AS. Muscle mass index as a predictor of longevity in older adults. Am J Med. 2014;127(6):547–553.

160. Wannamethee SG, Shaper AG, Lennon L, Whincup PH. Decreased muscle mass and increased central adiposity are independently related to mortality in older men. Am J Clin Nutr. 2007;86(5):1339–1346.

161. Bigaard J, Frederiksen K, Tjonneland A, et al. Body fat and fat-free mass and all-cause mortality. Obes Res. 2004;12(7):1042–1049.

162. Chuang SY, Chang HY, Lee MS, Chia-Yu Chen R, Pan WH. Skeletal muscle mass and risk of death in an elderly population. Nutr Metab Cardiovasc Dis. 2014;24(7):784–791.

163. Graf CE, Herrmann FR, Spoerri A, et al. Impact of body composition changes on risk of all-cause mortality in older adults. Clin Nutr. 2016;35(6):1499–1505.

164. Heymsfield SB, Gonzalez MC, Shen W, Redman L, Thomas D. Weight loss composition is one-fourth fat-free mass: A critical review and critique of this widely cited rule. Obes Rev. 2014;15(4):310–321.

165. Schwingshackl L, Dias S, Hoffmann G. Impact of long-term lifestyle programmes on weight loss and cardiovascular risk factors in overweight/obese participants: A systematic review and network meta-analysis. Syst Rev. 2014;3:130.

166. Chaston TB, Dixon JB, O'Brien PE. Changes in fat-free mass during significant weight loss: A systematic review. Int J Obes (Lond). 2007;31(5):743–750.

167. Davidson LE, Yu W, Goodpaster BH, et al. Fat-free mass and skeletal muscle mass five years after bariatric surgery. Obesity (Silver Spring). 2018;26(7):1130–1136.

168. Valera-Mora ME, Simeoni B, Gagliardi L, et al. Predictors of weight loss and reversal of comorbidities in malabsorptive bariatric surgery. Am J Clin Nutr. 2005;81(6):1292–1297.

169. Friedrich AE, Damms-Machado A, Meile T, et al. Laparoscopic sleeve gastrectomy compared to a multidisciplinary weight loss program for obesity—effects on body composition and protein status. Obes Surg. 2013;23(12):1957–1965.

170. Skinner JW, Otzel DM, Bowser A, et al. Muscular responses to testosterone replacement vary by administration route: A systematic review and meta-analysis. J Cachexia Sarcopenia Muscle. 2018;9(3):465–481.

171. Niskanen L, Laaksonen DE, Punnonen K, Mustajoki P, Kaukua J, Rissanen A. Changes in sex hormone-binding globulin and testosterone during weight loss and weight maintenance in abdominally obese men with the metabolic syndrome. Diabetes Obes Metab. 2004;6(3):208–215.

172. Heufelder AE, Saad F, Bunck MC, Gooren L. Fifty-two-week treatment with diet and exercise plus transdermal testosterone reverses the metabolic syndrome and improves glycemic control in men with newly diagnosed type 2 diabetes and subnormal plasma testosterone. J Androl. 2009;30(6):726–733.

173. Hoyos CM, Yee BJ, Phillips CL, Machan EA, Grunstein RR, Liu PY. Body compositional and cardiometabolic effects of testosterone therapy in obese men with severe obstructive sleep apnoea: A randomised placebo-controlled trial. Eur J Endocrinol. 2012;167(4):531–541.

174. Katznelson L, Robinson MW, Coyle CL, Lee H, Farrell CE. Effects of modest testosterone supplementation and exercise for 12 weeks on body composition and quality of life in elderly men. Eur J Endocrinol. 2006;155(6):867–875.

175. Hildreth KL, Barry DW, Moreau KL, et al. Effects of testosterone and progressive resistance exercise in healthy, highly functioning older men with low-normal testosterone levels. J Clin Endocrinol Metab. 2013;98(5):1891–1900.

176. Glintborg D, Vaegter HB, Christensen LL, et al. Testosterone replacement therapy of opioid-induced male hypogonadism improved body composition but not pain perception: A double-blind, randomized, and placebo-controlled trial. Eur J Endocrinol. 2020;182(6):539–548.

177. Aversa A, Bruzziches R, Francomano D, et al. Effects of testosterone undecanoate on cardiovascular risk factors and atherosclerosis in middle-aged men with late-onset hypogonadism and metabolic syndrome: Results from a 24-month, randomized, double-blind, placebo-controlled study. J Sex Med. 2010;7(10):3495–3503.

178. Permpongkosol S, Tantirangsee N, Ratana-olarn K. Treatment of 161 men with symptomatic late onset hypogonadism with long-acting parenteral testosterone undecanoate: Effects on body composition, lipids, and psychosexual complaints. J Sex Med. 2010;7(11):3765–3774.

179. Corona G, Giagulli VA, Maseroli E, et al. Testosterone supplementation and body composition: Results from a meta-analysis study. Eur J Endocrinol. 2016;174(3):R99–R116.

180. Hackett G, Cole N, Bhartia M, Kennedy D, Raju J, Wilkinson P. Testosterone replacement therapy improves metabolic parameters in hypogonadal men with type 2 diabetes but not in men with coexisting depression: The BLAST study. J Sex Med. 2014;11(3):840–856.

181. Groti Antonič K, Antonič B, Žuran I, Pfeifer M. Testosterone treatment longer than 1 year shows more effects on functional hypogonadism and related metabolic, vascular, diabetic and obesity parameters (results of the 2-year clinical trial). Aging Male. 2020 [Epub ahead of print]; DOI: 10.1080/13685538.2020.1793132.

182. Groti K, Zuran I, Antonic B, Forsnaric L, Pfeifer M. The impact of testosterone replacement therapy on glycemic control, vascular function, and components of the metabolic syndrome in obese hypogonadal men with type 2 diabetes. Aging Male. 2018;21(3):158–169.

183. Kelly DM, Jones TH. Testosterone: A metabolic hormone in health and disease. J Endocrinol. 2013;217(3):R25–R45.

184. Corona G, Giagulli VA, Maseroli E, et al. Testosterone supplementation and body composition: Results from a meta-analysis of observational studies. J Endocrinol Invest. 2016;39(9):967–981.

185. Sørensen TIA, Frederiksen P, Heitmann BL. Levels and changes in body mass index decomposed into fat and fat-free mass index: Relation to long-term all-cause mortality in the general population. Int J Obes (Lond). 2020 [Epub ahead of print]; DOI: 10.1038/s41366-020-0613-8.

186. Howard EE, Margolis LM, Berryman CE, et al. Testosterone supplementation up-regulates androgen receptor expression and translational capacity during severe energy deficit. Am J Physiol Endocrinol Metab. 2020 [Epub ahead of print]; DOI: 10.1152/ajpendo.00157.2020.

187. Singal AG, Higgins PD, Waljee AK. A primer on effectiveness and efficacy trials. Clin Transl Gastroenterol. 2014;5(1):e45.

188. Cohen AT, Goto S, Schreiber K, Torp-Pedersen C. Why do we need observational studies of everyday patients in the real-life setting? Eur Heart J Suppl. 2015;17(suppl D):D2–D8.

189. Cox JL, Pieper K. Harnessing the power of real-life data. Eur Heart J Suppl. 2015;17(suppl_D):D9–D14.

190. Hall KD, Sanghvi A, Göbel B. Proportional Feedback Control of Energy Intake During Obesity Pharmacotherapy. Obesity (Silver Spring). 2017;25(12):2088–2091.

191. Ward ZJ, Bleich SN, Cradock AL, et al. Projected U.S. state-level prevalence of adult obesity and severe obesity. N Engl J Med. 2019;381(25):2440–2450.

192. Williamson K, Nimegeer A, Lean M. Rising prevalence of BMI ≥40 kg/m(2): A high-demand epidemic needing better documentation. Obes Rev. 2020;21(4):e12986.

193. Fildes A, Charlton J, Rudisill C, Littlejohns P, Prevost AT, Gulliford MC. Probability of an obese person attaining normal body weight: Cohort study using electronic health records. Am J Public Health. 2015;105(9):e54–e59.

194. Gómez-Ambrosi J, Andrada P, Valentí V, et al. Dissociation of body mass index, excess weight loss and body fat percentage trajectories after 3 years of gastric bypass: Relationship with metabolic outcomes. Int J Obes (Lond). 2017;41(9):1379–1387.

195. Sherf-Dagan S, Zelber-Sagi S, Buch A, et al. Prospective longitudinal trends in body composition and clinical outcomes 3 years following sleeve gastrectomy. Obes Surg. 2019;29(12):3833–3841.

196. Toro-Ramos T, Goodpaster BH, Janumala I, et al. Continued loss in visceral and intermuscular adipose tissue in weight-stable women following bariatric surgery. Obesity (Silver Spring). 2015;23(1):62–69.

197. Wang C, Cunningham G, Dobs A, et al. Long-term testosterone gel (AndroGel) treatment maintains beneficial effects on sexual function and mood, lean and fat mass, and bone mineral density in hypogonadal men. J Clin Endocrinol Metab. 2004;89(5):2085–2098.

198. Jardi F, Laurent MR, Kim N, et al. Testosterone boosts physical activity in male mice via dopaminergic pathways. Sci Rep. 2018;8(1):957.

199. Amanatkar HR, Chibnall JT, Seo BW, Manepalli JN, Grossberg GT. Impact of exogenous testosterone on mood: A systematic review and meta-analysis of randomized placebo-controlled trials. Ann Clin Psychiatry. 2014;26(1):19–32.

200. Spitzer M, Basaria S, Travison TG, Davda MN, DeRogatis L, Bhasin S. The effect of testosterone on mood and well-being in men with erectile dysfunction in a randomized, placebo-controlled trial. Andrology. 2013; 1(3):475–482.

201. Wang C, Alexander G, Berman N, et al. Testosterone replacement therapy improves mood in hypogonadal men—A clinical research center study. J Clin Endocrinol Metab. 1996;81(10):3578–3583.

202. Jockenhovel F, Minnemann T, Schubert M, et al. Comparison of long-acting testosterone undecanoate formulation versus testosterone enanthate on sexual function and mood in hypogonadal men. Eur J Endocrinol. 2009;160(5):815–819.

203. Jockenhovel F, Minnemann T, Schubert M, et al. Timetable of effects of testosterone administration to hypogonadal men on variables of sex and mood. Aging Male. 2009;12(4):113–118.

204. O'Connor DB, Archer J, Wu FC. Effects of testosterone on mood, aggression, and sexual behavior in young men: A double-blind, placebo-controlled, cross-over study. J Clin Endocrinol Metab. 2004;89(6):2837–2845.

205. Saad F, Aversa A, Isidori AM, Gooren LJ. Testosterone as potential effective therapy in treatment of obesity in men with testosterone deficiency: A review. Curr Diabetes Rev. 2012;8(2):131–143.

206. Kalinchenko SY, Tishova YA, Mskhalaya GJ, Gooren LJ, Giltay EJ, Saad F. Effects of testosterone supplementation on markers of the metabolic syndrome and inflammation in hypogonadal men with the metabolic syndrome: The double-blinded placebo-controlled Moscow study. Clin Endocrinol (Oxf). 2010;73(5):602–612.

207. Frühbeck G, Toplak H, Woodward E, Yumuk V, Maislos M, Oppert JM. Obesity: The gateway to ill health—An EASO position statement on a rising public health, clinical and scientific challenge in Europe. Obesity facts. 2013;6(2):117–120.

Abbreviations Used

AHEAD = Action for Health in Diabetes
BMD = bone mineral density
BMI = body mass index
CARDIA = Coronary Artery Risk Development in Young Adults
CI = confidence interval
CIMT = carotid intima-media thickness
CV = cardiovascular
CVD = cardiovascular disease
DALYs = disability-adjusted life years
DPE = diet plus exercise
ED = erectile dysfunction
EMAS = European Male Aging Study
FFM = fat-free mass
FMD = flow mediated dilatation
HbA$_{1c}$ = hemoglobin A1c
HDL = high-density lipoprotein cholesterol
HOMA-IR = Homeostatic Model Assessment of Insulin Resistance
HORMA = Hormonal Regulators of Muscle and Metabolism in Aging
HR = hazard ratio
IIEF-EF = International Index of Erectile Function, Erectile Function Domain
ILI = intensive lifestyle intervention
LAGB = laparoscopic adjustable gastric banding
LDL = low-density lipoprotein cholesterol
MetS = metabolic syndrome
MI = myocardial infarction
MMAS = Massachusetts Male Aging Study
MrOS = Osteoporotic Fractures in Men
PCa = prostate cancer
RCT = randomized controlled trial
RWE = real-world evidence
RYGB = roux-en-Y gastric bypass
T2DM = type 2 diabetes mellitus
TD = testosterone deficiency
TEAAM = Testosterone's Effects on Atherosclerosis Progression in Aging Men
TTh = testosterone therapy
WC = waist circumference

13

Design and Conduct of a Real-World Single-Center Registry Study on Testosterone Therapy of Men with Hypogonadism

Karim Sultan Haider,[1] Ahmad Haider,[1] Gheorghe Doros,[2] and Farid Saad[3,4,*]

Abstract

Aims: Despite the prevalence of hypogonadism (testosterone deficiency [TD]) and widespread use of testosterone therapy (TTh), the effectiveness and safety of long-term testosterone use remains highly contested. Over the past 15 years, we have conducted a registry study of men with TD with a focus on several health outcomes associated with TTh.

Design: Observational patient disease registry study.

Materials and Methods: Noninterventional disease registry with prospective longitudinal data on a large sample of adult hypogonadal men ($n = 858$) who were treated in a single Urology Clinic. The registry evaluates men with symptomatic TD during a urological exam of patients who have not been previously treated with TTh. There were no inclusion/exclusion criteria. All hormone assays are carried out in a single laboratory. Standard-of-care treatment of each patient is the sole responsibility of the attending clinician. The registry data consist of comprehensive medical records and questionnaire data collected during patient visits. The registry has a dedicated statistician to ensure adequate statistical analyses of all outcome measures assessed.

Main Outcome Measures: We measured the following parameters: height, weight, waist circumference, hemoglobin, hematocrit, fasting glucose, glycated hemoglobin, insulin, systolic and diastolic blood pressure, heart rate, lipids (total cholesterol, low-density lipoprotein, high-density lipoprotein, triglycerides), highly sensitive C-reactive protein, and total testosterone (T). We assessed quality of life, erectile and urinary function. Clinical parameters were measured two to four times a year. Data are analyzed in regular intervals.

Results: As of 2019, 858 men have been enrolled, of whom 85 patients exhibited primary hypogonadism, and the remaining 773 exhibited secondary or functional hypogonadism. Findings from this registry study on the benefit of TTh on anthropometric parameters, cardiometabolic function, diabetes, and prostate health have been reported.

Conclusions: This registry study has provided real-world clinical evidence and produced new important findings regarding the effectiveness and safety of long-term TTh in hypogonadal men.

Keywords: hypogonadism; real-world evidence; long-term therapy; testosterone; observational study

[1]Private Urology Practice, Bremerhaven, Germany.
[2]Department of Epidemiology and Biostatistics, Boston University School of Public Health, Boston, Massachusetts, USA.
[3]Gulf Medical University School of Medicine, Ajman, United Arab Emirates.
[4]Dresden International University, Dresden, Germany.

*Address correspondence to: Farid Saad, DVM, PhD, Hinsbleek 1, Hamburg 22391, Germany, Email: farid.saad@bayer.com

Introduction

Clinical evidence suggests that testosterone therapy (TTh) is a long-term, if not lifelong, treatment. Although a number of randomized controlled trials (RCTs) have been carried out in hypogondal men receiving TTh, most of these trials are of very short duration ranging from 1 to 36 months.[1] To date, there are only three prospective RCTs with a duration of 3 years.[2–4] Two of those clinical trials were not restricted to hypogonadal men,[2,4] and one trial included a group of men receiving a combination of T and finasteride, and only 24 men each received testosterone (T) or placebo.[3] Other long-term studies with 42 and 60 months' duration were not placebo-controlled.[5,6]

Many RCTs on TTh screen a large number of men, exceeding thousands of patients, in their recruitment process after establishing substantial lists of inclusion and exclusion criteria. This results in exclusion of thousands of patients producing study populations that significantly differ from the patient populations often presenting in physicians' offices and clinics in their everyday practice.

Although RCTs are considered the gold standard of clinical research, they are not entirely free from all forms of bias.[7] In addition, the high associated costs of long-term RCTs, especially those that are expected to recruit a large number of patients, make such trials prohibitive to execute, and therefore, such trials have yet to surface in the TTh field.

Recently, increased attention has focused on observational, so-called "real-life" or "real-world" studies reflecting daily clinical practice.[8] Indeed, relevant clinical information had been attained from large observational studies that had contributed to the advancement of clinical research. Such trials provide additional knowledge to RCTs.

In the early 2000s, urologists became aware of the concept of the metabolic syndrome, a cluster of cardiometabolic risk factors, since they are managing patients with such risk factors. In fact, the relationship between metabolic syndrome and androgen deficiency was recognized as early as 1990.[9] Further, studies conducted in the field of erectile dysfunction (ED) that were triggered by the introduction of phosphodiesterase type 5 inhibitors showed that ED was an early predictor of cardiovascular events.[10]

The absence of long-term RCTs in hypogonadal men to investigate the effects of long-term TTh and the concept that TTh requires a long duration to produce the expected clinical outcomes due to the pathophysiology of hypogonadism and the remodeling and repair in response to androgen treatment necessitated new approaches to investigating TTh in men with TD. Our registry study was initiated in 2004 with the objective of investigating long-term effectiveness and safety of a novel depot injection of testosterone undecanoate (TU) in otherwise unselected, adult patients with symptomatic hypogonadism. Patients were considered symptomatic if they had at least moderate symptoms on the Aging Males' Symptoms (AMS) Scale[11] and T levels below 12.1 nmol/L. At that time, it had became routine in our urological office to also measure parameters that may not always be assessed by urologists but were related to the metabolic syndrome (e.g., weight, waist circumference [WC], body mass index [BMI], lipid profiles, glucose levels, and insulin), a common condition in the vast majority of our patients. In this communication, we wish to provide details of our registry study and summaries of major findings reported from this registry.

There is an ongoing discussion about testosterone deficiency (TD) due to organic (classical or pathological) hypogonadism arising from disorders of the hypothalamus, pituitary, or testes, or functional hypogonadism due to obesity and comorbidities.[12] Whether this is clinically relevant or an academic discussion remains to be seen. There is recent evidence suggesting that obesity may lead to hypothalamic inflammation,[13] which, in turn, leads to suppression of testosterone production.[14] This would mean that functional hypogonadism is in reality secondary hypogonadism. Zitzmann et al. have shown that there is little difference in response to TTh regardless of whether a patient is diagnosed with primary, secondary, or functional hypogonadism.[15]

Materials and Methods

The "Ethical guidelines as formulated by the German 'Ärztekammer' (the German Medical Association) for observational studies in patients receiving standard treatment" were followed. After receiving a detailed and informative explanation regarding the nature and the purpose of the study, all subjects provided written consent, regardless whether or not they decide for TTh.

Patients who displayed or reported symptoms or who requested to have their testosterone levels measured are routinely screened for TD (hypogonadism). Men with two total testosterone measurements ≤12.1 nmol/L (350 ng/mL) were informed about their laboratory results during a personal consultation. They are then offered treatment and informed about different testosterone preparations, including transdermal gels and short-acting injections. The majority of patients opted for treatment with TU 1000 mg injections (Nebido®; Bayer AG, Berlin, Germany) in 12-week intervals after an initial 6-week interval as one of the treatment options.

All patients were informed that they had the option to receive or not receive testosterone medication based on their own level of understanding of the benefits of this medication to their overall health. Patients were encouraged to continue to follow up with their urologist to treat their urological complaints and/or routine check-ups, irrespective of the choice to receive or not to receive TTh. The patients were given ample time to think through which option to choose or to consider obtaining a second opinion before their next appointment. Patients who opted to undergo TTh made their decision based on a number of reasons, including well-known effects of TTh on increased vitality, energy and sexual function, as well as improved mood. More recently, an increasing number of patients with type 2 diabetes were referred to our clinic by a local diabetes center after they had seen beneficial changes in many of their patients receiving testosterone at our clinic. Additional referrals come from local orthopedists who refer patients with osteoporosis, especially younger men, with a suspicion of hypogonadism. Most patients in our clinic opted for TU 1000 mg injectable over transdermal gels for convenience, as it is only one injection every quarter instead of daily self-administration.

Patients who opted not to be treated with testosterone were concerned about adverse cardiovascular effects of testosterone, the increased risk for prostate cancer, as well as negative effects on liver metabolism, in many cases after consultation with their general practitioners (GPs). Most patients presenting with hypogonadal symptoms exhibited overweight, obesity, and/or poor lifestyle habits. These patients are encouraged to improve their lifestyles and start exercising through an eductional program that was devised for this study. Patients were provided with an educational pamphlet (Supplementary Appendix SA1), including exercise suggestions as well as dietary recommendations and daily routine recommendations.

Patients were asked to fill and complete the following three questionnaires:

1. The AMS scale.[16]
2. The International Prostate Symptom Score (IPSS).[17]

3. The International Index of Erectile Function—Erectile Function Domain (IIEF-EF 5 + 1).[18]

At each visit, all patients are asked to complete a form for current changes in their medication, medical incidences, or other major events that have occurred since their last visits. In addition, blood pressure (BP) and heart rate are measured in each patient. Blood samples are taken from each patient and sent to a commercial laboratory (Synlab, Hamburg, Germany). The parameters are measured, and the methods are summarized in Table 1. Urine samples are also obtained from each patient. Weight and WC are measured in each patient. All patients receive an ultrasound examination (Samsung Ultrasound System H60) of the kidneys, testes, and the bladder, including measurement of residual bladder voiding volume and suprapubically of the prostate. If the ultrasound is unable to calculate the testes volume, a Prader orchidometer is used to estimate the testicular volume. A digital rectal examination (DRE) followed by a transrectal ultrasound examination of the prostate are performed in each patient. TU (1000 mg) injection is administered in the clinic by slowly injecting the medication with a duration of at least 3 min, administered by use of a 20G needle into the relaxed gluteus medius muscle of the patient. The length of the needle is usually 40 mm; however, in very obese patients, we may select a needle with a 60 or 70 mm length. The patient can choose between receiving the injection in a recumbent position and in a standing position with the leg on the injection side slightly bent to relax the gluteal muscle. The injection area is then gently massaged for about 15 sec. There is a 100% adherence to TTh, as every single injection is applied in our office and documented accordingly. TTh was temporarily interrupted in patients diagnosed with prostate cancer, but it resumed between 1 and 3 years after radical prostatectomy. There were no dropouts during the entire observation time.

Only patients who completed 2 years of treatment are included in the registry. The dropout rate during the first 2 years is estimated in a magnitude of 5%. Reasons for discontinuation of TTh are that patients' expectations were not met by the treatment during this time, and there were a few men who withdrew their consent to use their data for analysis.

Patient educational support

As stated earlier, all patients with overweight and obesity are encouraged to modify their lifestyles and

Table 1. Laboratory Methods

Parameter	Device/manufacturer	Method	Kit	Intra assay variation (%)	Inter assay variation (%)	Description
Total Testosterone	Alinity i-Module/Abbott	CMIA	2nd Generation Testosterone Reagent Kit	2.8	3.1	
Hemoglobin	CELL DYN RUBY/Abbott	Photometry		0.3	1.0	Utilization of multi-angle polarized scatter separation technology, laser flow cytometry, integral reticulocyte analysis, and nuclear optical count.
Leukocytes	CELL DYN RUBY/Abbott	Flow cytometry		1.3	1.6	Utilization of multi-angle polarized scatter separation technology, laser flow cytometry, integral reticulocyte analysis, and nuclear optical count.
Erythrocytes	CELL DYN RUBY/Abbott	Flow cytometry		0.8	0.9	Utilization of multi-angle polarized scatter separation technology, laser flow cytometry, integral reticulocyte analysis, and nuclear optical count.
Thrombocytes (Platelets)	CELL DYN RUBY/Abbott	Flow cytometry		1.3	2.6	Utilization of multi-angle polarized scatter separation technology, laser flow cytometry, integral reticulocyte analysis, and nuclear optical count.
MCV	CELL DYN RUBY/Abbott	Flow cytometry		0.5	0.3	Utilization of multi-angle polarized scatter separation technology, laser flow cytometry, integral reticulocyte analysis, and nuclear optical count.
Hematocrit	BC-3000Plus/Mindray	Calculated		0.5	1.5	The machine uses the impedance method to determine WBCs, RBCs, and PLTs. It does not directly measure the hematocrit, but rather calculates hematocrit from measurements of individual RBCs sizes and counts. The hematocrit of the original sample is calculated from the number of cells (rbcs) by using the following equation: $Hct = number\ of\ RBCs \times MCV/10$.
Hematocrit	PowerSpin™ BX Centrifuge/UNICO	Microhematocrit		1.0	1.0	$12,000g$, 5 min
ALT	Alinity c-Module/Abbott	Enzymatic (NADH)	Alinity c Activated Alanine Aminotransferase Reagent Kit	0.7	0.9	The reaction is monitored by measuring the rate of decrease in absorbance at 340nm due to the oxidation of NADH to NAD.
AST	Alinity c-Module/Abbott	Enzymatic (NADH)	Alinity c Activated Aspartate Aminotransferase Reagent Kit	0.3	0.6	The reaction is monitored by measuring the rate of decrease in absorbance at 340nm due to the oxidation of NADH to NAD.
GGT	Alinity c-Module/Abbott	Enzymatic	Alinity c Gamma-Glutamyl Transferase Reagent Kit	0.4	1.1	The rate of the absorbance increase at 412nm is directly proportional to the GGT in the sample.
Bilirubin (Total)	Alinity c-Module/Abbott	Photometric color-test	Alinity c Total Bilirubin Reagent Kit	0.7	1.3	Total (conjugated and unconjugated) bilirubin couples with a diazo reagent in the presence of a surfactant to form azobilirubin. The increase in absorbance at 548nm due to azobilirubin is directly proportional to the total bilirubin concentration.
LDL	Alinity c-Module/Abbott	Enzymatic color-test	Alinity c Direct LDL Reagent Kit	0.7	1.5	The Alinity c Processing Module uses photometric detection technology to measure sample absorbance for the quantification of analyte concentration after an enzymatically catalyzed reaction in a buffer solution.
HDL	Alinity c-Module/Abbott	Enzymatic color-test	Alinity c Ultra HDL Reagent Kit	0.6	1.1	The Alinity c Processing Module uses photometric detection technology to measure sample absorbance for the quantification of analyte concentration after an enzymatically catalyzed reaction in a buffer solution.
Cholesterol	Alinity c-Module/Abbott	Enzymatic color-test	Alinity c Cholesterol Reagent Kit	0.7	1.0	The Alinity c Processing Module uses photometric detection technology to measure sample absorbance for the quantification of analyte concentration after an enzymatically catalyzed reaction in a buffer solution.

(continued)

Table 1. (Continued)

Parameter	Device/manufacturer	Method	Kit	Intra assay variation (%)	Inter assay variation (%)	Description
Triglycerides	Alinity c-Module/Abbott	Enzymatic color-test	Alinity c Triglyceride Reagent Kit	0.5	0.8	The Alinity c Processing Module uses photometric detection technology to measure sample absorbance for the quantification of analyte concentration after an enzymatically catalyzed reaction in a buffer solution.
PSA	Alinity i-Module/Abbott	CMIA	Alinity I Total PSA Reagent Kit	3.1	3.3	
Creatinine	Alinity c-Module/Abbott	Enzymatic color-test	Alinity c Creatinine (Enzymatic) Reagent Kit	0.6	2.4	At an alkaline pH, creatinine in the sample reacts with picrate to form a creatinine-picrate complex. The rate of increase in absorbance at 500 nm due to the formation of this complex is directly proportional to the concentration of creatinine in the sample.
Insulin—C-Peptide	Atellica® Solution/Siemens	CLIA		1.12	6.5	HPLC, short for high-performance liquid chromatography, is a form of column chromatography (laboratory technique used to separate mixtures) used frequently in biochemistry and analytical chemistry. It involves passing a mixture that contains the and "analyte" through a column (stationary phase), by a liquid (mobile phase) at high pressure. Cation exchange chromatography is a process that allows the separation of the mixture based on the charge properties of the molecules in the mixture. Cation exchange chromatography retains analyte molecules based on coulombic (ionic) interactions. The stationary phase surface displays negatively charged functional groups that interact with positively charged cations in the mixture.
HBA1c	TOSOH (HLC-723 series)/ Bioscience	HPLC		0.33	0.50	
Glucose	Alinity c-Module/Abbott	Enzymatic (HK/G6PDH)	Alinity c Glucose Reagent Kit	0.65	1.51	Glucose is phosphorylated by HK in the presence of ATP a magnesium ions to produce G-6-P and ADP. G-6-PDH specifically oxidizes G-6-P to 6-phosphogluconate with the concurrent reduction of NAD to NADH. One micromole of NADH is produced for each micromole of glucose consumed. The NADH produced absorbs light at 340 nm and can be detected spectrophotometrically as an increased absorbance.
CRP	Alinity c-Module/Abbott	Immunoturbidimetric	Ality c CRP Vario Reagent Kit	0.8	0.8	When an antigen-antibody reaction occurs between CRP in a sample and anti-CRP antibody, which has been absorbed to latex particles, agglutination results. This agglutination is detected as an absorbance change (572 nm), with the rate of change being proportional to the quantity of CRP in the sample.

ADP, adenosine diphosphate; ALT, alanine transaminase (formerly GPT, glutamate pyruvate transaminase); AST, aspartate transaminase (formerly GOT, glutamate oxaloacetate transaminase); ATP, adenosine triphosphate; CLIA, chemiluminescent immunoassay; CMIA, chemiluminescent micropartide immunoassay; CRP, C-reactive protein; G-6-P, glucose-6-phosphate; G-6-PDH, glucose-6-phosphate dehydrogenase; GGT, gamma-glutamyl transferase; HDL, high-density lipoprotein; HK, hexokinase; HPLC, high-performance liquid chromatography; LDL, low-density lipoprotein; NAD, nicotinamide adenine dinucleotide; NADH; nicotinamide adenine dinucleotide reduced; PSA, prostate-specific antigen; RBC, red blood cell; WBC, white blood cell; PLT, platelet.

increase their physical activity to improve their quality of life. Patients are provided with an education pamphlet (Supplementary Appendix SA1) with exercise suggestions and nutritional recommendations. Patients with diabetes are encouraged to regularly check with their diabetologist. Patients with diabetes are treated in a local diabetes center and participate in a mandatory educational program for diabetes consisting of a certified educational course on diabetes, including information on lifestyle changes to prevent progression of diabetes. Patients who do not achieve the target HbA_{1c} after $\sim$2–3 years are asked to attend the educational courses again. Whenever an adaptation of medication is necessary, educational material and support are provided to patients who undergo medication changes. Patients in whom a secondary disease or comorbidity occurs as a result of their diabetes are provided educational materials and support regarding such comorbidities.

Assessment and follow-up

Patients receiving TTh return every 3 months for their next injection. Patients who opted not to be treated with testosterone are encouraged to visit our office between two and four times each year, depending on their medical complaints (e.g., prostatic diseases or ED). At each follow-up visit, anthropometric parameters, BP, and blood chemistry measurements are repeated.

Questions are asked about change of medication prescribed by their GPs, visits to other specialists, etc. and the answers are entered into their patient records. All electronic patient records are transferred into the registry database. Data reported by the commercial clinical laboratory in conventional units are converted to SI units. All other calculations are listed in Table 2.[19-23]

Statistical methods

Patients who opted to be treated with testosterone return quarterly for TU injections, whereas those who opted not to be treated return at least biannually for a routine visit. Data in both groups of patients are averaged across each year of patients participating in the study. The yearly data obtained are used to assess differences between patients treated with tesosterone and those who were not treated, while adjusting for possible confounding.

Adjusted multivariable analyses

In adjusted multivariable analyses, changes from baseline in parameters (weight, WC, etc.) are analyzed by using a mixed model for repeated measures in terms of treatment, visit, and treatment-by-visit interaction as fixed factors and age, WC, weight, systolic and diastolic BP, TC, high-density lipoprotein (HDL), low-density lipoprotein (LDL), triglycerides (TG), AMS,

Table 2. Calculated Parameters

Calculated parameter	Algorithm or method
BMI	Body mass in weight (kg) divided by the square of the body height (m)
Non-HDL cholesterol	Total cholesterol minus HDL cholesterol
Remnant cholesterol	Total cholesterol minus LDL cholesterol minus HDL cholesterol
HOMA-IR	Fasting insulin (U/L)×fasting glucose (mmol/L)/22.5
HOMA-beta	20×Fasting insulin (U/L)/fasting glucose (mmol/L) −3.5
HOMA2-IR	By use of the HOMA2 calculator provided by the Oxford University: www.dtu.ox.ac.uk/homacalculator/download.php
HOMA2_%S	By use of the HOMA2 calculator provided by the Oxford University: www.dtu.ox.ac.uk/homacalculator/download.php
HOMA2_%B	By use of the HOMA2 calculator provided by the Oxford University: www.dtu.ox.ac.uk/homacalculator/download.php
Matsuda index (ISI)	By use of the web calculator for Matsuda index: http://mmatsuda.diabetes-smc.jp/MIndex.html
Increment AUC glucose	By use of the web calculator for Matsuda index: http://mmatsuda.diabetes-smc.jp/MIndex.html
Increment AUC C-peptide	By use of the web calculator for Matsuda index: http://mmatsuda.diabetes-smc.jp/MIndex.html
IGI	By use of the web calculator for Matsuda index: http://mmatsuda.diabetes-smc.jp/MIndex.html
Disposition index	By use of the web calculator for Matsuda index: http://mmatsuda.diabetes-smc.jp/MIndex.html
MCH	(hemoglobin/erythrocytes)×10
MCHC	(Hemoglobin/hematocrit)×100
Pulse pressure	Systolic BP minus diastolic BP
RPP	Systolic BP x heart rate/100
VAI	According to the equation published by Amato et al0.[19]
ABSI	According to the equation published by Krakauer and Krakauer[20]
LAP	According to the equation published by Kahn[21]
FLI	According to the equation published by Bedogni et al.[22]
eGFR	According to the equation published by the Modification of Diet in Renal Disease Study Group[23]

ABSI, A Body Shape Index; eGFR, estimated glomerular filtration rate; FLI, Fatty Liver Index; HOMA-IR, homeostasis model assessment of insulin resistance; IGI, insulinogenic index; ISI, insulin sensitivity index; LAP, lipid accumulation product; MCH, mean corpuscular hemoglobin; MCHC, mean corpuscular hemoglobin concentration; RPP, rate pressure product; VAI, visceral adiposity index.

glucose, and baseline values of the analysis parameter as covariates. Baseline parameter values are the values recorded before the first TU injection. A random effect is included in the model for the intercept. Adjusted mean differences between treatment groups at each time point and across time within each treatment group are estimated by using estimate statements in SAS PROC MIXED, Version 9.3 (2011) provided by SAS Institute, Inc., Cary, North Carolina.

Propensity matching analyses

For some analyses, we used propensity matching. Our general strategy for propensity matching of those on active treatment to those who remained untreated included calculating propensity score based on logistic regression model and selecting matching pairs (or one to many) based on the score. The matching was performed by "nearest neighbor" selection with caliper set to a fraction of standard deviation (SD) of the propensity score. Several scenarios were considered. We first attempted to create propensity score based on the following variables: age, WC, weight, SBP and DBP, TC, HDL, LDL, TG, AMS, and glucose. That model discriminated between active drugs and those who remained untreated too well, resulting in a very small overlap of propensity score distributions. We then created propensity score based on the following variables: age, BMI, and WC. The 1:1 matching was done by choosing the nearest neighbor match with the caliper set to 0.2 SD of the propensity score. In addition, we explored a 1:1 matching setting caliper to 0.5 SD and 1:2 matching with 0.2 SD and 0.5 SD calipers. These additional scenarios did not result in noticeable gain of the matched sample. Analyses were performed by using SAS 9.3 software (SAS Institute, Cary, North Carolina).

Results

Table 3 describes the baseline characteristics, comorbidities, and concomitant medications of all patients (T-treated or -untreated), categorized into patients with functional hypogonadism and those with primary hypogonadism. Men with primary hypogonadism were younger than men with functional hypogonadism. Forty-seven (61.8%) of men with primary hypogonadism had Klinefelter's syndrome. Most of these patients had been referred by orthopedists with a suspicion of hypogonadism, because they had presented with back pain and osteoporosis at a young age, with the youngest of these patients being 33 years old.

Results from this registry study were published since 2007, partly pooled with a parallel registry of a similar design.[24–28] Table 4 shows the bibliography of papers published from this registry. So far, six papers were published in journals of Endocrinology, five in Urology, four in Andrology, four in Obesity, three in General Medicine, three in Diabetes, and two in Cardiology.

Of note, the benefits of long-term effects of TTh in hypogonadal patients were exemplified by reduced body weight (Fig. 1A), WC (Fig. 1B), and BMI (Fig. 1C).[28] More importantly, the impact of long-term TTh on obesity in comparison with untreated controls is shown in Figure 2.[29] These findings were not observed in prior studies, because there were no long-term studies with TTh before this registry. Moreover, our recent publication that one third of men with TD and type 2 diabetes experience remission of diabetes is of great clinical importance (Fig. 3).[30]

The findings from this registry study have contributed important clinical knowledge regarding treatment of TD and the beneficial health effects that were not seen in short-term studies. In terms of safety of TTh, reductions in mortality, myocardial infarctions, strokes, and prostate cancer became apparent after less than 8 years of follow-up,[31,32] and those early results were confirmed and became more robust with continued observation time (Fig. 4).[33]

Discussion

Our registry is the first observational study carried out over more than 15 years in a single urological practice. Since the initiation of the study in 2004, all patients have been under the care of the same urologist (A.H.) so that investigator bias can be excluded. Because there are no randomized, placebo-controlled studies exceeding 3 years' duration, the registry revealed new insights that had been unpredictable in the field of androgen therapy.

One unexpected finding was that men with hypogonadism undergoing TTh lose weight. This became apparent for the first time when 5-year data were analyzed.[34] The weight loss is slow but progressive and usually remains below 5% in the first year of TTh.[34] Also, men who are obese lose more weight than men who are overweight who lose more weight than men of normal weight.[29] In almost all RCTs, obesity was not an inclusion criterion and populations were mixed regarding their baseline BMI, which may explain why weight loss was not described in

Table 3. Baseline Characteristics, Comorbidities, and Concomitant Medication at Baseline in Men with Functional Hypogonadism and in Men with Primary Hypogonadism

	All functional hypogonadism (n=773)	Functional hypogonadism treated (n=380)	Functional hypogonadism untreated (n=393)	p-Value between groups	All primary hypogonadism (n=85)	Primary hypogonadism treated (n=76)	Primary hypogonadism untreated (n=9)	p-Value between groups
Mean baseline age (years)	61.5±6.1	59.1±6.3	63.8±4.8	<0.0001	52.3±96.1	51.0±8.8	63.0±3.0	0.0001
Mean follow-up (years)	9.0±2.5	8.7±2.7	9.4±2.3		7.8±1.9	8.0±1.8	6.8±2.2	
Median follow-up (years)	10	10	10		9	9	7	
Testosterone								
Total testosterone (nmol/L)	9.6±1.4	9.6±1.5	9.7±1.1	0.1580	9.3±1.7	9.3±1.7	9.5±1.1	0.7288
Anthropometric parameters								
Weight (kg)	100.7±16.4	106.3±17.1	95.2±13.5	<0.0001	97.8±14.7	97.0±14.2	104.3±18.4	0.1606
Waist circumference (cm)	110.4±12.5	110.1±13.1	110.8±11.8	0.4078	105.4±12.1	102.7±7.7	128.3±18.3	<0.0001
BMI (kg/m²)	32.5±5.7	34.2±5.4	30.8±5.5	<0.0001	30.0±5.1	29.4±4.5	34.5±7.2	0.0040
Height (cm)	176.6±3.3	176.3±3.0	176.9±3.7	0.0177	181.2±4.7	181.8±4.5	176.4±4.4	0.0010
Waist:height ratio	0.63±0.07	0.62±0.07	0.63±0.07	0.6295	0.58±0.08	0.57±0.05	0.73±0.12	<0.0001
VAI	4.6±2.4	5.0±2.5	4.2±2.2	<0.0001	4.5±1.4	4.5±1.3	4.3±2.1	0.6531
Normal weight (proportion), n (%)	56 (7.2)	19 (5.0)	37 (9.4)	<0.0001	8 (9.4)	8 (10.5)	0 (0.0)	0.1110
Overweight (proportion), n (%)	246 (31.8)	85 (22.4)	161 (41.0)	<0.0001	42 (49.4)	38 (50.0)	4 (44.4)	0.1110
Obesity (proportion), n (%)	471 (60.9)	276 (72.7)	195 (49.6)	<0.0001	35 (41.2)	30 (39.5)	5 (55.5)	0.1110
Obesity class I (proportion), n (%)	0	99 (26.1)	132 (33.6)	<0.0001	22 (25.9)	21 (27.6)	1 (11.1)	0.1110
Obesity class II (proportion), n (%)	164 (21.2)	118 (31.1)	46 (11.7)	<0.0001	7 (8.2)	5 (6.6)	2 (22.2)	0.1110
Obesity class III (proportion), n (%)	76 (9.8)	59 (15.5)	17 (4.3)	<0.0001	6 (7.1)	4 (5.3)	2 (22.2)	0.1110
Glycemic control								
Fasting glucose (mmol/L)	6.2±1.2	6.5±1.4	5.8±0.7	<0.0001	5.7±0.9	5.6±0.9	6.4±0.8	0.0161
HbA1c (%)	7.0±1.9	8.0±2.1	6.3±1.4	<0.0001	6.2±1.6	6.0±1.5	7.2±1.7	0.0288
Fasting insulin (μU/mL)	25.9±6.6	26.4±8.4	25.3±2.9	0.1468	27.9±3.8	29.8±3.6	26.3±3.4	0.1361
HOMA-IR	8.7±2.3	10.1±2.1	7.2±1.3	<0.0001	9.6±2.7	11.5±2.9	8.1±1.5	0.0350
BP and hemodynamic parameters								
Systolic BP (mmHg)	148.8±16.7	155.7±16.4	142.2±14.0	<0.0001	137.3±14.2	136.6±13.9	143.1±16.3	0.1918
Diastolic BP (mmHg)	87.1±11.9	92.9±11.8	81.6±9.0	<0.0001	81.7±10.1	81.4±9.5	84.8±14.4	0.3392
Heart rate (bpm)	77.5±4.5	78.3±3.9	76.8±4.8	<0.0001	76.9±3.9	76.5±3.8	80.2±3.9	0.0065
Pulse pressure (mmHg)	61.6±8.1	62.7±8.4	60.6±7.8	0.0004	55.5±6.8	55.2±6.9	58.3±4.9	0.1945
RPP	11537±1658	12172±1741	10923±1309	<0.0001	10577±1444	10467±1393	11503±1620	0.0412
Lipids								
Total cholesterol (mmol/L)	7.3±1.4	8.0±1.1	6.6±1.3	<0.0001	7.1±0.9	7.1±0.8	7.1±1.3	0.8395
HDL cholesterol (mmol/L)	1.1±0.4	1.0±0.3	1.2±0.5	<0.0001	1.0±0.3	0.9±0.3	1.2±0.4	0.0014
LDL cholesterol (mmol/L)	3.9±1.2	4.3±0.9	3.5±1.4	<0.0001	4.0±0.9	4.1±0.9	3.3±0.6	0.0094
Triglyceride (mmol/L)	3.1±0.6	3.2±0.6	3.0±0.5	<0.0001	2.8±0.4	2.8±0.4	3.0±0.6	0.2977
Non-HDL cholesterol (mmol/L)	6.1±1.5	6.9±1.1	5.4±1.4	<0.0001	6.2±0.9	6.2±0.8	5.9±1.6	0.02404
Remnant cholesterol (mmol/L)	2.2±1.0	2.6±1.0	1.9±0.9	<0.0001	2.2±0.8	2.1±0.7	2.5±1.3	0.1302
LAP (cm×mmol/L)	143.7±60.3	149.6±67.4	138.0±51.9	0.0075	115.6±46.0	107.0±34.4	188.1±67.4	<0.0001
Questionnaires								
AMS	46.5±10.0	53.0±9.5	40.3±5.6	<0.0001	47.8±9.6	49.1±9.3	36.6±2.8	0.0001
IPSS	5.9±3.1	7.1±3.6	4.8±1.9	<0.0001	3.4±3.0	3.1±3.0	5.9±0.8	0.0084
IIEF-EF	18.6±4.9	17.4±5.8	19.8±3.4	<0.0001	18.7±5.8	18.7±6.0	18.0±3.6	0.7249
Prostate parameters								
Prostate volume (mL)	33.7±8.0	32.2±9.3	35.2±6.1	<0.0001	22.8±10.5	20.9±9.3	39.1±4.6	<0.0001
PSA (ng/mL)	2.3±1.2	2.1±1.0	2.5±1.3	<0.0001	1.2±1.3	0.9±0.9	3.7±1.5	<0.0001

(continued)

Table 3. (Continued)

	All functional hypogonadism (n = 773)	Functional hypogonadism treated (n = 380)	Functional hypogonadism untreated (n = 393)	p-Value between groups	All primary hypogonadism (n = 85)	Primary hypogonadism treated (n = 76)	Primary hypogonadism untreated (n = 9)	p-Value between groups
Erythropoiesis								
Hemoglobin (g/dL)	14.6±0.6	14.4±0.7	14.7±0.5	**<0.0001**	14.7±0.5	14.7±0.5	14.9±0.7	0.1605
Hematocrit (%)	45.0±2.0	44.1±2.2	45.8±1.3	**<0.0001**	44.9±1.9	44.8±1.9	46.4±1.1	**0.0101**
Inflammatory markers								
CRP (mg/dL)	3.5±5.4	5.7±6.9	1.4±1.3	**<0.0001**	3.4±5.0	3.4±5.2	2.6±2.7	0.6370
Liver function								
AST (U/L)	33.2±13.9	40.0±15.2	26.6±8.1	**<0.0001**	34.1±12.2	33.2±12.3	42.3±7.1	**0.0314**
ALT (U/L)	38.8±13.6	42.9±15.1	30.8±8.5	**<0.0001**	36.1±13.1	34.9±13.1	46.2±6.6	**0.0127**
AST:ALT ratio	0.90±0.12	0.93±0.15	0.86±0.05	**<0.0001**	0.96±0.16	0.96±0.17	0.91±0.04	0.3881
FLI	86.8±13.0	89.4±11.9	84.1±13.5	**<0.0001**	80.7±13.4	79.1±13.1	94.6±5.2	**0.0007**
Renal function								
Creatinine	0.96±0.15	0.92±0.15	1.00±0.14	**<0.0001**	0.90±0.09	0.88±0.07	1.02±0.16	**<0.0001**
eGFR	81.4±12.6	85.7±11.8	77.3±12.0	**<0.0001**	90.1±10.2	91.7±8.4	76.1±13.8	**<0.0001**
Comorbidities at baseline, n (%)								
Type 2 diabetes	345 (44.6)	173 (45.5)	172 (43.8)	0.6226	11 (12.9)	5 (6.6)	6 (66.7)	**<0.0001**
Type 1 diabetes	21 (2.7)	21 (5.5)	0 (0.0)	**<0.0001**	0 (0.0)	0 (0.0)	0 (0.0)	1.0
Hypertension	664 (85.9)	362 (95.3)	302 (76.8)	**<0.0001**	56 (65.9)	52 (68.4)	4 (44.4)	**0.0014**
Prior cardiovascular disease[a]	217 (28.1)	99 (26.1)	118 (30.0)	0.2191	9 (10.6)	4 (5.3)	5 (55.6)	**<0.0001**
Prior myocardial infarction	105 (13.6)	64 (16.8)	41 (10.4)	**0.0093**	6 (7.1)	3 (3.9)	3 (33.3)	**0.0011**
Prior stroke	55 (7.1)	24 (6.3)	31 (7.9)	0.3953	0 (0.0)	0 (0.0)	0 (0.0)	1.0
Prior coronary artery disease	143 (18.5)	53 (13.9)	90 (22.9)	**0.0014**	6 (7.1)	3 (3.9)	3 (33.3)	**0.0011**
ED	744 (96.3)	354 (93.2)	390 (99.2)	**<0.0001**	72 (84.7)	63 (82.9)	9 (100.1)	**0.0411**
Osteoporosis	59 (7.6)	26 (6.8)	33 (8.4)	0.4157	46 (54.1)	46 (60.5)	0 (0.0)	**0.0006**
Concomitant medication, n (%)								
Antidiabetic medication	362 (46.8)	190 (50.0)	172 (43.8)	0.0825	11 (12.9)	5 (6.6)	6 (66.7)	**<0.0001**
Antihypertensive medication	364 (47.1)	223 (58.7)	141 (35.9)	**<0.0001**	14 (16.5)	10 (13.2)	4 (44.4)	**0.0013**
Statins	414 (53.6)	189 (49.7)	225 (57.3)	**0.0362**	15 (17.6)	10 (13.2)	5 (55.6)	**0.0016**
PDE5 inhibitors	184 (23.8)	97 (25.5)	87 (22.1)	<0.01	15 (17.6)	12 (15.8)	3 (33.3)	0.1917
Alpha-blockers	366 (47.3)	168 (44.2)	197 (50.1)	0.1498	13 (15.3)	5 (6.6)	8 (88.9)	**<0.0001**
5-α-reductase inhibitors	43 (5.6)	10 (2.6)	33 (8.4)	**0.0005**	3 (3.5)	0 (0.0)	3 (33.3)	**<0.0001**
Klinefelter's syndrome	0 (0.0)	0 (0.0)	0 (0.0)	1.0	47 (55.3)	47 (61.8)	0 (0.0)	**0.0004**
Smoking	289 (37.4)	145 (38.3)	144 (36.6)	0.6425	42 (49.4)	37 (48.7)	5 (55.6)	0.6966

p-values in bold are statistically significant.

Data are shown as means ± SD.

[a]Cardiovascular disease was defined as prior myocardial infarction, stroke, or diagnosis of coronary artery disease.

AMS, Aging Males' Symptoms; ED, erectile dysfunction; IIEF-EF, International Index of Erectile Function—Erectile Function Domain; IPSS, International Prostate Symptom Score; SD, standard deviation.

Table 4. Bibliography

Papers published on registry study until July 8, 2020

1. F Saad, L Gooren, A Haider, A Yassin
An exploratory study of the effects of 12 month administration of the novel long-acting testosterone undecanoate on measures of sexual function and the metabolic syndrome
Arch Androl. 2007;53(6):353–357.[a]

2. A Haider, LJ Gooren, P Padungtod, F Saad
Concurrent improvement of the metabolic syndrome and lower urinary tract symptoms upon normalisation of plasma testosterone levels in hypogonadal elderly men
Andrologia. 2009;41(1):7–13.

3. A Haider, LJ Gooren, P Padungtod, F Saad
Beneficial effects of 2 years of administration of parenteral testosterone undecanoate on the metabolic syndrome and on non-alcoholic liver steatosis and C-reactive protein
Horm Mol Biol Clin Invest. 2010;1(1):27–33.

4. A Haider, LJ Gooren, P Padungtod, F Saad
A safety study of administration of parenteral testosterone undecanoate to elderly men over minimally 24 months
Andrologia. 2010;42(6):349–355.

5. A Haider, W Kurtz, EJ Giltay, LJ Gooren, F Saad
Administration of testosterone to elderly hypogonadal men with Crohn's disease improves their Crohn's Disease Activity Index: A pilot study
Horm Mol Biol Clin Invest. 2010;2(3):287–292.

6. A Haider, LJ Gooren, P Padungtod, F Saad
Improvement of the metabolic syndrome and of non-alcoholic liver steatosis upon treatment of hypogonadal elderly men with parenteral testosterone undecanoate
Exp Clin Endocrinol Diabetes. 2010;118(3):167–171.

7. F Saad, A Haider, EJ Giltay, LJG Gooren
Age, obesity and inflammation at baseline predict the effects of testosterone administration on the metabolic syndrome
Horm Mol Biol Clin Invest. 2011;6(1):193–199.

8. F Saad, A Haider, G Doros, A Traish
Long-term treatment of hypogonadal men with testosterone produces substantial and sustained weight loss
Obes 2013;21(10):1975–1981.

9. A Haider, A Yassin, G Doros, F Saad
Effects of long-term testosterone therapy on patients with "diabesity": Results of observational studies of pooled analyses in obese hypogonadal men with type 2 diabetes
Int J Endocrinol. 2014;2014:683515.[a]

10. A Haider, F Saad, G Doros, L Gooren
Hypogonadal obese men with and without diabetes mellitus type 2 lose weight and show improvement in cardiovascular risk factors when treated with testosterone: An observational study
Obes Res Clin Pract. 2014;8(4):e339–e349.

11. A Haider, U Meergans, A Traish, F Saad, G Doros, P Lips, L Gooren
Progressive improvement of T-scores in men with osteoporosis and subnormal serum testosterone levels upon treatment with testosterone over six years
Int J Endocrinol. 2014;2014:496948.

12. AM Traish, A Haider, G Doros, F Saad
Long-term testosterone therapy in hypogonadal men ameliorates elements of the metabolic syndrome: An observational, long-term registry study
Int J Clin Pract. 2014;68(3):314–329.

13. A Haider, M Zitzmann, G Doros, H Isbarn, P Hammerer, A Yassin
Incidence of prostate cancer in hypogonadal men receiving testosterone therapy: Observations from 5-year median followup of 3 registries
J Urol. 2015;193(1):80–86.[a]

14. F Saad, A Yassin, A Haider, G Doros, L Gooren
Elderly men over 65 years of age with late-onset hypogonadism benefit as much from testosterone treatment as do younger men
Korean J Urol. 2015;56(4):310–317.[a]

(*continued*)

Papers published on registry study until July 8, 2020

15. M Nasser, A Haider, F Saad, W Kurtz, G Doros, M Fijak, L Vignozzi, L Gooren
Testosterone therapy in men with Crohn's disease improves the clinical course of the disease: Data from long-term observational registry study
Horm Mol Biol Clin Invest. 2015;22(3):111–117.

16. A Haider, A Yassin, KS Haider, G Doros, F Saad, G Rosano
Men with testosterone deficiency and a history of cardiovascular diseases benefit from long-term testosterone therapy: Observational, real-life data from a registry study
Vasc Health Risk Manag. 2016:12(6):251–261.[a]

17. F Saad, A Yassin, G Doros, A Haider
Effects of long-term treatment with testosterone on weight and waist size in 411 hypogonadal men with obesity classes I-III: Observational data from two registry studies
Int J Obes. 2016;40(1):162–170.[a]

18. F Saad, A Haider, L Gooren
Hypogonadal men with psoriasis benefit from long-term testosterone replacement therapy—A series of 15 case reports
Andrologia. 2016;48(3):341–346.

19. AM Traish, A Haider, KS Haider, G Doros, F Saad
Long-term testosterone therapy improves cardiometabolic function and reduces risk of cardiovascular disease in men with hypogonadism: A real-life observational registry study setting comparing treated and untreated (control) groups
J Cardiovasc Pharmacol Therap. 2017;22(5):414–433.

20. KS Haider, A Haider, G Doros, A Traish
Long-term testosterone therapy improves urinary and sexual function, and quality of life in men with hypogonadism: Results from a propensity matched subgroup of a controlled registry study
J Urol. 2018;199(1):257–265.

21. M Hanefeld, A Haider, M Zitzmann, F Saad
Remission of type 2 diabetes after long-term testosterone therapy
Diabetes, Stoffwechsel und Herz. 2018;27(1):33–37

22. F Saad, G Doros, KS Haider, A Haider
Hypogonadal men with moderate-to-severe lower urinary tract symptoms have a more severe cardiometabolic risk profile and benefit more from testosterone therapy than men with mild lower urinary tract symptoms
Investig Clin Urol. 2018;59(6):399–409.

23. X Zhang, Y Zhong, F Saad, K Haider, A Haider, X Xu
Clinically occult prostate cancer cases may distort the effect of testosterone replacement therapy on risk of PCa
World J Urol. 2019;37(10):2091–2097.

24. F Saad, M Caliber, G Doros, KS Haider, A Haider
Long-term treatment with testosterone undecanoate injections in men with hypogonadism alleviates erectile dysfunction and reduces risk of major adverse cardiovascular events, prostate cancer, and mortality
Aging Male. 2020;23(1):81–92.

25. X Zhang, Y Zhong, F Saad, KS Haider, A Haider, A Clendenin, X Xu
Testosterone therapy may reduce prostate cancer risk due to testosterone deficiency at a young age via stabilizing serum testosterone levels
Aging Male. 2020;23(2):112–118.

26. F Saad, G Doros, KS Haider, A Haider
Differential effects of 11 years of long-term injectable testosterone undecanoate therapy on anthropometric and metabolic parameters in hypogonadal men with normal weight, overweight and obesity in comparison with untreated controls: Real-world data from a controlled registry study
Int J Obes. 2020;44(6):1264–1278.

27. KS Haider, A Haider, F Saad, G Doros, M Hanefeld, S Dhindsa, P Dandona, A Traish
Remission of type 2 diabetes following long-term treatment with injectable testosterone undecanoate in patients with hypogonadism and type 2 diabetes: 11-year data from a real-world registry study
Diabetes Obes Metab. 2020;22(11):2055–2068.

Papers published on registry study until July 22, 2020.
[a]Papers reporting pooled analyses from the current registry study in combination with parallel registry studies

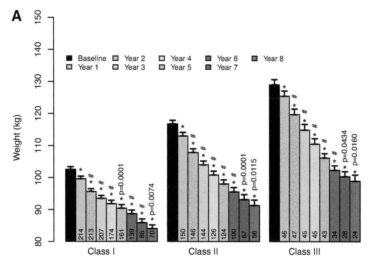

* p<0.0001 vs. baseline; # p<0.0001 vs. previous year; all other p values indicate comparison to previous

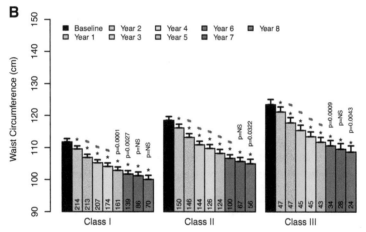

* p<0.0001 vs. baseline; # p<0.0001 vs. previous year; all other p values indicate comparison to previous

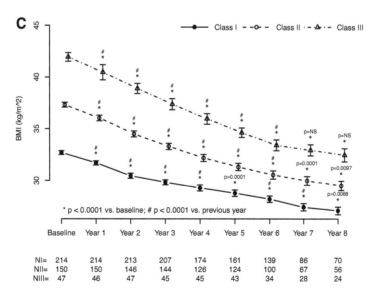

* p < 0.0001 vs. baseline; # p < 0.0001 vs. previous year

FIG. 1.   Reductions of **(A)** weight, **(B)** waist circumference, and **(C)** BMI in 411 hypogonadal men receiving long-term testosterone treatment. All values are shown as mean ± SE. From: Saad et al.[28] BMI, body mass index; SE, standard error.

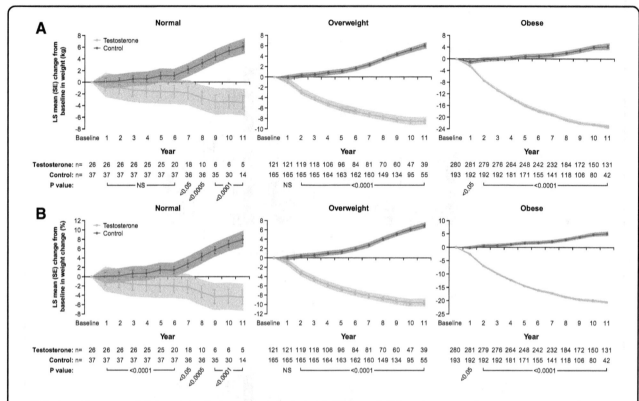

FIG. 2. Changes of **(A)** weight (kg), **(B)** weight (%), **(C)** BMI, and **(D)** waist circumference in men with testosterone deficiency and normal weight, overweight, and obesity after treatment with testosterone undecanoate injections, compared with untreated men (Control). Data from: Saad et al.[29]

those trials. However, more recently, our results were confirmed in a small RCT with 2 years' duration in men with obesity and type 2 diabetes.[35] Another controlled study in mostly obese men treated with testosterone after an ischemic stroke also resulted in profound weight loss after 2 years, of which most was maintained over 5 years whereas patients who discontinued TTh after 2 years regained all the weight they had previously lost at 5 years.[36] Francomano demonstrated progressive reductions in weight and WC over 5 years in obese men with metabolic syndrome compared with an untreated control group.[6] Hackett et al. could show that a reduction in WC was progressive over 5 years in the follow-up of a study in men with type 2 diabetes mellitus (T2DM) that had started as an RCT.[37] The magnitude of weight loss is clearly a function of treatment duration[38] but may also depend on formulation and the route of administration with testosterone injections having a greater effect than topical preparations.[39]

Because the majority of our patients were overweight or obese, it was not surprising to see a substantial proportion of men with T2DM. Although some studies had shown benefits of treating men with TD and T2DM with testosterone, the fact that long-term TTh could lead to remission of T2DM in one third of the patients after a mean treatment duration of more than 8 years did come unexpectedly.[30] These profound improvements resulted in more referrals from diabetologists to our urological office for assessing TD and treating men with T2DM with TTh if indicated.

Another unexpected result was the improvement noted in patients with inflammatory bowel disease (IBD). After the local hospital had realized that a few men with Crohn's disease receiving TTh were benefiting from this treatment, they started assessing TD in these patients and referring men with TD to the urologist for TTh. Over time, 74 patients with Crohn's disease and two with ulcerative colitis were included in the

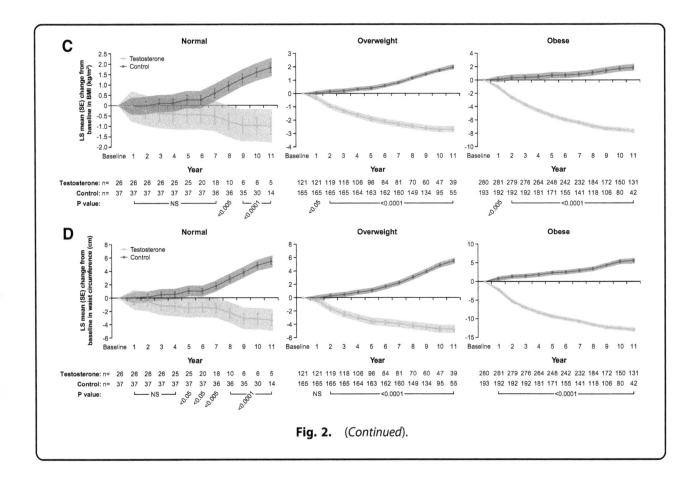

Fig. 2. (Continued).

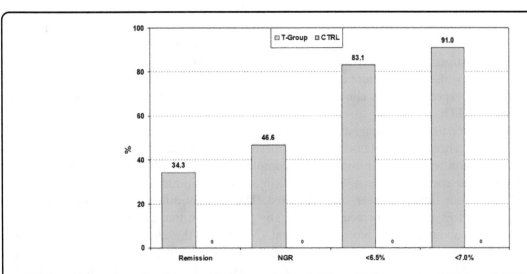

FIG. 3. Proportion of patients achieving remission, NGR, or HbA$_{1c}$ targets of 6.5% and 7.0%, respectively, in patients with testosterone deficiency and type 2 diabetes with (*n* = 178) and without (*n* = 178) testosterone therapy. From: Haider et al.[30] NGR, normal glucose regulation.

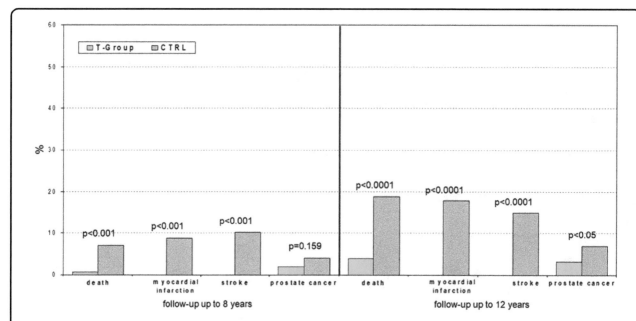

FIG. 4. Adverse events (%) in patients with testosterone deficiency following up to 8 years with ($n = 360$) and without ($n = 296$) testosterone therapy (left) and following up to 12 years with ($n = 412$) and without ($n = 393$) testosterone therapy (right). Data from: (left) Traish et al.[31]; Haider et al.[32] (right); Saad et al.[33] CTRL, control group; T-group, testosterone-treated group.

registry, and without exception all improved on TTh.[40] Suspecting that this effect could be of a more general nature in autoimmune diseases, we looked for other autoimmune diseases and identified 17 men with psoriasis whose response to TTh was very similar to that seen in IBD patients.[41] The anti-inflammatory effects of testosterone have recently been discussed in a comprehensive review,[42] however testosterone is rarely used to clinically treat inflammatory diseases. As more evidence becomes available, we expect that this clinical area will be the new front of TTh.

Because considerable concerns arose suggesting that TTh may cause prostate cancer or activate occult prostate cancer, much attention was paid to prostate examinations. Patients' prostate-specific antigen (PSA) levels were measured up to four times per year, and transrectal ultrasound and DREs were performed at least twice a year. Decisions about prostate biopsies were always made by the same clinician (A.H.) so that investigator bias can be excluded. With the long-term follow-up, a better understanding of the relationship between TTh and prostate cancer became available. Not only was it reassuring to demonstrate that there was no increased risk of prostate can-

cer in men receiving TTh,[25] but we also noted that prostate cancer always occurred during the first 18 months of TTh[43] and the hypothesis was supported that maintaining stable testosterone levels could be protective.[44]

It should be noted that the UK Androgen Study reported the 25 years' experience with TTh of a single center in the United Kingdom with various androgen preparations, also concluding that long-term TTh was safe with regard to prostate and cardiovascular function.[45]

We firmly believe that the use of the three-monthly TU injections is essential in our registry, as it allows for complete control of medication adherence. Every single injection is administered in our office and documented. This level of adherence cannot be achieved with any preparation that is self-administered by the patient. Moreover, the intramuscular route of administration excludes any potential problems with absorption that may be experienced with transdermal application, particularly in patients with obesity.[46] The superior effectiveness of intramuscular compared with transdermal TTh has been demonstrated by Skinner et al. and is consistent with our own clinical experience.[39] Therefore, it may not be possible to extrapolate results from our registry study to the use of other testosterone preparations.

An interesting development in the field was that TTh affects many medical specialties. Originally, testosterone was believed to primarily play a role in sexual function and used in endocrinology, urology, andrology, and sexual medicine to treat patients with sexual dysfunction and infertility. TTh has now made its way into diabetology, cardiology, gastroenterology, dermatology, psychology, and the emerging field of obesity, which, in turn, affects almost all medical disciplines.

It is rewarding to note that other researchers have expressed an interest in using our data for their own analyses, and collaborations have been established with Texas A&M University in College Station, TX, USA, and University Hospitals Birmingham NHS Foundation Trust, Good Hope Hospital, Birmingham, United Kingdom.

Limitations and strengths

As with all observational studies and registries, randomization of patients is neither expected nor feasible, in particular in an office setting where patients expect to be treated. We must note that a substantial proportion of patients opted against TTh. By adjusting for baseline differences between groups or performing propensity matching, the best possible measures have been taken to achieve robust results. A limitation of our study is that we do not have information on adherence to concomitant medication or to the lifestyle changes recommended to our patients. Other limitations of the study are the lack of untreated patients in IBD, psoriasis, type 1 diabetes, and Klinefelter's syndrome for ethical considerations. We have not attempted to include a trial registration, because duration and clinical significance of the study exceeded expectations by far.

The strengths of the study are its long duration, the real-life patient population that was only selected for the presence of symptomatic TD, and the fact that there is no investigator bias in our setting, which was managed exclusively by a single urologist (A.H.). This has resulted in trustful patient–physician relationships, in many cases developed over decades. Another strength of this registry study is the large number of patients recruited concomitant with the highest possible level of medication adherence. Because injections of TU have to be applied in the physician's office, every single administration is documented.

Outlook

As the study is ongoing, we will continue to perform further analyses. These may include studying additional subgroups as well as other aspects such as the impact of concomitant medications, for instance in patients with T2DM, hypertension, and dyslipidemia.

In summary, our registry study has provided new insights in the field of TTh, particularly in regard to the time course of treatment and patients' and physicians' expectations. Beyond confirming the safety of TTh, we provided further evidence that TTh can reduce mortality and major adverse cardiovascular events. The registry is ongoing and will continue to deliver long-term real-world data.

Acknowledgments

The authors thank all patients who participated in the study. The work described in this article received partial financial support for data entry and statistical analyses from Bayer AG, Berlin, Germany, manufacturer of the testosterone preparation used in this study.

Author Contributions

K.S.H. and A.H. treated the patients and performed the data entry. A.H. and F.S. designed the study and collected the data. GD performed the statistical analyses. K.S.H., A.H., and F.S. interpreted the data and wrote and reviewed the article.

References

1. Corona G, Giagulli VA, Maseroli E, et al. Testosterone supplementation and body composition: Results from a meta-analysis study. Eur J Endocrinol. 2016;174(3):R99–R116.

2. Snyder PJ, Peachey H, Hannoush P, et al. Effect of testosterone treatment on bone mineral density in men over 65 years of age. J Clin Endocrinol Metab. 1999;84(6):1966–1972.

3. Amory JK, Watts NB, Easley KA, et al. Exogenous testosterone or testosterone with finasteride increases bone mineral density in older men with low serum testosterone. J Clin Endocrinol Metab. 2004;89(2):503–510.

4. Basaria S, Harman SM, Travison TG. Et al. Effects of testosterone administration for 3 years on subclinical atherosclerosis progression in older men with low or low-normal testosterone levels. J Am Med Assoc. 2015;314(6):570–581.

5. Wang C, Cunningham G, Dobs A, et al. Long-term testosterone gel (AndroGel) treatment maintains beneficial effects on sexual function and mood, lean and fat mass, and bone mineral density in hypogonadal men. J Clin Endocrinol Metab. 2004;9(5):2085–2098.

6. Francomano D, Ilacqua A, Bruzziches R, Lenzi A, Aversa A. Effects of 5-year treatment with testosterone undecanoate on lower urinary tract symptoms in obese men with hypogonadism and metabolic syndrome. Urology 2014;83(1):167–174.

7. Kaptchuk TJ. The double-blind, randomized, placebo-controlled trial: Gold standard or golden calf? J Clin Epidemiol. 2001;54(6):541–549.

8. Cohen AT, Goto S, Schreiber K, Torp-Pedersen C. Why do we need observational studies of everyday patients in the real-life setting? Eur Heart J Suppl. 2015;17(Suppl. D):D2–D8.

9. Seidell JC, Björntorp P, Sjöström L, Kvist H, Sannerstedt R. Visceral fat accumulation in men is positively associated with insulin, glucose and C-peptide levels, but negatively with testosterone levels. Metabolism. 1990;39(9):897–901.

10. Zhao B, Hong Z, Wei Y, Yu D, Xu J, Zhang W. Erectile sysfunction predicts cardiovascular events as an independent risk factor: A systematic review and meta-analysis. J Sex Med. 2019;16(7):1005–1017.

11. Heinemann LAJ, Saad F, Heinemann K, Thai DM. Can results of the Aging Males' Symptoms (AMS) scale predict those of screening scales for androgen deficiency? Aging Male. 2004;7(3):211–218.

12. Yeap BB, Wu FCW. Clinical practice update on testosterone therapy for male hypogonadism: Contrasting perspectives to optimize care. Clin Endocrinol. 2019(1);90:56–65.

13. Jais A, Brüning JC. Hypothalamic inflammation in obesity and metabolic disease. J Clin Invest. 2017;127(1):24–32.

14. Morelli A, Sarchielli E, Comeglio P, et al. Metabolic syndrome induces inflammation and impairs gonadotropin-releasing hormone neurons in the preoptic area of the hypothalamus in rabbits. Mol Cell Endocrinol. 2014;382(1):107–119.

15. Zitzmann M, Nieschlag E, Traish A, Kliesch S. Testosterone treatment in men with classical vs. functional hypogonadism: A 9-year registry. J Endocr Soc. 2019;3(Suppl. 1):SUN-222.

16. Heinemann LAJ, Zimmermann T, Vermeulen A, Thiel C, Hummel W. A new 'aging males' symptoms' rating scale. Aging Male. 1999;2:105–114.

17. Barry MJ, Fowler Jr FJ, O'Leary MP, et al. The American Urological Association Symptom Index for Benign Prostatic Hyperplasia. The Measurement Committee of the American Urological Association. J Urol. 1992; 148(5):1549–1557.

18. Cappelleri JC, Rosen RC, Smith MD, Mishra A, Osterloh IH. Diagnostic evaluation of the erectile function domain of the International Index of Erectile Function. Urol. 1999;54:346–351.

19. Amato MC, Giordano C, Galia M, et al. Visceral Adiposity Index. A reliable indicator of visceral fat function associated with cardiometabolic risk. Diabetes Care. 2010;33(4):920–922.

20. Krakauer NY, Krakauer JC. A new body shape index predicts mortality hazard independently of body mass index. PLoS ONE. 2012;7(7): e39504.

21. Kahn HS. The "lipid accumulation product" performs better than the body mass index for recognizing cardiovascular risk: A population-based comparison. BMC Cardiovasc Disorders. 2005;5:26.

22. Bedogni G, Bellentani S, Miglioli L, et al. The Fatty Liver Index: A simple and accurate predictor Sof hepatic steatosis in the general population. BMC Gastroenterol. 2006;6:33.

23. Levey AS, Bosch JP, Lewis JB, et al. A more accurate method to estimate glomerular filtration rate from serum creatinine: A new prediction equation. Ann Int Med. 1999;130(6):461–470.

24. Haider A, Yassin A, Doros G, Saad F. Effects of long-term testosterone therapy on patients with "diabesity": Results of observational studies of pooled analyses in obese hypogonadal men with type 2 diabetes. Int J Endocrinol. 2014;2014:683515.

25. Haider A, Zitzmann M, Doros G, Isbarn H, Hammerer P, Yassin A. Incidence of prostate cancer in hypogonadal men receiving testosterone therapy: Observations from 5-year median followup of 3 registries. J Urol. 2015; 193(1):80–86.

26. Saad F, Yassin A, Haider A, Doros G, Gooren L. Elderly men over 65 years of age with late-onset hypogonadism benefit as much from testosterone treatment as do younger men. Korean J Urol. 2015;56(4): 310–317.

27. Haider A, Yassin A, Haider KS, Doros G, Saad F, Rosano G. Men with testosterone deficiency and a history of cardiovascular diseases benefit from long-term testosterone therapy: Observational, real-life data from a registry study. Vasc Health Risk Manag. 2016;12(6): 251–261.

28. Saad F, Yassin A, Doros G, Haider A. Effects of long-term treatment with testosterone on weight and waist size in 411 hypogonadal men with obesity classes I-III: Observational data from two registry studies. Int J Obes. 2016;40(1):162–170.

29. Saad F, Doros G, Haider KS, Haider A. Differential effects of 11 years of long-term injectable testosterone undecanoate therapy on anthropometric and metabolic parameters in hypogonadal men with normal weight, overweight and obesity in comparison with untreated controls: Real-world data from a controlled registry study. Int J Obes. 2020;44(6): 1264–1278.

30. Haider KS, Haider A, Saad F, et al. Remission of type 2 diabetes following long-term treatment with injectable testosterone undecanoate in patients with hypogonadism and type 2 diabetes: 11-year data from a real-world registry study. Diabetes Obes Metab. 2020;22(11):2055–2068.

31. Traish AM, Haider A, Haider KS, Doros G, Saad F. Long-term testosterone therapy improves cardiometabolic function and reduces risk of cardiovascular disease in men with hypogonadism: A real-life observational registry study setting comparing treated and untreated (control) groups. J Cardiovasc Pharmacol Therap. 2017;22(5):414–433.

32. Haider KS, Haider A, Doros G, Traish A. Long-term testosterone therapy improves urinary and sexual function, and quality of life in men with hypogonadism: Results from a propensity matched subgroup of a controlled registry study. J Urol. 2018;199(1):257–265.

33. Saad F, Caliber M, Doros G, Haider KS, Haider A. Long-term treatment with testosterone undecanoate injections in men with hypogonadism alleviates erectile dysfunction and reduces risk of major adverse cardiovascular events, prostate cancer, and mortality. Aging Male. 2020; 23(1):81–92.

34. Saad F, Haider A, Doros G, Traish A. Long-term treatment of hypogonadal men with testosterone produces substantial and sustained weight loss. Obesity. 2013;21(10):1975–1981.

35. Groti Antonič K, Antonič B, Žuran I, Pfeifer M. Continuation of testosterone treatment beyond one year results in more profound benefits— Glycemic efficacy and metabolic profile in obese hypogonadal males with type 2 diabetes in a two-year clinical trial. Aging Male. 2020. DOI: 10.1080/13685538.2020.1793132.

36. Morgunov LY, Denisova A, Rozhkova TI, Stakhovskaya LV, Skvortsova VI. Hypogonadism and its treatment following ischaemic stroke in men with type 2 diabetes mellitus. Aging Male. 2020;23(1):71–80.

37. Hackett G, Cole N, Mulay A, Strange RC, Ramachandran S. Long-term testosterone therapy in type 2 diabetes is associated with decreasing waist circumference and improving erectile function. World J Men's Health. 2020;38(1):68–77.

38. Corona G, Giagulli VA, Maseroli E, et al. Testosterone supplementation and body composition: Results from a meta-analysis of observational studies. J Endocrinol Invest. 2016;39(9):967–981.

39. Skinner JW, Otzel DM, Bowser A, et al. Muscular responses to testosterone replacement vary by administration route: A systematic review and meta-analysis. J Cachexia Sarcopenia Muscle 2018;9(3):465–481.

40. Nasser M, Haider A, Saad F, et al. Testosterone therapy in men with Crohn's disease improves the clinical course of the disease: Data from long-term observational registry study. Horm Mol Biol Clin Invest. 2015; 22(3):111–117.

41. Saad F, Haider A, Gooren L. Hypogonadal men with psoriasis benefit from long-term testosterone replacement therapy—A series of 15 case reports. Andrologia. 2016; 48(3):341–346.

42. Traish A, Bolanos J, Nair S, Saad F, Morgentaler A. Do androgens modulate the pathophysiological pathways of inflammation? Appraising the contemporary evidence. J Clin Med. 2018;7:549.

43. Zhang X, Zhong Y, Saad F, Haider K, Haider A, Xu X. Clinically occult prostate cancer cases may distort the effect of testosterone replacement therapy on risk of PCa. World J Urol. 2019;37(10):2091–2097.

44. Zhang X, Zhong Y, Saad F, et al. Testosterone therapy may reduce prostate cancer risk due to testosterone deficiency at a young age via stabilizing serum testosterone levels. Aging Male. 2020;23(2): 112–118.

45. Carruthers M, Cathcart P, Fennelly MR. Evolution of testosterone treatment over 25 years: Symptom responses, endocrine profiles and cardiovascular changes. Aging Male. 2015;18(4):217–227.

46. Winter A, Marte A, Kelly M, Funaro M, Schlegel P, Paduch D. Predictors of poor response to transdermal testosterone therapy in men with metabolic syndrome. J Urol. 2014;4S(Suppl.):e528.

Abbreviations Used

AMS = Aging Males' Symptoms
BMI = body mass index
DRE = digital rectal examination
ED = erectile dysfunction
GP = general practitioner
HDL = high-density lipoprotein
IBD = inflammatory bowel disease
LDL = low-density lipoprotein
RCTs = randomized controlled trials
T2DM = type 2 diabetes mellitus
TD = testosterone deficiency
TG = triglyceride
TTh = testosterone therapy
TU = testosterone undecanoate
WC = waist circumference

14

Testosterone Therapy Reduces Cardiovascular Risk Among Hypogonadal Men: A Prospective Cohort Study in Germany

Xiao Zhang,[1] Ke Huang,[2,3] Farid Saad,[4] Karim Sultan Haider,[5] Ahmad Haider,[5] and Xiaohui Xu[1,*]

Abstract

Background: Low testosterone level has been associated with predictors of cardiovascular disease (CVD); however, controversies exist regarding the role of testosterone therapy, a treatment to improve testosterone levels, in preventing cardiovascular risk. Longitudinal studies with a large sample size and long follow-up duration are limited.

Materials and Methods: We conducted a prospective cohort study using data from 602 hypogonadism men free of CVDs at study baseline from a registry study in Germany who were eligible for testosterone therapy, with an age range of 31–74 years and a follow-up duration of up to 12 years. Receiving testosterone therapy or not was based on the patient's own choice at study entry. Patients who decided to take testosterone therapy were classified as treatment group (n = 325), and the rest were classified as the control group (n = 277). We compared the Framingham Global CVD Risk Score between the treatment and control groups over time and cardiovascular incidence during the follow-up period. We adjusted for baseline characteristics between the treatment and control groups in the mixed-effect model examining the longitudinal effect of testosterone treatment on the risk score, and we applied propensity score matching to control for confounders.

Results: We found that the control group had an overall increasing risk score and decreasing testosterone level over time. For the treatment group with improved testosterone level and lipid and glucose profiles, the risk score decreased before 24 months, and it became stable later on. After propensity score matching, there were 0 cardiovascular events in the treatment group and 45 in the control group.

Conclusions: Low testosterone level is associated with higher cardiovascular risk. Long-term testosterone therapy reduces cardiovascular events among hypogonadal men. Clinicians should be informed of this association when assessing a male patient's cardiovascular risk and ensure timely treatment if needed.

Keywords: hypogonadism; testosterone; Framingham Risk Score; cardiovascular risk

Introduction

Cardiovascular disease (CVD) is a major cause of morbidity and the leading cause of death globally.[1] Smoking, increased blood glucose, low-density lipoprotein (LDL) cholesterol, and blood pressure are major risk factors for CVD.[2] Multivariate risk prediction algorithms incorporating these risk factors has been developed to conveniently evaluate an individual's risk of developing future CVD events, including the widely used Framingham Global CVD Risk Score calculated

[1]Department of Epidemiology and Biostatistics, School of Public Health, Texas A&M University, College Station, Texas, USA.
[2]Department of Statistics, Texas A&M University, College Station, Texas, USA.
[3]Department of Statistics, University of California, Riverside, California, USA.
[4]Research Department, Gulf Medical University, Ajman, United Arab Emirates.
[5]Private Urology Practice, Bremerhaven, Germany.

*Address correspondence to: Xiaohui Xu, Department of Epidemiology and Biostatistics, School of Public Health, Texas A&M University, MS 1266, 212 Adriance Lab Road, College Station, TX 77843-1266, USA, Email: xiaohui.xu@tamu.edu

based on age, gender, total cholesterol, smoking status, high-density lipoprotein (HDL) cholesterol, and systolic blood pressure.[3,4]

Studies have recently been focused on the role of testosterone in cardiovascular risk among men, as it is the most abundant male hormone that is critical in maintaining normal glucose and lipid metabolism in men. It has been suggested that testosterone may limit vascular inflammation and cytokine activity underpinning the atherosclerosis process, and the morphological changes in the walls of the arteries might be due to metabolic syndrome resulting from testosterone deficiency.[5,6] Studies have shown that low testosterone levels were associated with higher carotid intima media thickness,[7–9] which is a surrogate marker of atherosclerosis that is closely related to abnormal glucose metabolism and lipid profile as well as a strong predictor of future clinical ischemic cardiac and cerebrovascular events.[10–12]

Although low testosterone level has been closely associated with predictors of CVD, controversies exist regarding the role of exogenous testosterone therapy, a treatment to improve testosterone levels, in preventing cardiovascular risk. One of the earliest randomized controlled trials, the testosterone in older men trial, was terminated because of the higher number of cardiovascular events in the intervention group compared with the placebo group.[13] However, study subjects in this trial were elderly men aged 65 years or older with a high prevalence of preexisting heart disease, obesity, diabetes, and hypertension, and "with no standard indication for testosterone therapy".[14] In addition, these elderly men had limitations in mobility, who were more likely to have clinical or subclinical cardiovascular conditions than those who did not have these limitations.

A recent study reviewed seven systematic reviews that included a total of 94 randomized controlled trials and investigated the association between exogenous testosterone and cardiovascular events.[15] Six of them showed no association, and one showed a significant increased risk for CVD associated with exogenous testosterone. The authors pointed out that because of limited sample sizes and short follow-up periods, these trials were underpowered to detect a true difference in cardiovascular risk between treatment and control groups. More evidence from well-designed studies with eligible participants, large sample sizes, and sufficient follow-up time are needed before a determination on the safety of testosterone therapy can be made.

In this study, we conducted a prospective cohort study by using data from 602 hypogonadism men of a registry study conducted in Germany who were eligible for testosterone therapy, with an age range of 31–74 years and a follow-up duration of up to 12 years. Receiving testosterone therapy or not was based on the patient's own choice at study entry. Patients who decided to take testosterone therapy were classified as the treatment group ($n = 325$), and the rest were classified as the control group ($n = 277$).

We investigated the association between testosterone therapy and cardiovascular risk by comparing the Framingham Global CVD Risk Score[3] between the treatment and control groups over time and cardiovascular incidence during the follow-up period. We controlled for baseline health condition and medication use between the treatment and control groups in the mixed-effect model examining the longitudinal effect of testosterone treatment on the Framingham Global CVD Risk Score, and we applied propensity score matching to control for confounders when comparing the incidence between the two groups. We hypothesize that treatment groups are more likely to have improvement in Framingham Global CVD Risk Score and fewer cardiovascular events as compared with the control group.

Materials and Methods
Study population

We used de-identifiable data from a registry study in Germany. Eight hundred five men were recruited from one urology center in Bremerhaven, Germany from 2004, where they had sought medical consultation for various urological complaints, including sexual dysfunction. Hypogonadism diagnosis was confirmed if they had total testosterone level ≤12.1 nmol/L (∼350 ng/dL) and symptoms as assessed by the Aging Males' Symptoms scale. We have chosen the threshold of 12.1 nmol/L, which is ∼350 ng/dL based on our own clinical experience and that was confirmed by Bhasin et al.[16] After excluding patients who had prior cardiovascular events, a total of 602 patients were included in the study. Among prostate cancer patients, measurements after cancer diagnosis have also been removed for the analysis. Ethical guidelines formulated by the German Ärztekammer (German Medical Association) for observational studies in patients receiving standard treatment were followed.

After receiving an explanation about the nature and the purpose of the study, all patients provided written consent to be included in the registry and had their data analyzed. Participants were followed up annually or semi-annually for updates in serum testosterone level, prostate-specific antigen (PSA) levels, height, weight, body mass index (BMI), waist circumference, blood pressure, lipid profile, glucose, and several other physical, laboratory, and imaging test results. Details on lab measurements have been described elsewhere.[17]

Treatment assignment

Patients with PSA <4 ng/mL were given the option of testosterone therapy. Hematocrit and other parameters were measured, and the laboratory cut-off was used as an inclusion criterion. Receiving testosterone therapy or not was based on the patient's own choice at the beginning of the study. Patients who decided to take testosterone therapy were classified as treatment group ($n = 325$), and the rest were classified as control group (277). As previously described,[18,19] patients on testosterone therapy received injections of 1000 mg of testosterone undecanoate with the second injection 6 weeks after the first injection, followed by 12-week intervals throughout the observation time. Since every injection was administered and documented in the urology office, the adherence to testosterone was 100%.

Cardiovascular outcome ascertainment

Cardiovascular events, including myocardial infarction and stroke occurring during follow-up, were recorded. Cardiovascular events were partly reported in the form of "physician letters" from the hospital or the cardiologist/neurologist/family physician, partly by patients themselves or relatives. The latter usually occurs when already scheduled patient visits have to be postponed due to an event. The Framingham Global CVD Risk Score was calculated for each patient at each visit. Details on score calculation have been described elsewhere.[3] Higher score indicates higher 10-year risk/probability of developing future cardiovascular events.

Statistical analysis

In the descriptive analysis, baseline characteristics, follow-up, comorbidity condition, and medication use between the treatment and control groups were compared by using t-test or chi-square test. Line charts were used to compare the mean risk score, lipid profile, glucose, circumference, and BMI changes over time between the two groups.

A mixed-effect model with a random intercept as the random effect, and follow-up time, treatment and their interaction as fixed effects were fitted to assess the testosterone therapy effect on longitudinal changes of the Framingham Global CVD Risk Score, adjusting for baseline risk score, age at study entry, family history of CVD, smoking, alcohol consumption, baseline total cholesterol, baseline HDL, type 2 diabetes (yes/no), and hypertension (yes/no), after considering collinearity.

In addition, CVD incidence rates of the two groups were compared after propensity score matching on baseline risk score, LDL, hypertension, HbA1c, family history of CVD, and alcohol consumption to balance the baseline health condition between treatment and groups.

All analyses were performed with R version 3.3.3. Tests results were considered statistically significant at $\alpha = 0.05$.

Results

After excluding patients with prior CVD events, a total of 602 patients were included in the study, of whom 277 received testosterone therapy. The mean age of total participants is 60 years, and the median follow-up is 8 years. Baseline characteristics, health condition, and medication use between the treatment and control groups are presented in Table 1. Age at study entry, follow-up period, lipid panel, glucose profile, alcohol consumption, smoking status, comorbidity condition, medication use, and family history of CVD were statistically significantly different between the two groups.

Results from the mixed-effect model are shown in Table 2. Overall, after adjusting for confounders, in the control group, for a 1-month increase in time, the Framingham Global CVD Risk Score increased by 0.02; in the treatment group, for a 1-month increase in time, the risk score increased by $0.02 - 0.01 = 0.01$. Before 24 months, for a 1-month increase, risk score in the control group increased by 0.03 and decreased by 0.03 ($0.03 = 0.028 - 0.057$) in the treatment group; after 24 months, for a 1-month increase, risk score in the control group increased by 0.03 and increased by 0.01 ($0.01 = 0.027 - 0.014$) in the treatment group.

As shown in Figures 1 and 2, testosterone level in the control group was decreasing over time, together with increased Framingham Global CVD Risk Score; whereas in the treatment group, testosterone level was increasing over time, along with decreased Framingham Global CVD Risk Score and improved lipid profile, glucose, BMI, and waist circumference. In a *post hoc* analysis among patients with metabolic syndrome, we noticed improved lipid profile and glucose

Table 1. Baseline Characteristics and Mean Follow-Up of Patients, by Treatment Group

Characteristics	Control (n = 277) Mean ± SE	Range	Treatment (n = 325) Mean ± SE	Range	p
Age at study entry (years)	63.63 ± 4.78	45–74	56.69 ± 7.73	31–71	<0.001
Testosterone (nmol/L)	9.68 ± 1.11	5.9–11.79	9.69 ± 1.42	0.8–12.13	<0.855
PSA (ng/mL)	2.45 ± 1.35	0.2–7.9	1.65 ± 0.93	0.08–3.87	<0.001
Total cholesterol (mg/dL)	249.49 ± 46.09	173–388	297.88 ± 38.09	202–423	<0.001
LDL (mg/dL)	131.56 ± 49.97	55–246	159.21 ± 30.96	82–229	<0.001
HDL (mg/dL)	47.49 ± 19.15	16–93	38.31 ± 11.78	15–88	<0.001
Glucose (mmol/L)	5.74 ± 0.56	5.11 ± 9.32	6.14 ± 1.15	4.88–9.99	<0.001
HbA1c (%)	6.11 ± 1.29	4.3–9.3	7.04 ± 1.79	4.1–13.4	<0.001
Systolic blood pressure (mmHg)	135.57 ± 9.76	115–181	147.63 ± 16.29	120–188	<0.001
Diastolic blood pressure (mmHg)	77.94 ± 7.17	66–121	87.51 ± 10.58	68–121	<0.001
BMI (kg/m2)	29.72 ± 3.88	22.2–44.1	32.15 ± 5.22	21.91–46.51	<0.001
Follow-up (years)	8.08 ± 1.93	1–12	7.60 ± 2.86	1.25-11.75	0.016

	n	%	n	%	
Alcohol consumption	129	46.60	111	34.20	0.003
Smoker	82	29.60	135	41.50	0.003
Type 2 diabetes	105	37.90	92	28.30	0.016
Hypertension	186	67.10	289	88.95	<0.001
Anti-diabetic use	105	37.90	101	31.10	0.094
Anti-hypertensive use	31	11.20	117	36.00	<0.001
Statin use	149	53.80	97	29.80	<0.001
Family history of CVD	31	11.20	73	22.50	<0.001

BMI, body mass index; CVD, cardiovascular disease; HbA1c, hemoglobin A1c; HDL, high-density lipoprotein; LDL, low-density lipoprotein; PSA, prostate specific antigen; SE, standard error.

panel among those who received testosterone therapy and an opposite situation in the control group (data not shown).

After propensity score matching, there were 232 participants in the treatment group and 212 participants in the control group. Forty-five CVD events were in the control group, and 0 events were in the treatment group. The incidence in the control group is 0.00219 whereas that in the treatment group is 0 (Table 3). The difference is statistically significant (Fisher's exact,

$p < 0.0001$). In the *post hoc* analysis, we also examined all-cause mortality in the two groups (Table 4), and we found that the control group has a significantly higher mortality rate as compared with the treatment group.

Discussion

This prospective cohort study using data from a registry study conducted in Germany demonstrated that hypogonadal men who did not receive testosterone therapy were more likely to experience an increase in

Table 2. Coefficients from Random-Effect Model Investigating the Effect of Testosterone Therapy on the Longitudinal Changes of the Framingham Global Cardiovascular Disease Risk Score

Variable	Overall Coefficient	95% CI	Before 24 months Coefficient	95% CI	After 24 months Coefficient	95% CI
Month	0.024	(0.02, 0.03)	0.028	(0.02, 0.03)	0.027	(0.026, 0.028)
Treatment	1.795	(1.61, 1.98)	1.544	(1.33, 1.75)	1.881	(1.64, 2.12)
Month*treatment	−0.011	(−0.013, −0.010)	−0.057	(−0.07, −0.05)	−0.014	(−0.02, −0.01)
Baseline risk score	0.077	(0.05, 0.10)	0.247	(0.22, 0.28)	0.055	(0.03, 0.08)
Age at study entry	0.289	(0.28, 0.30)	0.245	(0.23, 0.26)	0.290	(0.27, 0.30)
BMI	0.066	(0.05, 0.08)	0.046	(0.03, 0.06)	0.069	(0.05, 0.09)
Smoker	4.000	(3.92, 4.08)	3.515	(3.39, 3.63)	4.082	(3.92, 4.25)
Alcohol	−0.175	(−0.28, −0.07)	−0.366	(−0.49, −0.24)	−0.082	(−0.12, 0.03)
Type 2 diabetes	2.599	(2.44, 2.76)	2.221	(2.04, 2.40)	2.726	(2.56, 2.89)
Hypertension	0.371	(0.22, 0.52)	0.475	(0.31, 0.64)	0.173	(0.01, 0.33)
Total cholesterol	0.025	(0.02, 0.03)	0.018	(0.016, 0.020)	0.022	(0.020, 0.023)
HDL	−0.080	(−0.082, −0.077)	−0.065	(−0.07, −0.06)	−0.078	(−0.080, −0.075)
Family history of CVD	0.043	(−0.12, 0.21)	0.131	(−0.04, 0.30)	0.005	(−0.17, 0.18)

CI, confidence interval.

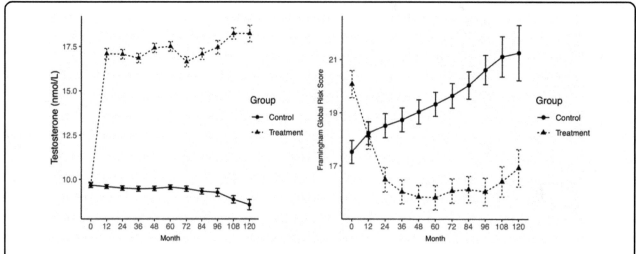

FIG. 1. Framingham global cardiovascular disease risk score and testosterone level changes over time, by treatment group.

the Framingham Global CVD Risk Score later on, whereas patients who received testosterone therapy were more likely to experience a significant decrease in risk score at an early phase of treatment and became relatively stable afterward. After propensity score matching, the treatment group had 0 cardiovascular events as compared with 45 incident cases in the control group. The adjusted incidence rate in the control group is 0.00219, which is statistically significantly higher than the treatment group.

It has been suggested that testosterone is closely associated with surrogate markers of CVD (e.g., cholesterol level, waist circumference, fasting glucose, blood pressure).[20,21] Monroe and Dobs reviewed articles regarding the relationship between endogenous testosterone and lipid profile and found endogenous testosterone to be inversely associated with LDL cholesterol, triglyceride, and total cholesterol, but positively associated with HDL cholesterol in cross-sectional and prospective observational studies.[22] Corona et al. conducted a systematic review and found that men with metabolic syndrome were likely to benefit from testosterone therapy.[23] This is consistent with our findings that patients with metabolic syndrome in the treatment group experienced elevated testosterone level as well as improved lipid and glucose profile during the study period.

Low testosterone level among hypogonadal men may affect lipid metabolism by upregulating the genes involved in HDL cholesterol clearance and decreasing triglyceride uptake,[22,24] resulting in central

obesity and adverse lipid profiles. The excess lipid accumulation due to abnormal lipid metabolism then forms the plaque in the walls of the arteries, the first step of atherosclerosis that may eventually lead to cardiovascular or cerebrovascular events if no action is taken. Recent evidence shows that oxidative stress and inflammation induced by elevated cholesterol level, high glucose, and hypertension may also contribute to the progression of atherosclerosis.[25,26]

In addition, as a predictor for atherosclerosis related to testosterone and future cardiovascular or cerebrovascular events, carotid intima-media thickness is also found to be associated with endogenous testosterone levels. This is because carotid intima–media thickening is a complex process, depending on a variety of factors including blood pressure, glycemic control, and lipid metabolism,[2,27] which are closely related to testosterone levels. Vikan et al., Soisson et al., Koskenvuo et al., and Kwon et al. reported an inverse association between testosterone and carotid intima–media thickness.[7–9,28] Our previous studies also suggested the beneficial effect of testosterone therapy on cardiometabolic function in aging men.[18,29]

Testosterone therapy that maintains normal testosterone level may improve lipid profile and glucose management and, therefore, reduce cardiovascular risk and mortality. Though the beneficial effect of testosterone therapy on cardiovascular health and potential underlying mechanisms have been reported in previous studies,[30–32] findings in clinical trials have been inconsistent.

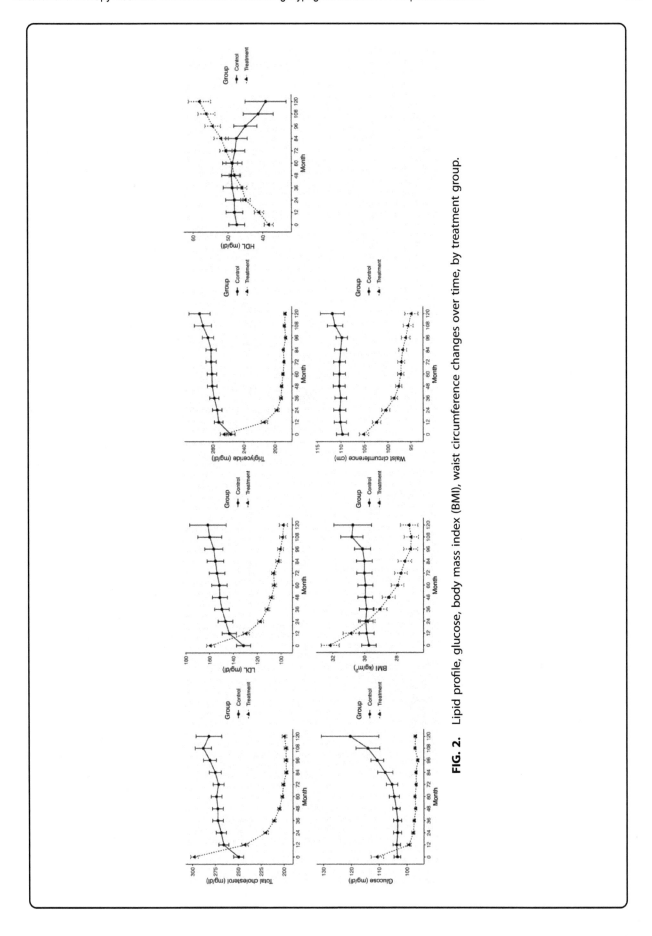

FIG. 2.   Lipid profile, glucose, body mass index (BMI), waist circumference changes over time, by treatment group.

Table 3. Cardiovascular Incidence, by Treatment Group

	CVD events	Total participants	Total person month	Incidence rate*
Before matching				
Treatment	0	325	29,631	0
Control	52[a]	277	26,874	0.00193
After matching				
Treatment	0	232	18,645	0
Control	45[b]	212	20,520	0.00219

*Incidence rate difference between the treatment and control group is statistically significant different from 0 ($p < 0.0001$, Fisher's exact test).

[a]Thirty cases of myocardial infarctions, 21 cases of strokes, and 1 case of both myocardial infarction and stroke.

[b]Twenty-five cases of myocardial infarctions, 19 cases of strokes, and 1 case of both myocardial infarction and stroke.

Testosterone's Effects on Atherosclerosis Progression in Aging Men (TEAAM) ($n = 308$, 3-year follow-up)[33] and the Testosterone Trials (TTrials) ($n = 138$, 1-year follow-up)[34] are two randomized clinical trials (RCTs) that investigated the effect of exogenous testosterone administration on cardiovascular function in older men with low testosterone levels. TTrials found among hypogonadal men that 1-year testosterone treatment was associated with a greater increase of coronary artery noncalcified plaque volume as compared with the placebo group. TEAAM found among older men with low or low-normal testosterone levels, after 3 years' treatment, that no significance difference in either common carotid artery intima–media thickness or coronary artery calcium changes was observed in the testosterone treatment group versus placebo group.

Though considered as the gold standard for causal inference, due to the highly restrictive inclusion and exclusion criteria, findings from RCTs cannot be easily generalized to the real-world scenarios. In addition, with a relatively shorter follow-up period and small-moderate sample sizes, these RCTs might be underpowered to detect the true effect of testosterone therapy on cardiovascular risk. This was also mentioned in Gagliano-Jucá and Basaria's recent review study on

Table 4. All-Cause Mortality, by Treatment Group

	Death	Total participants	Total person month	Mortality rate*
Before matching				
Treatment	8	325	29,634	0.00003
Control	35	277	27,432	0.00128
After matching				
Treatment	5	232	18,666	0.00027
Control	30	212	20,874	0.00144

*Mortality rate difference between the treatment and control group is statistically significant different from 0 ($p < 0.0001$, Fisher's exact test).

the evidence from epidemiologic studies regarding the cardiovascular safety of testosterone therapy.[35] They believe no trials of testosterone replacement therapy published to date were designed or adequately powered to assess cardiovascular events.

A large RCT (a planned sample of ∼6000 men, with 5-year treatment duration) that is currently recruiting will be powered to evaluate the effect of testosterone therapy on the incidence of major adverse cardiovascular events and efficacy measures in hypogonadal men (TRAVERSE study, NCT03518034). However, it still takes time to collect essential data before any analysis. Until then, well-designed observational studies with a sufficient sample size and a longer follow-up period may be able to provide convincing evidence in a more naturalistic setting. A multi-national, prospective study ($n = 999$) that used real-world data from the Registry of Hypogonadism in Men study assessed cardiovascular safety of testosterone therapy.[36] The authors found no increased cardiovascular risk in the treatment group, which is in line with our study findings.

Our study is a prospective cohort study with a relatively large sample size, long follow-up duration, and wide age range. All participants were hypogonadal and, therefore, had indication for testosterone treatment at the time of study. We used the Framingham Global CVD Risk Score, which well predicts the risk of future cardiovascular events.[3,37] As compared with the older versions of Framingham Risk Score,[38,39] this global risk score was derived based on a larger number of events, incorporated multiple risk factors as continuous variables instead of categorical variables, and replaced the disease-specific algorithms with a single general CVD prediction tool, which may increase the prediction precision as well as simplify risk prediction in office-based practices.[3]

In this study, we observed a protective effect of treatment on cardiovascular events, which are consistent with previous observational studies that used Framingham study-based Risk Score as the outcome variable. Lee et al. found a significant negative correlation between total testosterone level and the Framingham Risk Score among 308 patients with sexual dysfunction.[40] Chock and colleagues identified that 1479 veterans had previous total plasma testosterone checked in 2008 and reported a negative association between both total testosterone and free testosterone levels and the Framingham Risk Score.[41] We used repeated measurements of testosterone level and, therefore, were able to examine the effect of treatment on the longitudinal changes of the risk scores over time.

However, limitations of this study should be noted. First, though we have controlled for multiple covariates unevenly distributed in the two treatment groups due to the nature of observational study, there is always a confounding issue. Nevertheless, the effect of residual confounding would be minimal as we adjusted for major confounders in the model.

Second, the potential association between testosterone and cardiovascular risk may be curvilinear,[42] and treatment effect may only work when the individual's testosterone is supplemented and maintained at normal level.[14,21,42,43] We did not differentiate the treatment effects in this study. Besides, our results can only be related to this type of testosterone therapy, given the various treatment patterns available. Future studies may take this into account and compare the treatment effect difference when testosterone has not yet been elevated to normal level, in the normal level, and above normal level, and also consider the effect of other testosterone treatment methods.

Third, the Framingham Risk Score may overestimate cardiovascular risk in the European population.[4] Future studies comparing prediction abilities of different tools among populations with diverse makeup are needed.

Lastly, though low testosterone is a risk factor for CVD because it contributes to abnormal lipid metabolism and is physiologically plausible, it may be also reasonable to suggest that testosterone is a consequence of abnormal lipid metabolism. Low testosterone leads to excess fat accumulation, and overweight and obesity in turn worsen hypogonadism, similar to a vicious cycle.[44] However, the focus of this study is not to find out which comes first. We expected clinicians to be informed of this potential association and break the vicious cycle to prevent future cardiovascular events from happening.

Conclusions

In this longitudinal study, we found that low testosterone level was associated with impaired lipid and glucose profile and higher Framingham Global CVD Risk Score among hypogonadal men. Long-term testosterone therapy may improve lipid and glucose profile and reduce Framingham Global CVD Risk Score. Clinicians should be informed of this association when assessing the male patient's cardiovascular risk and make sure timely treatment if needed.

Authors' Contributions

X.Z.: conceptualization, visualization, writing—original draft preparation, writing—reviewing and editing.

K.H.: data curation, methodology, software, formal analysis visualization. F.S.: writing—reviewing and editing. K.S.H.: writing—reviewing and editing. A.H.: writing—reviewing and editing. X.X.: resources, supervision, conceptualization, visualization, writing—reviewing and editing, project administration.

References

1. CDC. Know the facts about: Heart disease. Natl Cent Chronic Dis Prev Heal Promot. 2008:1–2. Available at www.cdc.gov/nchs/ (accessed February 14, 2019).
2. Herrington W, Lacey B, Sherliker P, Armitage J, Lewington S. Epidemiology of atherosclerosis and the potential to reduce the global burden of atherothrombotic disease. Circ Res. 2016;118(4):535–546.
3. D'Agostino RB, Vasan RS, Pencina MJ, et al. General cardiovascular risk profile for use in primary care: The Framingham heart study. Circulation. 2008;117(6):743–753.
4. Lloyd-Jones DM. Cardiovascular risk prediction: Basic concepts, current status, and future directions. Circulation. 2010;121(15):1768–1777.
5. Malkin CJ, Pugh PJ, Jones RD, Jones TH, Channer KS. Testosterone as a protective factor against atherosclerosis—Immunomodulation and influence upon plaque development and stability. J Endocrinol. 2003;178(3):373–380.
6. Traish AM, Abdou R, Kypreos KE. Androgen deficiency and atherosclerosis: The lipid link. Vascul Pharmacol. 2009;51(5–6):303–313.
7. Vikan T, Johnsen SH, Schirmer H, Njølstad I, Svartberg J. Endogenous testosterone and the prospective association with carotid atherosclerosis in men: The Tromsø study. Eur J Epidemiol. 2009;24(6):289–295.
8. Soisson V, Brailly-Tabard S, Empana JP, et al. Low plasma testosterone and elevated carotid intima-media thickness: Importance of low-grade inflammation in elderly men. Atherosclerosis. 2012;223(1):244–249.
9. Kwon H, Lee D-G, Kang HC, Lee JH. The relationship between testosterone, metabolic syndrome, and mean carotid intima-media thickness in aging men. Aging Male. 2014;17(4):211–215.
10. Lorenz MW, Markus HS, Bots ML, Rosvall M, Sitzer M. Prediction of clinical cardiovascular events with carotid intima-media thickness: A systematic review and meta-analysis. Circulation. 2007;115(4):459–467.
11. Nezu T, Hosomi N, Aoki S, Matsumoto M. Carotid intima-media thickness for atherosclerosis. J Atheroscler Thromb. 2016;23(1):18–31.
12. O'Leary DH, Kronmal RA, Polak JF, Manolio TA, Burke GL, Wolfson SK. Carotid-artery intima and media thickness as a risk factor for myocardial infarction and stroke in older adults. N Engl J Med. 2002;340(1):14–22.
13. Basaria S, Coviello AD, Travison TG, et al. Adverse events associated with testosterone administration. N Engl J Med. 2010;363(2):109–122.
14. Loo SY, Chen BY, Yu OHY, Azoulay L, Renoux C. Testosterone replacement therapy and the risk of stroke in men: A systematic review. Maturitas. 2017;106(August):31–37.
15. Onasanya O, Iyer G, Lucas E, Lin D, Singh S, Alexander GC. Association between exogenous testosterone and cardiovascular events: an overview of systematic reviews. Lancet Diabetes Endocrinol. 2016;4(11):943–956.
16. Bhasin S, Pencina M, Jasuja GK, et al. Reference ranges for testosterone in men generated using liquid chromatography tandem mass spectrometry in a community-based sample of healthy nonobese young men in the framingham heart study and applied to three geographically distinct cohorts. J Clin Endocrinol Metab. 2011;96(8):2430–2439.
17. Sultan K, Haider A, Doros G, Saad F. Design and conduct of a real-world single-center registry study on testosterone therapy of men with hypogonadism. Androg Clin Res Ther. 2020;1(1):1–17.
18. Traish AM, Haider A, Haider KS, Doros G, Saad F. Long-term testosterone therapy improves cardiometabolic function and reduces risk of cardiovascular disease in men with hypogonadism. J Cardiovasc Pharmacol Ther. 2017;22(5):414–433.
19. Haider KS, Haider A, Doros G, Traish A. Long-term testosterone therapy improves urinary and sexual function, and quality of life in men with hypogonadism: Results from a propensity matched subgroup of a controlled registry study. J Urol. 2018;199(1):257–265.
20. Saad F, Haider A, Doros G, Traish A. Long-term treatment of hypogonadal men with testosterone produces substantial and sustained weight loss. Obesity. 2013;21(10):1975–1981.

21. Deng C, Zhang Z, Li H, Bai P, Cao X. Analysis of cardiovascular risk factors associated with serum testosterone levels according to the US 2011–2012 National Health and Nutrition Examination Survey. Aging Male. 2019; 22(2):121–128.
22. Monroe AK, Dobs AS. The effect of androgens on lipids. Curr Opin Endocrinol Diabetes Obes. 2013;20(2):132–139.
23. Corona G, Maseroli E, Rastrelli G, et al. Cardiovascular risk associated with testosterone-boosting medications: A systematic review and meta-analysis. Expert Opin Drug Saf. 2014;13(10):1327–1351.
24. Schleich F, Legros JJ. Effects of androgen substitution on lipid profile in hypogonadal men. Rev Med Liege. 2003;58(11):681–689.
25. Varghese JF, Patel R, Yadav UCS. Novel insights in the metabolic syndrome-induced oxidative stress and inflammation-mediated athero-sclerosis. Curr Cardiol Rev. 2017;14(1):4–14.
26. Alexopoulos N, Katritsis D, Raggi P. Visceral adipose tissue as a source of inflammation and promoter of atherosclerosis. Atherosclerosis. 2014; 233(1):104–112.
27. Wang CF, Lv GP, Zang DW. Risk factors of carotid plaque and carotid common artery intima-media thickening in a high-stroke-risk population. Brain Behav. 2017;7(11):1–9.
28. Koskenvuo M, Pöllänen P, Huhtaniemi I, et al. Increased carotid athero-sclerosis in andropausal middle-aged men. J Am Coll Cardiol. 2005;45(10): 1603–1608.
29. Saad F, Caliber M, Doros G, Haider KS, Haider A. Long-term treatment with testosterone undecanoate injections in men with hypogonadism allevi-ates erectile dysfunction and reduces risk of major adverse cardiovascular events, prostate cancer, and mortality. Aging Male. 2020;23(1):81–92.
30. Kelly DM, Jones TH. Testosterone and cardiovascular risk in men. In: Cardiovascular Issues in Endocrinology. Front Horm Res. 2014;43:1–20.
31. Jones Th, Kelly D. Randomized controlled trials—Mechanistic studies of testosterone and the cardiovascular system. Asian J Androl. 2018;20(2):120.
32. Kilby EL, Kelly DM, Jones TH. Testosterone stimulates cholesterol clearance from human macrophages by activating LXRα. Life Sci. 2021;269:119040.
33. Basaria S, Harman SM, Travison TG, et al. Effects of testosterone admin-istration for 3 years on subclinical atherosclerosis progression in older men with lower low-normal testosterone levels: A randomized clinical trial. JAMA. 2015;314(6):570–581.
34. Budoff MJ, Ellenberg SS, Lewis CE, et al. Testosterone treatment and coronary artery plaque volume in older men with low testosterone. JAMA. 2017;317(7):708–716.
35. Gagliano-Jucá T, Basaria S. Testosterone replacement therapy and car-diovascular risk. Nat Rev Cardiol. 2019;16(9):555–574.
36. Maggi M, Wu FCW, Jones TH, et al. Testosterone treatment is not asso-ciated with increased risk of adverse cardiovascular events: results from the Registry of Hypogonadism in Men (RHYME). Int J Clin Pract. 2016; 70(10):843–852.
37. Towfighi A, Markovic D, Ovbiagele B. Utility of framingham coronary heart disease risk score for predicting cardiac risk after stroke. Stroke. 2012;43(11):2942–2947.
38. Wilson PW, D'Agostino RB, Levy D, Belanger AM, Silbershatz H, Kannel WB. Prediction of coronary heart disease using risk factor categories. Circulation. 1998;97(18):1837–1847.
39. Kannel WB, McGee D, Gordon T. A general cardiovascular risk profile: The Framingham Study. Am J Cardiol. 1976;38(1):46–51.
40. Lee WC, Kim MT, Ko KT, et al. Relationship between serum testosterone and cardiovascular disease risk determined using the Framingham risk score in male patients with sexual dysfunction. World J Mens Health. 2014;32(3):139–144.
41. Chock B, Lin TC, Li CS, Swislocki A. Plasma testosterone is associated with Framingham risk score. Aging Male. 2012;15(3):134–139.
42. Srinath R, Golden SH, Carson KA, Dobs A. Endogenous testosterone and its relationship to preclinical and clinical measures of cardiovascular disease in the atherosclerosis risk in communities study. J Clin Endocrinol Metab. 2015;100(4):1995–1995.
43. Anderson JL, May HT, Lappé DL, et al. Impact of testosterone replacement therapy on myocardial infarction, stroke, and death in men with low testosterone concentrations in an integrated health care system. Am J Cardiol. 2016;117(5):794–799.
44. Corona G, Mannucci E, Forti G, Maggi M. Hypogonadism, ED, metabolic syndrome and obesity: A pathological link supporting cardiovascular diseases. Int J Androl. 2009;32(6):587–598.

Abbreviations Used

BMI = body mass index
CI = confidence interval
CVD = cardiovascular disease
HbA1c = hemoglobin A1c
HDL = high-density lipoprotein
LDL = low-density lipoprotein
PSA = prostate specific antigen
SE = standard error

15

Testosterone Therapy in Men with Biochemical Recurrence and Metastatic Prostate Cancer: Initial Observations

Abraham Morgentaler,[1,*,i] Alejandro Abello,[1,ii] and Glenn Bubley[2]

Abstract

Introduction: Although prostate cancer (PCa) has long been considered an absolute contraindication for testosterone therapy (TTh), growing literature suggests TTh may be safely offered to men with localized PCa. We here present a single-center series of men treated with TTh for relief of symptoms, despite having more advanced disease, namely biochemical recurrence (BCR) or metastatic PCa (MET).

Methods: We identified men treated with TTh with BCR, MET, or adjuvant androgen deprivation therapy (ADT). Consent included risks of rapid PCa progression and death. Laboratory and clinical results were analyzed.

Results: Twenty-two men received TTh: 7 with BCR, 13 with MET, and 2 with adjuvant ADT. Median age was 70.5 years (range 58–94). Median TTh duration was 12 months (range 2–84) overall, including 20 months for BCR and 9.5 months for MET. Mean serum testosterone (T) increased from 210 to 1111 ng/dL. Median PSA (interquartile range) increased from 3.1 ng/mL (0.2–4.5) to 13.3 ng/mL (3.4–22) in the BCR group, 6.3 ng/mL (1.2–31) to 17.8 ng/mL (6.2–80.1) in the MET group, and <0.1 to 0.3 ng/mL in the ADT group. All patients reported symptom relief, especially improved vigor and well-being. Overall mortality was 13.6% and PCa-specific mortality was 4.5% during the period of TTh and 6 months after discontinuation. Seven of 10 with follow-up imaging within 12 months showed no progression. Five men have died: three during TTh and two succumbed at 2 years or longer after discontinuing TTh. One of the three deaths during TTh was PCa-specific. Three men developed significant bone pain at 7–41 months; two discontinued TTh and one continued, after focal radiation. There were no cases of rapid-onset complications, vertebral collapse, or pathological fracture.

Conclusions: These initial observations indicate TTh was not associated with precipitous progression of PCa in men with BCR and MET, suggesting a possible role for TTh in selected men with advanced PCa whose desire for improved quality of life is paramount.

Keywords: testosterone; prostate cancer; testosterone therapy; testosterone and prostate diseases; androgen deprivation therapy; hormone replacement therapy; metastatic prostate cancer and testosterone

Introduction

The diagnosis of prostate cancer (PCa) has been considered an absolute contraindication for testosterone (T) therapy (TTh) for decades, based on the belief that TTh "activates" PCa growth, first asserted by Huggins and Hodges.[1] In 1981, Fowler and Whitmore reported that 45 of 52 men with metastatic PCa who received testosterone demonstrated an "unfavorable

[1]Division of Urology, Department of Surgery, Beth Israel Deaconess Medical Center, Harvard Medical School, Boston, Massachusetts, USA.
[2]Division of Hematology and Oncology, Department of Medicine, Beth Israel Deaconess Medical Center, Harvard Medical School, Boston, Massachusetts, USA.
[i]ORCID ID (https://orcid.org/0000-0002-5925-4086).
[ii]ORCID ID (https://orcid.org/0000-0001-8302-2763).

*Address correspondence to: Abraham Morgentaler, MD, 200 Boylston Street, #309, Chestnut Hill, MA 02467, USA, Email: amorgent@bidmc.harvard.edu

response" within 30 days.[2] Since standard treatment for advanced PCa is to lower serum T with androgen deprivation therapy (ADT), it seemed logical that raising serum T promotes PCa growth. For these reasons it has been widely believed that raising testosterone is likely to cause rapid disease progression, morbidity, and death in men with PCa.

However, a growing literature has challenged this concept. Multiple case series have demonstrated low rates of PCa progression or recurrence in men after radical prostatectomy (RP),[3,4] radiation therapy,[5] and in men on active surveillance.[6,7] Population-based studies have failed to show that use of TTh is associated with worse PCa outcomes.[8] The apparent paradox whereby ADT causes disease regression in PCa yet TTh appears to not cause worse PCa outcomes is resolved by the saturation model,[9] describing a growth curve in which maximal androgenic stimulation of PCa is achieved at low serum T concentrations, with little to no additional stimulation occurring at higher serum T concentrations. There is extremely limited evidence regarding saturation in advanced PCa, consisting of absence of prostate-specific antigen (PSA) progression with TTh in a case report,[10] and an inverted U-curve in PCa cell lines *in vitro* exposed to progressively increasing androgen concentrations, with maximal growth achieved at near-physiological concentrations followed by growth inhibition at higher concentrations.[11] However, positive results from the use of bipolar androgen therapy (BAT) in men with castrate-resistant PCa,[12] and a modified BAT protocol (mBAT)[13] indicate that elevating serum testosterone is not necessarily harmful.

Whereas there has been growing evidence for the benefits of TTh in the general population of men with testosterone deficiency,[14] and moderate experience in men with PCa after definitive local therapy or with low-risk disease on active surveillance, there is scant published experience with use of TTh in men with nonlocalized PCa in clinical practice. We present in this study our initial observations of TTh in a set of men with advanced PCa treated with TTh. These men all specifically sought TTh, for a number of reasons, including prior experience with TTh, adverse experience with ADT, or belief that a robust serum T concentration would be beneficial for their health despite known concerns that TTh would hasten PCa growth.

Methods

We identified all men in the database at Men's Health Boston treated with TTh and with biochemical recurrence (BCR), metastatic PCa (MET), or who were treated with ADT for high risk of recurrence after definitive local treatment through end of June 2020. One man presented initially with BCR and eventually developed metastases: his results are included in both the BCR and MET groups for the relevant periods. Treatment with TTh was initiated in all cases at the patient's request to improve or optimize quality of life. All patients underwent extensive counseling and signed a consent form indicating their awareness that treatment could cause rapid disease progression, with associated morbidity and death. Relevant data were collected for PCa disease status and prior treatment. BCR was defined as PSA >0.2 ng/mL after surgery, or nadir +2 ng/mL after radiation or high-intensity focused ultrasound (HIFU).

All men in the study had previously consulted with an oncologist or urologist specializing in PCa and were aware of standard PCa-specific treatment options. All patients specifically requested TTh, many because of previous experience with TTh or due to symptoms that arose from ADT. There was no requirement to obtain psychological counseling. One patient with MET on ADT with bothersome sexual symptoms first underwent surgical placement of a penile prosthesis to address his erectile dysfunction. There was no protocol in place for cessation of TTh, although men understood they could discontinue treatment at any time and for any reason. Coordination of care was attempted whenever possible with local oncologists or urologists; however, in many cases patients were advised by their local physicians that they would not participate in a treatment regimen that included TTh. At each visit men affirmed they wished to continue with TTh, or it was discontinued.

Men were considered candidates for TTh if they had suggestive symptoms and total testosterone was <350 ng/dL or free testosterone <100 pg/mL. Treatment consisted of injections of testosterone cypionate at doses ranging from 100 to 200 mg weekly or in more recent years at high-dose treatment of 200–400 mg every 2 weeks. High-dose injections were used in the MET group based on data suggesting supraphysiological T concentrations may suppress PCa growth[11] and after publication of results of BAT in men with metastatic castrate-resistant PCa.[12] Topical gels and subcutaneous pellets were also used in standard doses to maintain normal serum T concentrations, and dosage was adjusted to optimize clinical response. An mBAT protocol was used in selected men with MET, consisting of repeated 12-week cycles during which high-dose (400 mg) testosterone cypionate intramuscular injections were given every 2 weeks for a total of 8 weeks, followed by 4 weeks of daily oral enzalutamide 80–160 mg.[13] None of the men in the MET group had castrate-resistant disease.

Monitoring for the BCR group included PSA at 3 months intervals for the first year, and then every 6 months. For MET group on TTh alone, PSA was obtained every 3 months, and for the mBAT group PSA was obtained every 3 months at the end of 4 weeks of antiandrogens. Follow-up imaging studies were obtained at 6-month intervals in men with MET, and at least annually in BCR. Follow-up for local patients was performed in the office every 3 months for the first year and then at least every 6 months. For patients living at a distance, follow-up visits were in person when possible, and through televisits at other times. Subjective response to treatment was based on structured discussions that addressed energy, mood, strength, and sexuality. No validated questionnaire was used.

The Memorial Sloan Kettering Cancer Center online tool was used to calculate PSA doubling times (https://www.mskcc.org/nomograms/prostate/psa_doubling_time). Prostate cancer-specific (PCS) mortality was defined as deaths occurring as a result of PCa during TTh or within 6 months of discontinuation of TTh. Overall mortality was defined as deaths from any cause during the period of TTh or within 6 months of its discontinuation.

Statistical analysis

We compared and summarized findings from BCR and metastatic groups. Medians and interquartile ranges (IQRs) were used to describe continuous variables based on small sample size and non-normally distributed variables. Ranges were presented for selected results. Percentages and proportions were used to describe categorical variables. We compare continuous variables between groups using Wilcoxon rank sum tests, and a p-value <0.05 was set to determine statistical significance. We used Stata 15® to perform the statistical analysis of the data. This study is reported under IRB # 2010-P-000241 from Beth Israel Deaconess Medical Center.

Results

Between 2005 through June 2020 a total of 22 men with advanced PCa received TTh, with 15 of these treated within the past 5 years. The study group comprised 13 men with MET, 7 men with BCR, and 2 men treated with adjuvant ADT after radiation deemed high risk.

For the entire group, the median age at TTh initiation was 71 years (range 58–94), median PSA was 2.52 (range 0.01–546), median Gleason score was 7 (range 6–9), and median baseline testosterone was 204 ng/dL (range 3–629). The median duration of TTh was 12.5 months (range 2–84). Duration of TTh was 6 months or greater in 19 men. Baseline characteristics for the BCR and MET groups are presented in Table 1, and individual case details, including response to TTh, are shown in Table 2. For the entire group, PCS mortality was 4.5% and overall mortality was 13.6%. Results for the BCR and MET groups are presented in Table 3.

BCR group

Median age for the seven men in the BCR group was 69.5 years (range 59–85). Primary treatment was RP in three and radiation therapy in four. Treatment of the radiation group was external beam radiotherapy (XRT) alone in two men, brachytherapy in one. One additional man first underwent two treatments with HIFU, followed by XRT when PSA continued to rise. Two of three men with BCR after RP developed rising PSA despite additional treatment with radiation. The third developed BCR 9 years after RP and did not

Table 1. Baseline Characteristics by Group

	BCR = 7	Metastatic = 14
Median age (IQR)	69.5 (59–85)	72.0 (66–74)
Median PSA (IQR)	3.14 (0.2–4.5)	4.1 (0.3–31)
Primary PCa treatment (%)		
Unknown	0%	7.7%
Brachytherapy	14.3%	0%
External beam radiation therapy	28.6%	23.1%
External beam radiation+HIFU	14.3%	7.7%
RP		
Proton therapy	42.9%	23.1%
ADT only	0%	7.7%
	0%	30.8%
Bone metastases (%)		
Yes	0%	71.4%
No	100%	28.6%
Nodal metastases (%)		
Yes	0%	50%
No	100%	50%
ADT (%)		
Yes	14.3%	50.0%
No	85.7%	50.0%
mBAT		
Yes	0%	57.1%
No	100%	42.9%

ADT, androgen deprivation therapy; BCR, biochemical recurrence; HIFU, high-intensity focused ultrasound; IQR, interquartile range; mBAT, modified BAT protocol; PCa, prostate cancer; PSA, prostate-specific antigen; RP, radical prostatectomy.

Table 2. Case Details

Age (years)	Disease status	Duration TTh (months)	Initial PCa Rx	Metastatic disease burden	Prior TTh	Hx ADT	Response to TTh	Comments
70	Met	14	Proton Tx	High	N	Y	Weakness improved and personality returned	Continues on TTh. Increased uptake bone scan without new lesions at 1 year
74	Met	10	ADT	Low	Y	Y	Strength, vigor, sexual function improved, and personality returned	Myocardial infarction at 6 months, died during TTh at 10 months from peptic ulcer disease
61	Met	41	RP	Low	N	N	Strength and sexuality improved	Discontinued TTh at 41 months due to increased hip pain, worsened bone scan
94	Met	11	ADT	High	N	Y	Strength and cognition improved	Died during TTh
76	Met	4	XRT	High	N	Y	Strength and vigor improved with TTh	Urinary retention at 3 months. Discontinued TTh on advice of local MD
68	Met	2	None	Low	N	N	Strength and vigor improved with TTh	Discontinued TTh on recommendation of local MD
73	Met	8	ADT	Low	N	Y	Vigor, walking, and sexual function improved	Continues TTh. New bone lesions at 10 months
75	Met	9	RP	High	N	Y	Vigor improved	Continues on TTh. XRT to new pelvic adenopathy at 6 months
63	Met	24	XRT	Low	N	Y	Strength improved and personality returned	Discontinued TTh when PNBx showed residual cancer
72	Met	8	ADT	High	N	Y	Strength and vigor improved	Discontinued TTh when needed XRT for back pain/metastases
71	Met	4	RP	Low	N	N	Strength, well-being, and sexuality improved	Continues on TTh. Bone scan unchanged at 12 months
60	Met	7	XRT	Low	Y	Y	Sense of well-being improved	TTh discontinued for rising PSA
66	Met	84	ADT	Low	N	Y	Sexual function and vigor improved	Died of myelofibrosis after 7 years TTh
67	Met	41	HIFU	Low	Y	Y	Strength and libido improved	Discontinued TTh when developed bone marrow replacement by PCa
59	BCR	63	RP	NA	Y	N	Vigor, mood, libido, and well-being improved	Continues on TTh
65	BCR	16	HIFU/XRT	NA	Y	Y	Strength, vigor, and libido improved	Bone metastases noted at 16 months, continued TTh
58	BCR	33	RP	NA	Y	N	Vigor and well-being improved	Discontinued TTh when PSA reached 20 ng/mL
61	BCR	48	RP	NA	Y	N	Well-being, strength, and sexual function improved	Continues on TTh
85	BCR	20	XRT	NA	N	Y	Cognition improved	Discontinued TTh when PSA reached 22 ng/mL
74	BCR	13	Brachy	NA	Y	N	Well-being and vigor improved	Continues on TTh
75	BCR	5	XRT	NA	N	Y	Cognition improved	Continues on TTh
69	Adjuvant ADT	16	XRT	NA	N	Y	Cognition improved	Continues on TTh without metastases
77	Adjuvant ADT	12	XRT	NA	N	Y	Well-being and vigor improved	Discontinued TTh on recommendation of local MD

TTh, testosterone therapy; XRT, external beam radiotherapy.

Table 3. Baseline and Follow-Up Variables While on Testosterone Therapy Between Metastatic and Biochemical Recurrence Groups

	BCR = 7	Metastatic = 14
Median baseline PSA, ng/dL (IQR)	3.1 (0.2–4.5)	6.3 (0.3–31)
Median follow-up PSA, ng/dL (IQR)	13.3 (3.4–22)	17.8 (6.2–80.1)
Median increase in PSA, ng/dL (IQR)	13.3 (2.8–19)	7.5 (2.35–83.7)
Median baseline T, ng/dL (IQR)	264 (202–470)	181 (21–333)
Median follow-up T, ng/dL (IQR)	1062 (980–1076)	1011 (724–1500)
Median increase in T, ng/dL (IQR)	613 (585–874)	879.5 (591–1241)
Median baseline hematocrit, % (IQR)	45.6 (39.2–49.5)	42 (40.5–44.2)
Median follow-up hematocrit, % (IQR)	46.5 (42–48.2)	47.2 (41.7–49.25)
Median hematocrit change, % (IQR)	−0.9 (-1.3–0.90)	4.8 (2.4–5.9)
Duration of TTH (IQR)	20 (13–48)	9.5 (7–24)

T, testosterone.

receive pelvic XRT. Five had previous experience with TTh for a diagnosis of T deficiency before developing BCR. None were castrate at time of initiation of TTh.

Baseline median PSA was 3.1 ng/mL (range 0.2–8.2 ng/mL). Median duration (IQR) of TTh was 20 months (13–48), and median (IQR) increase in PSA after TTh was 13.3 (2.8–19). Median PSA (IQR) doubling time was 8.9 months (7.1–14.0). One man with BCR developed metastases after 16 months of TTh with a baseline PSA of 32 ng/mL after two HIFU treatments for Gleason 8 disease. No other complications were observed in this group during TTh. One died of metastatic PCa 6 years after discontinuing TTh when his PSA exceeded 20 ng/mL after 33 months of TTh. Four men continue on TTh for up to 5 years without evidence of metastases, with a mean duration of 32.5 months. Overall and PCS mortality were 0% in this group.

MET group

Median age for the 14 men in the MET group was 72 years (range 60–94), and baseline median PSA was 6.3 ng/mL (range <0.1–546). Seven had bone metastases, three had pelvic adenopathy, and four had both. Five of the men with bone metastases had high disease burden. Seven men presented while on ADT and/or antiandrogen therapy, four had been previously treated with ADT, and three had never received ADT or antiandrogens. Men who presented on ADT or antiandrogen therapy were encouraged to undergo a trial of these medications before beginning TTh. Three did so, and

returned after minimum of 3 months still requesting initiation of TTh. Median duration of TTh was 9.5 months (IQR 7–24). Median PSA doubling time (IQR) was 4.4 months (2.4–8.3).

Eight men were treated with at least one cycle of mBAT and six received continuous TTh through injections, gels, or subcutaneous pellets.

Follow-up imaging was available for 10 men at 3–12 months after initiating TTh. Seven showed no progression and three showed progression, all with new foci of bone metastases.

Three men died during TTh: one from PCa at 95 years from PCa after 10 months TTh; one at 73 years from myelofibrosis, 7 years after beginning TTh; and one at 75 years after 10 months TTh from peptic ulcer disease. One additional man died of PCa, 2 years after discontinuing TTh. Complications during TTh included myocardial infarction (MI) at 6 months in a patient with three prior strokes, the most recent being 2 years before initiation of TTh; bone marrow replacement by PCa 3.5 years after first development of bone metastases; urinary retention with urosepsis 3 months after initiation of TTh; and a recurrent deep vein thrombosis 8 months after beginning TTh. There were no cases of pulmonary emboli, pathological fractures, or acute spinal cord compression. Of the 11 men still alive, 2 discontinued TTh due to PCa progression, 4 discontinued TTh on the recommendation of their local physicians, and 5 continued treatment with TTh. Overall mortality in this group was 21.4% and PCS mortality was 7.1%. Median baseline and final PSA values for BCR and MET groups are shown in Figure 1.

Adjuvant ADT

Two men with Gleason 8 PCa initially treated with ADT for high-risk disease after stereotactic radiation therapy treatment received TTh for a median of 14 months (12–16). One was treated for 9 months with combination leuprolide and enzalutamide, and developed impaired cognition, unusually slow speech and movements. Leuprolide was discontinued together with initiation of TTh, while continuing enzalutamide. The second patient was treated with leuprolide for 1 year, then discontinued due to disabling fatigue, and began TTh 5 months later. Mean testosterone levels increased from 50 to 854 ng/dL. Mean PSA increased from 0.01 to 0.3 ng/mL while on TTh. No adverse events were noted. The second patient discontinued TTh at 1 year at urging of his local

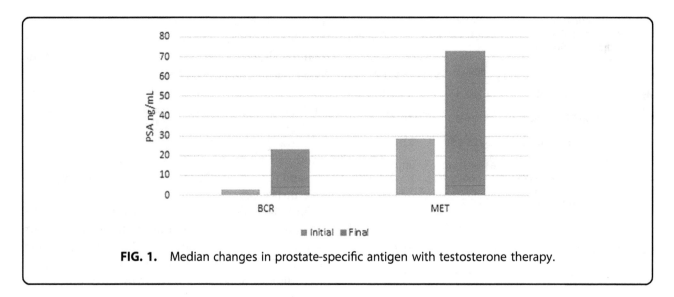

FIG. 1.   Median changes in prostate-specific antigen with testosterone therapy.

physician, and the first continues with TTh in combination with enzalutamide with greatly improved cognition and ease of movement.

Discussion

To the best of our knowledge this is the first reported clinical series in the PSA era of outcomes with TTh specifically in men with BCR or MET in a clinical setting, and not part of a formal trial. A total of 20 men with nonlocalized PCa and two receiving ADT deemed at high risk for metastases received TTh for up to 7 years with a median duration of >1 year, with considerable subjective improvement in quality of life, and without rapid progression, morbidity, or death. There was only one PCa-specific death during TTh, occurring 11 months after initiation of TTh in a 94-year-old man with diffuse metastases and initial PSA 546 ng/dL. Although this series of cases cannot establish safety of TTh in the setting of advanced PCa, these results do challenge the long-standing assumption that even transient exposure to increased serum T in a man with advanced PCa-with testosterone flare, for example, will rapidly precipitate morbidity or death.[15]

The original basis for the belief that TTh is dangerous for PCa arose from the work of Huggins and Hodges, who in 1941 concluded that "Testosterone injections cause activation of prostate cancer[1]" Contemporary review of their original data revealed it was based on erratic acid phosphatase data for only 14 days in a single hormonally intact individual.[16] Fowler and Whitmore reported 45 of 52 men who received TTh demonstrated an undefined "unfavorable result" within 30 days; however, all but four of these men had

already undergone castration or were on estrogen treatment to suppress serum T.[2] Of these four men, three demonstrated no unfavorable results despite daily injections of T propionate for 51, 55, and 310 days. The appearance of poor outcomes for men on ADT but not for men who were hormonally intact inspired the development of the saturation model, which demonstrates a finite capacity of androgens to stimulate PCa growth, with exquisite sensitivity to changes in androgen concentrations at low values, and then insensitivity once the saturation point is reached,[9] which appears to be ~ 250 ng/dL in men.[17,18] This study provides suggestive evidence for saturation in nonlocalized PCa, since men with BCR failed to demonstrate precipitous increases in PSA despite substantial periods of TTh.

There is scant literature regarding testosterone administration in men with advanced PCa in the PSA era. Leibowitz et al. reported results of a variety of strategies involving TTh in a mixed population of 96 men with PCa, of which it appears 31 likely had metastatic disease.[19] Clinical trials of BAT in men with castrate-resistant prostate cancer reported a PSA decline in 7 of 14 men, and evaluable disease was reduced in 5 of 10 men.[12] To optimize the duration of time on TTh, mBAT was developed[13] and was used in seven men in the MET group in this study.

There are several notable observations from this clinical series. First, there exists a set of men for whom quality of life is more important than duration of life. Each patient understood that their choice of TTh could cause immediate or hastened disease progression, morbidity, and death. Second, these men only continued TTh because it provided them with symptomatic benefits to a degree that made it worthwhile, in their estimation, to risk their lives. This defies a frequently made assertion that TTh provides only minimal symptomatic benefits.[20] Nearly all men experienced increased vigor. Sexual desire and ability were improved in many, and several were able to resume sexual activity after years without it, especially those on ADT. One man gained enough strength to give up the need for a walker. Several men and their partners noted a return of their "personality." One regained fluency of speech and brain processing that had been severely compromised by ADT. Further research in this area would benefit from use of validated instruments to address subjective response to treatment.

Arguably the most important observation from this study is that TTh was not associated with rapid disease progression. Among men with BCR, with median duration of 33 months of TTh, only one progressed to metastatic disease >5 years after beginning TTh. This compares with 3 years estimates of metastatic disease in men with BCR after RP of 14% for Gleason score 5–7 and 37% for Gleason score 8–10.[21] Hruby et al. reported that 70 of 538 men demonstrated biochemical failure after XRT for localized PCa with median follow-up of 50 months. Of these 70 men with biochemical failure, 13 had died and metastases were observed in 5 of the remaining 57 (8.8%).[22] Only 30% of men with MET demonstrated progression on follow-up imaging studies by 3–12 months. The overall survival of 79.6% (mortality 21.4%) in the MET group compares with median survival of 47.2 months in the ADT alone arm of the CHAARTED Trial.[23] The relevance of the short median PSA doubling times of 8.9 months in BCR and 4.4 months in MET is uncertain, as PSA doubling times are not usually determined in men receiving androgens, particularly since PSA expression is itself androgen-dependent.[24]

There are several important limitations to this study, including its retrospective nature, multiple forms of TTh treatment, and small sample size. In addition, PCa is a heterogenous disease, and this report includes those with Gleason scores ranging from 6 to 9, which may cloud interpretation of results. Nonetheless, these preliminary results indicate that TTh does not appear to cause precipitous PCa progression in men with BCR and MET. There may be a role for TTh in selected men with BCR, MET, or high-risk disease willing to accept the theoretical risk of hastened disease progression in return for enhanced quality of life.

Conclusion

TTh in men with BCR, MET, and high-risk PCa was associated with symptomatic benefits and low rates of complications, although interpretation of these results must be tempered by small sample size and a heterogeneous population. Well-designed prospective studies are needed to provide better evidence for the potential use of TTh in similarly affected individuals. In the meantime, these results may provide clinicians with a framework to counsel patients who prioritize quality of life over longevity.

Authors' Contributions

Data extraction by A.M.; data analysis and drafting of the article by A.A. and A.M.; critical revision of article for important intellectual content by A.A., G.B., and A.M.

References

1. Huggins C, Hodges CV. Studies on prostatic cancer. I. The effect of castration, of estrogen and of androgen injection on serum phosphatases in metastatic carcinoma of the prostate. Cancer Res. 1941;1:293–297.
2. Fowler JE, Whitmore Jr WF. The response of metastatic adenocarcinoma of the prostate to exogenous testosterone. J Urol. 1981;126:372–375.
3. Pastuszak AW, Pearlman AM, Lai WS, et al. Testosterone replacement therapy in patients with prostate cancer after radical prostatectomy. J Urol. 2013;190:639–644.
4. Ahlering TE, Huynh LM, Towe M, et al. Testosterone replacement therapy reduces biochemical recurrence after radical prostatectomy. BJUI. 2020; 126:91–96.
5. Pastuszak AW, Khanna A, Badhiwala N, et al. Testosterone therapy after radiation therapy for low, intermediate and high risk prostate cancer. J Urol. 2015;194:1271–1276.
6. Morgentaler A, Lipshultz LI, Avila D, Jr, et al. Testosterone therapy in men with untreated prostate cancer. J Urol 2011;185:1256–1261.
7. Kacker R, Mariam H, San Francisco IF, et al. Can testosterone therapy be offered to men on active surveillance for prostate cancer? Preliminary results. Asian J Androl. 2016;18:16–20.
8. Baillargeon J, Kuo YF, Fang X, Shahinian VB. Long-term exposure to testosterone therapy and the risk of high-grade prostate cancer. J Urol. 2015; 194:1612–1616.
9. Morgentaler A, Traish AM. Shifting the paradigm of testosterone and prostate cancer: The saturation model and the limits of androgen-dependent growth. Eur Urol. 2009;55(2):310–320.
10. Mathew P. Prolonged control of progressive castration-resistant metastatic prostate cancer with testosterone replacement therapy: The case for a prospective trial. Ann Oncol. 2008;19:395–403.
11. Song W, Khera M. Physiological normal levels of androgen inhibit proliferation of prostate cancer cells in vitro. Asian J Androl. 2014;16(6):864–868.
12. Schweizer MT, Antonarakis ES, Wang H, et al. Effect of bipolar androgen therapy for asymptomatic men with castration-resistant prostate cancer: Results from a pilot clinical study. Sci Transl Med. 2015;7(269):269ra2.
13. Morgentaler A. Strategies for testosterone therapy in men with metastatic prostate cancer in clinical practice: Introducing modified bipolar androgen therapy. Androgens. 2020;1:76–84.

14. Snyder PJ, Bhasin S, Cunningham GR, et al. Effects of testosterone treatment in older men. NEJM. 2016;374:611–624.

15. Krakowsky Y, Morgentaler A. Risk of testosterone flare in the era of the saturation model: One more historical myth. Eur Urol Focus. 2019;5:81–89.

16. Morgentaler A. Testosterone and prostate cancer: An historical perspective on a modern myth. Eur Urol. 2006;50:935–939.

17. Khera M, Bhattacharya RK, Blick G, et al. Changes in prostate specific antigen in hypogonadal men after 12 months of testosterone replacement therapy: Support for the prostate saturation theory. J Urol. 2011;186:1005–1011.

18. Morgentaler A, Benesh JA, Denes BS, et al. Factors influencing prostate-specific antigen response among men treated with testosterone therapy for 6 months. J Sex Med. 2014;11:2818–2825.

19. Leibowitz RL, Dorff TB, Tucker S, et al. Testosterone replacement in prostate cancer survivors with hypogonadal symptoms. BJU Int. 2010;105(10):1397–1401.

20. Kolata G. Testosterone Gel has modest benefits for men, study says. New York Times. 2016.

21. Darwish OM, Raj GV. Management of biochemical recurrence after primary localized therapy for prostate cancer. Front Oncol. 2012. [Epub ahead of print]; DOI: 10.3389/fonc.2012.00048.

22. Hruby G, Eade T, Keebone A, et al. Delineating biochemical failure with ^{68}Ga-PSMA-PET following definitive external beam radiation treatment for prostate cancer. Radiother Oncol. 2017;122:99–102.

23. Kyriakopoulos CE, Chen Y-H, Carducci MA, et al. Chemohormonal therapy in metastatic hormone-sensitive prostate cancer: Long-term survival analysis of the randomized phase III E3805 CHAARTED trial. J Clin Oncol. 2018;36:1080–1087.

24. Peter CA, Walsh PC. Effect of nafarelin acetate, a luteinizing-hormone-releasing hormone agonist, on benign prostatic hyperplasia. NEJM. 1987;317:599–604.

Abbreviations Used

ADT = androgen deprivation therapy
BAT = bipolar androgen therapy
BCR = biochemical recurrence
HIFU = high-intensity focused ultrasound
IQR = interquartile range
mBAT = modified BAT protocol
MET = metastatic PCa
PCa = prostate cancer
PCS = prostate cancer-specific
PSA = prostate-specific antigen
RP = radical prostatectomy
T = testosterone
TTh = testosterone therapy
XRT = external beam radiotherapy

16

Testosterone Therapy in Adult-Onset Testosterone Deficiency: Hematocrit and Hemoglobin Changes

Nathan Lorde,[1] Amro Maarouf,[1] Richard C. Strange,[2] Carola S. König,[3] Geoff Hackett,[4,i] Ahmad Haider,[5] Karim Sultan Haider,[5,ii] Pieter Desnerck,[6] Farid Saad,[7,8,iii] and Sudarshan Ramachandran[1–3,9,iv]

Abstract

Objective: Hematocrit (HCT)/hemoglobin (Hb) ratio in (%/g/dL) is around 3, with high fidelity between measured and derived Hb (applying the conversion using HCT) in various pathologies. We examined changes in HCT and Hb values and HCT/Hb, compared with baseline, in men with adult-onset testosterone deficiency (TD) given testosterone therapy (TTh).

Materials and Methods: Data were analyzed from an observational, prospective registry study at various time points in 353 men with adult-onset TD receiving testosterone undecanoate (median follow-up: 105 months). After establishing baseline HCT/Hb, we compared (cf. baseline) changes in HCT, Hb, and HCT/Hb at 12, 48, 72, and 96 months. Regression analyses determined predictors of HCT and Hb change.

Results: TTh was associated with ($p < 0.0001$) increases in median HCT and Hb; 44% to 49% and 14.5 to 14.9 g/dL at final assessment, respectively. Regression analyses showed that HCT change was associated with baseline HCT and testosterone levels, while Hb change was associated with baseline Hb, HCT, and testosterone levels. In the total cohort and subgroups, HCT/Hb increased significantly at all time points ($p < 0.0001$, cf. baseline) with over 90% of men demonstrating increases. Linear regression showed that the ratio of HCT change/Hb change (i.e., difference between HCT at the various time points and baseline value/difference between Hb at the various time points and baseline value), following TTh at each time point was higher than the baseline HCT/Hb ratio.

Conclusion: HCT increase was greater than we anticipated from the established HCT/Hb of 3. We speculate that increased erythrocyte life span with associated higher Hb loss via vesiculation could account for our observation. This could have a bearing when using HbA1c as an indicator in men with adult-onset TD on TTh.

Keywords: testosterone therapy; hematocrit; hemoglobin; adult-onset testosterone deficiency; erythrocyte life span

[1]Department of Clinical Biochemistry, University Hospitals Birmingham NHS Foundation Trust, West Midlands, England, United Kingdom.
[2]Institute for Science and Technology in Medicine, Keele University, Staffordshire, United Kingdom.
[3]Department of Mechanical and Aerospace Engineering, Brunel University London, United Kingdom.
[4]School of Health and Life Sciences, Aston University, Birmingham, United Kingdom.
[5]Praxis Dr. Haider, Bremerhaven, Germany.
[6]Department of Engineering, University of Cambridge, Cambridge, United Kingdom.
[7]Medical Affairs Andrology, Bayer AG, Berlin, Germany.
[8]Gulf Medical University School of Medicine, Ajman, UAE.
[9]Department of Clinical Biochemistry, University Hospitals of North Midlands, Staffordshire, United Kingdom.
[i]ORCID ID (https://orcid.org/0000-0003-2274-111X).
[ii]ORCID ID (https://orcid.org/0000-0003-4396-9324).
[iii]ORCID ID (https://orcid.org/0000-0002-0449-6635).
[iv]ORCID ID (https://orcid.org/0000-0003-2299-4133).

*Address correspondence to: Sudarshan Ramachandran, FRCPath, Department of Clinical Biochemistry, University Hospitals Birmingham NHS Foundation Trust, Good Hope Hospital, Rectory Road, Sutton Coldfield, West Midlands B75 7RR, United Kingdom, Email: sud.ramachandran@heartofengland.nhs.uk

Introduction

Adult-onset testosterone deficiency (TD) is defined by low serum testosterone levels and associated symptoms and signs.[1] The condition is common, with a prevalence of 6–12% in the general male population and even higher at 40% in men with type 2 diabetes (T2DM).[2,3] A meta-analysis of pooled observational studies demonstrated increased all-cause and cardiovascular mortality in men with adult-onset TD.[4] Longitudinal studies by Muraleedharan et al.[5] and Hackett et al.,[6,7] having demonstrated increased mortality in men with T2DM and low serum testosterone, showed a reduction in all-cause mortality following testosterone therapy (TTh). A few studies[8–10] have suggested increased TTh-associated cardiovascular disease (CVD) and, despite the methodology being criticized,[11] organizations such as the U.S. Food and Drug Administration have expressed concerns.[12] Reassuringly, a meta-analysis of interventional studies concluded that appropriate TTh was not associated with increased risk of CVD, and in some subpopulations, a beneficial effect was possible.[13] Thus, guidelines by the British Society for Sexual Medicine[3] and International Society for Sexual Medicine[14] suggest that men with a serum total testosterone (TT) <8 nmol/L or free testosterone <0.180 nmol/L usually require TTh, while men with serum TT between 8 and 12 nmol/L may, depending on symptoms, be considered for a TTh trial.

Despite the accumulating safety data,[11,13] it is important that vigilance is maintained, especially for factors associated with CVD. This must be extended to subgroups as heterogeneity may be evident in adult-onset TD.[15] An elevated hematocrit (HCT) appears the most frequent adverse effect of TTh.[16,17] The relationship between HCT, atherogenesis, and mortality is not well understood, with many conflicting studies.[18–23] Interestingly, one of these showed a U-shaped association between HCT and mortality, suggesting a complex nonlinear relationship.[22] Currently, monitoring of HCT is recommended during TTh, with guidelines setting differing HCT thresholds (50–54%) above which change in management is recommended.[1,3,24–26]

The mechanism of testosterone-induced erythrocytosis has not been fully elucidated. While some early studies suggested indirect bone marrow action via erythropoietin activity,[27,28] these findings have not always been evident.[29] A more recent study in 2016 by Dhindsa et al. showed that TTh in men with hypogonadotropic hypogonadism increased HCT and this was associated with a rise in erythropoietin, expression of ferroportin and transferrin receptor-2, as well as suppression of hepcidin.[30] Testosterone leading to direct stimulation of bone marrow erythroblast synthesis and iron incorporation into the erythroblasts via circulating soluble transferrin receptor (sTfr), which is involved in the intracellular transport of iron and chiefly found within erythroblasts, have also been considered as possible mechanisms.[31–33] However, Coviello et al. were unable to demonstrate sTfr correlating with testosterone levels.[29]

Another putative mechanism for the observed erythrocyte increase associated with TTh could arise from a decrease in degradation. Following TTh, changes in lipid membrane composition of the erythrocyte have been observed, thereby perhaps enhancing erythrocyte flexibility and thus survival.[34] Interestingly, in healthy subjects, about 20% of erythrocyte hemoglobin (Hb) appears to be shed via vesiculation, a phenomenon that increases during the second half of the erythrocyte life span.[35,36] Thus, in the event of increased erythrocyte life span with a consequent greater Hb loss, an increased HCT/Hb ratio may be expected. In most individuals, the HCT (percentage) appears about three times the Hb (g/dL), with high fidelity between measured and derived (from HCT) Hb values.[36] Furthermore, sensitivity, specificity, and positive predictive values (except in anemia) remained high, irrespective of age, gender, renal function, and hydration status.[37–39]

In this analysis, we aim to characterize Hb and HCT changes (absolute values and the ratio) associated with TTh in men with adult-onset TD, using data from an observational registry study[40] at various time points (0, 12, 48, 72, and 96 months). First, the aim was to report changes in HCT and Hb, and second, to examine the HCT/Hb ratio at each time point (in the total cohort and in subgroup-stratified baseline characteristics).

Materials and Methods

The data used were from an observational, prospective, cumulative registry study[40] of 353 men [median age (IQR): 60.0 (55.0, 64.0), median follow-up (IQR): 105 (78, 141) months] with adult-onset TD (serum TT ≤12.1 nmol/L) given testosterone undecanoate (TU) 1000 mg/12 weeks following an initial 6-week interval). Data were collected at a minimum of 6-month intervals. The database also contained 384 men [median age (IQR): 64.0 (60.0, 67.0), median follow-up (IQR): 114 (96, 126) months] who opted against TTh due to financial constraints and/or negative perceptions of

TTh. The main analyses studied changes in HCT, Hb, and HCT/Hb ratios after 12 (353 men), 48 (313 men), 72 (279 men), and 96 (207 men) months of TTh with the number of patients decreasing in view of the study design. The baseline characteristics of the 353 men commenced on TU are shown in Table 1 and footnotes. The German Medical Association's ethical guidelines for observational studies were adhered to with every participant consenting to be included and having his data analyzed. Following review, ethics committees in Germany and England stated that formal approval was not required. Institutional review board statement for University Hospitals Birmingham was received.

Serum TT (trough) levels were measured using an immunoassay (Abbott Architect). Hb levels were checked using photometry (CELL DYN Ruby/Abbott) and HCT was estimated using Microhematocrit (Mindray 3000 Plus).

Statistical methods

The baseline HCT and Hb values were not normally distributed with both skewness and kurtosis evident ($p < 0.0001$ when considered in combination), hence nonparametric tests were used to compare changes in HCT, Hb values, and HCT/Hb ratios between baseline and fixed time points during treatment. Sign-rank tests were carried out to compare changes in HCT and Hb values between baseline and at fixed time points during treatment. Factors associated with change in HCT and Hb during follow-up were studied using multiple regression. HCT/Hb ratios were calculated for each individual, and changes between the baseline values and those obtained after 12, 48, 72, and 96 months of TTh were compared using sign-rank tests. Finally, the associations between (1) baseline HCT and Hb, and (2) changes in HCT and changes in Hb were studied using linear regression, with scatterplots with trend lines visually reinforcing the findings.

Results

Table 1 shows that serum TT levels increased ($p < 0.0001$, sign-rank test) from baseline (median: 10.05 nmol/L) to 16.64, 16.99, 15.95, 16.99, and 18.72 nmol/L at 12, 48, 72, 96 months, and final assessment, respectively, in the men receiving TTh. In the men not receiving TTh, median serum TT was 9.71 and 8.32 nmol/L at baseline and final assessment, respectively. HCT or Hb did not increase during follow-up in the 384 men not opting for TTh; median (IQR) HCT = 46 (45–47) % and median (IQR) Hb = 14.7 (14.3–15.1) g/dL at baseline; median (IQR) HCT = 46 (45–47) % and median (IQR) Hb = 14.5 (14.2–15.0) g/dL at final assessment. In contrast, TTh was associated with an increase ($p < 0.0001$, sign-rank test) in both HCT and Hb values in the 353 treated men;

Table 1. Hematocrit and hemoglobin values at baseline and fixed time points (12, 48, 72, and 96 months of testosterone therapy) in the total cohort and subgroups stratified by smoking and type 2 diabetes

	Pre-TTh	12 months TTh	48 months TTh	72 months TTh	96 months TTh
			Median (IQR)		
Total cohort, n	353	353	313	279	207
TT (nmol/L)	10.05 (9.36–10.75)	16.64 (14.91–19.07)	16.99 (15.94–19.07)	15.95 (14.91–17.68)	16.99 (15.95–18.38)
Hb (g/dL)	14.5 (14.1–14.9)	14.7 (14.3–15.3)	14.8 (14.6–15.3)	14.9 (14.6–15.3)	15.1 (14.7–15.3)
HCT (%)	44 (43–46)	46 (45–48)	48 (47–49)	48 (47–49)	48 (47–49)
Cohort categorized by baseline characteristics					
Current smokers, n	135	135	119	103	88
Hb (g/dL)	14.6 (14.2–15.1)	14.9 (14.5–15.4)	15.0 (14.6–15.3)	15.1 (14.7–15.3)	15.2 (14.7–15.4)
HCT (%)	44 (43–45)	47 (45–49)	48 (47–49)	48 (47–49)	48 (47–49)
Nonsmokers, n	218	218	194	176	119
Hb (g/dL)	14.5 (14.1–14.8)	14.7 (14.3–15.2)	14.8 (14.6–15.3)	14.8 (14.6–15.3)	15.0 (14.7–15.3)
HCT (%)	44 (43–46)	46 (45–48)	48 (47–49)	48 (47–49)	48 (47–48)
Men with T2DM, n	148	148	121	100	74
Hb (g/dL)	14.6 (14.2–14.9)	14.8 (14.5–15.3)	14.9 (14.7–15.3)	15.0 (14.7–15.3)	15.2 (14.8–15.3)
HCT (%)	45 (44–46)	46 (45–48)	48 (47–49)	48 (47–49)	48 (47–49)
Men without T2DM, n	205	205	192	179	133
Hb (g/dL)	14.3 (14.1–14.8)	14.7 (14.3–15.3)	14.8 (14.5–15.2)	14.8 (14.5–15.3)	15.0 (14.6–15.3)
HCT (%)	44 (42–45)	46 (44–48)	48 (47–49)	48 (47–49)	48 (47–49)

Baseline characteristics of the 353 men not shown in the above table; median (IQR). Age: 60 (55, 64) years, follow-up: 105 (78, 141) months. Waist circumference: 108 (100, 114) cm. Serum TT: 10.05 (9.36, 10.75) nmol/L. HbA1c: 8.15 (5.8, 8.9)%, total cholesterol: 7.7 (7.2, 8.6) mmol/L, triglycerides: 3.2 (2.8, 3.5) mmol/L. Systolic blood pressure: 158 (141, 167) mmHg, diastolic blood pressure: 94 (83, 98) mmHg.

Hb, hemoglobin; HCT, hematocrit; T2DM, type 2 diabetes; TT, total testosterone; TTh, testosterone therapy.

median (IQR) HCT = 44 (43–46) % and median (IQR) Hb = 14.5 (14.1–14.9) g/dL at baseline; median (IQR) HCT = 49 (48–50) % and median (IQR) Hb = 14.9 (14.7–15.3) g/dL at final assessment. Table 1 demonstrates HCT and Hb levels at baseline and the fixed time points during follow-up in the total cohort on TTh, as well as subgroups based on baseline characteristics (smoking status and T2DM). Both HCT and Hb increased significantly at each time point ($p < 0.0001$, sign-rank test) compared with baseline in the total cohort as well as subgroups.

Separate multiple regression analyses showed that change in HCT at final assessment was associated with baseline HCT (coefficient $[c] = -0.95$, 95% confidence intervals $[CI] = -1.05$ to -0.87, $p < 0.001$) and baseline TT ($c = -0.11$, 95% CI = -0.21 to -0.016, $p = 0.023$), while change in Hb at final assessment was associated with baseline Hb ($c = -0.53$, 95% CI = -0.60 to -0.46, $p < 0.001$), baseline HCT ($c = 0.021$, 95% CI = -0.40 to -0.0018, $p = 0.032$), baseline TT ($c = -0.026$, 95% CI = -0.048 to -0.0043, $p = 0.019$), and follow-up ($c = 0.0035$, 95% CI = 0.0025–0.0044, $p < 0.001$). Age, smoking status, and T2DM were not associated with change in either HCT or Hb.

Table 2 shows the median calculated HCT/Hb ratio in the total cohort and subgroups (stratified by median baseline age, Hb, HCT, serum TT, as well as smoking and diabetes status). The baseline HCT/Hb ratio was 3.03 in the total cohort. The HCT/Hb ratio increased significantly ($p < 0.0001$, sign-rank test) at every time point (sign-rank test, $p < 0.0001$) compared with baseline in the total cohort of men on TTh and all the subgroups (Table 2). Table 2 also presents the number (and %) of men with increasing and decreasing HCT/Hb ratio. After 48, 72, and 96 months of TTh, >90% of men had an increasing HCT/Hb ratio.

We now wish to confirm the increased HCT/Hb ratio during TTh by studying the association between the change in HCT and change in Hb. A scatter plot demonstrating the association between baseline HCT and Hb ($c = 3.03$, 95% CI = 2.75–3.31) is shown (Fig. 1). We then determined the association between change in HCT and change in Hb after 48 (Fig. 2), 72, and 96 months of TTh (12-month follow-up data were omitted as the HCT continued to rise after that time point). Figure 2 (footnote table) shows the results of the linear regression; the c and intercept values were higher than those obtained from the linear regression between baseline HCT and Hb, with no overlap between the 95% CI seen in Figure 1 (footnote table).

These data and plots reinforce the findings presented in Table 2: an increase in the HCT/Hb ratio occurs in men with adult-onset TD on TTh.

Although we focused on the HCT/Hb ratio following TTh, we also had data on the 384 men who opted against TTh. The median HCT remained 48% at all time points studied [baseline (384 men), 12 months (383 men), 48 months (367 men), 72 months (342 men), 96 months (283 men), and final assessment]. Interestingly there was a slight reduction in Hb during follow-up: 14.7 g/dL (baseline), 14.7 g/dL (12 months), 14.6 g/dL (48 months), 14.6 g/dL (72 months), 14.6 g/dL (96 months), and 14.5 g/dL (final assessment). Thus, unlike in the cohort on TTh where both HCT and Hb increased at all time points, in the men opting against TTh, any change in the median HCT/Hb ratios appeared driven by changes in Hb: 3.13 (baseline), 3.13 (12 months), 3.13 (48 months), 3.11 (72 months), 3.15 (96 months), and 3.16 (final assessment). As the baseline characteristics of the cohorts (men on TTh and men opting against TTh) varied, we avoided intercohort comparisons.

Discussion

In this study, we characterized the changes in HCT and Hb associated with TTh (TU) in men with adult-onset TD. At the final assessment, median HCT and Hb increased 5% and 0.4 g/dL, respectively. We also presented the changes in HCT and Hb at fixed time points (12, 48, 72, and 96 months) with the changes appearing to plateau after 48 months of treatment. The HCT/Hb ratio of 3.03 at baseline (Table 2 and Fig. 1) was similar to the numeral 3.0 that is often quoted in the literature.[37–39] However, while on TTh, the HCT/Hb ratio significantly increased with the ratios increasing in >90% of men on TTh for 48, 72, and 96 months. The change in HCT/change in Hb ratio was also significantly greater while on TTh (Fig. 2).

Studies determining the long-term effects of TTh on both HCT and Hb are scarce. Wang et al. studied HCT and Hb concentrations in 123 men after 36 months of treatment with long-term testosterone gel.[41] HCT and Hb levels appeared to show a dose-related increase over 12 months before plateauing. Aversa et al. showed in an randomized-controlled trial (RCT) that TU (40 men with the metabolic syndrome or adult-onset TD) led to HCT and Hb increases after 12 and 24 months. HCT and Hb increased from baseline figures of 44.0 ± 3.0% and 14.9 ± 1.2 g/dL by 3.5 ± 3.0% and

Table 2. Hematocrit/hemoglobin ratios at baseline and after 12, 48, 72, and 96 months of testosterone therapy together with the proportion of men with increasing/decreasing ratios at each time point

	Baseline HCT/Hb ratio Median (IQR)	12 months TU HCT/Hb ratio Median (IQR)	Increase (%)	Decrease (%)	48 months TU HCT/Hb ratio Median (IQR)	Increase (%)	Decrease (%)	72 months TU HCT/Hb ratio Median (IQR)	Increase (%)	Decrease (%)	96 months TU HCT/Hb ratio Median (IQR)	Increase (%)	Decrease (%)
Total cohort	3.03 (2.97–3.10)	3.15 (3.07–3.22)	276/353 (78.2%)	33/353 (9.3%)	3.22 (3.14–3.29)	301/313 (96.2%)	9/313 (2.9%)	3.20 (3.14–3.27)	264/279 (94.6%)	15/279 (5.4%)	3.20 (3.12–3.24)	198/207 (95.7%)	9/207 (4.3%)
Age <60 years	3.02 (2.96–3.11)	3.15 (3.06–3.22)	128/170 (75.3%)	16/170 (9.4%)	3.22 (3.15–3.29)	151/157 (96.2%)	6/157 (3.8%)	3.20 (3.14–3.27)	138/145 (95.2%)	7/145 (4.8%)	3.20 (3.11–3.25)	106/108 (98.1%)	2/108 (1.9%)
Age ≥60 years	3.03 (2.97–3.10)	3.15 (3.07–3.22)	148/183 (80.9%)	17/183 (9.3%)	3.22 (3.14–3.29)	150/156 (96.2%)	3/156 (1.9%)	3.21 (3.15–3.27)	126/134 (94.0%)	8/134 (6.0%)	3.20 (3.12–3.24)	92/99 (92.9%)	7/99 (7.1%)
Hb <14.5 g/dL	3.05 (2.95–3.12)	3.17 (3.09–3.22)	143/172 (83.1%)	13/172 (7.6%)	3.24 (3.20–3.31)	150/153 (98.0%)	3/153 (2.0%)	3.24 (3.20–3.31)	127/131 (96.9%)	4/131 (3.1%)	3.22 (3.19–3.27)	102/105 (97.1%)	3/105 (2.9%)
Hb ≥14.5 g/dL	3.03 (2.98–3.09)	3.12 (3.05–3.20)	133/181 (73.5%)	20/181 (11.0%)	3.18 (3.10–3.24)	151/160 (94.4%)	6/160 (3.8%)	3.18 (3.08–3.24)	137/148 (92.6%)	11/148 (7.4%)	3.14 (3.06–3.20)	96/102 (94.1%)	6/102 (5.9%)
Hct <44%	2.95 (2.90–3.01)	3.14 (3.05–3.22)	104/113 (92.0%)	6/113 (5.3%)	3.24 (3.19–3.31)	109/110 (99.1%)	1/110 (0.9%)	3.25 (3.19–3.31)	98/98 (100.0%)	0/98 (0.0%)	3.22 (3.18–3.27)	89/89 (100.0%)	0/89 (0.0%)
Hct ≥44%	3.08 (3.01–3.14)	3.15 (3.08–3.22)	172/240 (71.7%)	27/240 (11.3%)	3.20 (3.13–3.27)	192/203 (94.6%)	8/203 (3.9%)	3.20 (3.11–3.24)	166/181 (91.7%)	15/181 (8.3%)	3.16 (3.08–3.24)	109/118 (92.4%)	9/118 (7.6%)
TT <10.05 nmol/L	3.08 (2.97–3.15)	3.17 (3.09–3.25)	120/159 (75.5%)	19/159 (11.9%)	3.24 (3.18–3.29)	121/125 (96.8%)	3/125 (2.4%)	3.22 (3.17–3.29)	102/107 (95.3%)	5/107 (4.7%)	3.22 (3.14–3.27)	67/67 (100.0%)	0/67 (0.0%)
TT ≥10.05 nmol/L	3.02 (2.96–3.08)	3.13 (3.06–3.20)	156/194 (80.4%)	14/194 (7.2%)	3.21 (3.14–3.27)	180/188 (95.7%)	6/188 (3.2%)	3.20 (3.12–3.27)	162/172 (94.2%)	10/172 (5.8%)	3.18 (3.09–3.24)	131/140 (93.6%)	9/140 (6.4%)
Smokers	3.02 (2.95–3.09)	3.15 (3.07–3.25)	104/135 (77.0%)	19/135 (14.1%)	3.22 (3.17–3.29)	117/119 (98.3%)	1/119 (0.8%)	3.24 (3.16–3.29)	102/103 (99.0%)	1/103 (1.0%)	3.20 (3.14–3.24)	86/88 (97.7%)	2/88 (2.3%)
Nonsmokers	3.05 (2.98–3.12)	3.15 (3.07–3.20)	172/218 (78.9%)	14/218 (6.4%)	3.22 (3.14–3.27)	184/194 (94.8%)	8/194 (4.1%)	3.20 (3.13–3.27)	162/176 (92.0%)	14/176 (8.0%)	3.19 (3.08–3.24)	112/119 (94.1%)	7/119 (5.9%)
Men with T2DM	3.05 (2.99–3.15)	3.14 (3.06–3.20)	107/148 (72.3%)	20/148 (13.5%)	3.20 (3.13–3.27)	116/121 (95.9%)	3/121 (2.5%)	3.20 (3.12–3.26)	94/100 (94.0%)	6/100 (6.0%)	3.18 (3.08–3.24)	68/74 (91.9%)	6/74 (8.1%)
Men without T2DM	3.02 (2.96–3.09)	3.15 (3.08–3.22)	169/205 (82.4%)	13/205 (6.3%)	3.22 (3.17–3.28)	185/192 (96.4%)	6/192 (3.1%)	3.22 (3.15–3.28)	170/179 (95.0%)	9/179 (5.0%)	3.20 (3.13–3.25)	130/133 (97.7%)	3/133 (2.3%)

HCT/Hb ratios were significantly higher ($p < 0.0001$, sign-rank test) after 12, 48, 72, and 96 months of TTh than baseline values in the total cohort and subgroups (age, Hb, HCT, and TT stratified by median baseline values and smoking and T2DM status).

TU, testosterone undecanoate.

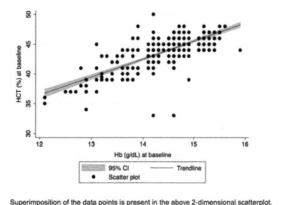

Superimposition of the data points is present in the above 2-dimensional scatterplot.

Linear regression analysis between HCT and Hb at baseline.

	c (95% CI), p	Intercept (95% CI), p	
Dependent variable: Baseline HCT (%)			n=353
Independent variable: Baseline Hb (g/dL)	3.03 (2.75, 3.31), p<0.001	0.13 (-3.90, 4.17), p=0.95	R²=0.56

FIG. 1. A scatter plot and trend line demonstrating the association between HCT and Hb at baseline. HCT, hematocrit; Hb, hemoglobin.

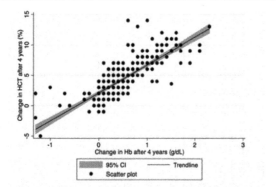

Superimposition of the data points is present in the above 2-dimensional scatterplot.

Linear regression analyses between change in HCT (dependent variables) and change in Hb (independent variables) at 48 (scatterplot presented above), 72 and 96 months.

	c (95% CI), p	Intercept (95% CI), p	
Dependent variable: HCT (%) - 48 months			n=313
Independent variable: Hb (g/dL) - 48 months	4.60 (4.21, 5.00), p<0.001	2.10 (1.82, 2.37), p<0.001	R²=0.56
Dependent variable: HCT (%) - 72 months			n=279
Independent variable: Hb (g/dL) - 72 months	5.13 (4.70, 5.56), p<0.001	1.77 (1.45, 2.08), p<0.001	R²=0.56
Dependent variable: HCT (%) - 96 months			n=207
Independent variable: Hb (g/dL) - 96 months	4.56 (4.09, 5.04), p<0.001	1.99 (1.59, 2.38), p<0.001	R²=0.64

FIG. 2. A scatter plot and trend line demonstrating the association between change in HCT and Hb after 48 months of TTh. TTh, testosterone therapy.

1.4 ± 1.05 g/dL (12 months) and $3.1 \pm 3.5\%$ and -0.3 ± 1.1 g/dL (24 months), respectively.[42] The results after 24 months are similar to our results. We showed a similar pattern after 12, 48, 72, and 96 months, an increase in HCT being a common effect of TU.[42]

An increase in erythropoiesis is a possible mechanism for the increased HCT and Hb. This could occur with increased erythropoietin and/or direct stimulation of bone marrow erythroblasts, as well as iron incorporation into erythrocytes.[27,28,31–33] Lundby et al. treated eight healthy subjects with baseline HCT of $42.0\% \pm 3.0\%$ and Hb of 14.2 ± 6.2 g/dL with erythropoietin, which stimulates the erythroid precursor cells located in the bone marrow.[43] After 12 weeks of treatment, the HCT and Hb concentrations increased to $49.0\% \pm 3.0\%$ and 17.1 ± 5.1 g/dL.[43] Their observed increase in Hb in comparison with HCT in this situation appears much higher than our own study observations, although subjects were given supplemental iron before and throughout follow-up, which may have influenced outcomes. The role of the androgen receptor CAG repeat polymorphism in mediating TTh-associated HCT change was studied by Stanworth et al. in the TIMES2 substudy.[44] It was noted that neither androgen CAG repeats nor change in serum TT levels was associated with change in HCT. Interestingly, in contrast to our findings, baseline HCT appeared positively correlated with change in HCT.[44] We cannot explain the varied findings observed; even after 12 months of follow-up (as in the TIMES2 study), the association between change in HCT and baseline HCT was negative ($c = -0.63$, 95% CI $= -0.72$ to -0.53, $p < 0.001$, $n = 346$). It must also be stated that changes in fluid status (5 cases of peripheral edema in the 23 men experiencing adverse cardiovascular events that led to the trial being discontinued prematurely) in men on TTh, as suggested by the Testosterone in Older Men with Mobility Limitations (TOM) trial, do not provide an explanation for the changes in HCT, Hb, and HCT/Hb ratio seen in our study following TTh.[8]

Our results suggest that the association between TTh and increased HCT and Hb, in addition to erythropoiesis, may also be mediated by other mechanisms. One mechanism could involve an increase in the life span of the erythrocyte associated with TTh in men with adult-onset TD. Erythrocytes are usually destroyed by macrocytes via erythrophagocytosis in the splenic and hepatic sinusoids after around 120 days, although variation in this duration can occur.[45] It has been suggested that oxidative stress, by damaging the cell membrane and cytoplasm of the erythrocyte, shortens life span.[46,47] However, mechanisms such as eryptosis (considered a suicidal cell death due to hyperosmolarity, oxidative stress, and exposure to xenobiotics) may occur, although earlier than erythrophagocytosis.[48] The process of erythrophagocytosis appears mediated by a dynamic balance between phosphatidylserine (prophagocytic)[45] on the inner layer of the cell membrane and the membrane protein CD47 (antiphagocytic).[49] Angelova et al. studied the impact of TTh on erythrocytes and found compositional changes in the cell membrane.[34] This change may possibly lead to lengthening the erythrocyte life span. Around 20% of Hb is lost from erythrocytes via vesiculation, which removes damaged membrane constituents.[36,50,51] As this appears to be a gradual process,[51] increased life span would lead to greater Hb loss.

Thus, we can speculate that reduced degradation of erythrocytes, possibly associated with TTh due to changes in membrane structure, could result in an increased HCT and increased HCT/Hb ratio, as observed in our analysis. In the event of the above phenomena, it is important to consider the clinical implications as increased erythrocyte life span may result in HbA1c values that do not represent the glycemic status of the patient. The testosterone for diabetes mellitus (T4DM) RCT showed that TTh (TU) treatment and lifestyle measures in 504 obese/overweight men with impaired glucose tolerance or newly diagnosed T2DM aged 50–74 years over a 24-month period (compared with 503 men on placebo and lifestyle measures) were associated with significantly lower glucose values (2-h glucose tolerance test).[52] Interestingly, however, no difference in HbA1c between the two study arms was observed. The authors of the T4DM trial speculated whether increased erythrocyte longevity could have contributed to this finding.[52] It must be noted that unlike our longitudinal study where no man was seen to have an HCT >52%, 22% (106 men) of the men on TU (1% (6 men) in the placebo group) had at least a single HCT ≥54%.[52] It must be stated that TU was discontinued in only 23 men due to two HCT values ≥54%.[52] Change in Hb has not yet been reported by the T4DM investigators.

An increase in viscosity associated with higher HCT is likely to affect blood flow and perfusion.[16] This effect would be dependent on many factors such as erythrocyte age, deformability, and morphological changes associated with glycemic status.[16] Thus, the optimal HCT

may vary for the various conditions leading to increased HCT, as they may have differing effects on the condition of the erythrocyte.

Our longitudinal registry study has strengths and weaknesses. Compliance was absolute as the TU was administered in the practice. Follow-up was relatively long, and data on HCT and Hb were almost complete. We did not have data on erythrocyte count or estrogen levels, which could be related to erythrocytosis.[53] It must be emphasized that our findings are perhaps specific for the cohort studied and TU therapy. The effects could be different with other testosterone preparations with varying half-lives.[17] Finally, our findings were observational and did not investigate mechanisms of TTh-associated erythrocytosis.

Conclusion

In this longitudinal study of 353 men with adult-onset TD treated with TU, we studied the changes in HCT and Hb at fixed follow-up time points: 12, 48, 72, and 96 months. Both HCT and Hb increased at every time point (c.f. baseline) in the total cohort and subgroups based on baseline characteristics. Baseline HCT and Hb levels were inversely associated with change in HCT and Hb, respectively, at all the time points studied. At baseline, the HCT/Hb ratio of 3.03 (95% CI: 2.97–3.10) was similar to the expected value of 3.0. Importantly, the median HCT/Hb ratio increased in the total cohort and selected subgroups following TU, with over 90% of the men demonstrating an increase in value. We suggest that the increase in the ratio may be due to the increased erythrocyte life span as speculated by the investigators of the T4DM study.[52] It is essential that the effects of the TTh-associated changes in HCT, Hb, and HCT/Hb ratio on outcomes such as erythrocyte life span, blood flow characteristics such as peak systolic velocity, CVD, and mortality be evaluated via prospective studies.[16,54]

Authors' Contributions

N.L., A.M., C.S.K., and S.R.: design of study, data analysis, and preparation of the article. R.C.S. and G.H.: preparation of the article. A.H. and K.S.H.: patient recruitment, data collection, and preparation of the article. P.D.: transposing the data and maintaining the database. F.S.: maintaining the database, design of study, and preparation of the article.

References

1. Dohle G, Arver S, Bettocchi C, Jones T, Kliesch S. EAU guidelines on male hypogonadism. 2018. http://uroweb.org/guideline/male-hypogonadism/
2. Kapoor D, Aldred H, Clark S, Channer KS, Jones TH. Clinical and biochemical assessment of hypogonadism in men with type 2 diabetes: Correlations with bioavailable testosterone and visceral adiposity. Diabetes Care. 2007;30(4):911–917.
3. Hackett G, Kirby M, Edwards D, et al. British Society for Sexual Medicine guidelines on adult testosterone deficiency, with statements for UK practice. J Sex Med. 2017;14(12):1504–1523.
4. Araujo AB, Dixon JM, Suarez EA, Murad MH, Guey LT, Wittert GA. Clinical review: Endogenous testosterone and mortality in men: A systematic review and meta-analysis. J Clin Endocrinol Metab. 2011;96(10):3007–3019.
5. Muraleedharan V, Marsh H, Kapoor D, Channer KS, Jones TH. Testosterone deficiency is associated with increased risk of mortality and testosterone replacement improves survival in men with type 2 diabetes. Eur J Endocrinol. 2013;169(6):725–733.
6. Hackett G, Heald AH, Sinclair A, Jones PW, Strange RC, Ramachandran S. Serum testosterone, testosterone replacement therapy and all-cause mortality in men with type 2 diabetes: Retrospective consideration of the impact of PDE5Inhibitors and statins. Int J Clin Pract. 2016;70(3):244–253.
7. Hackett G, Jones PW, Strange RC, Ramachandran S. Statin, testosterone and phosphodiesterase 5-inhibitor treatments and age related mortality in diabetes. World J Diabetes. 2017;8(3):104–111.
8. Basaria S, Coviello AD, Travison TG, et al. Adverse events associated with testosterone administration. N Engl J Med. 2010;363(2):109–122.
9. Vigen R, O'Donnell CI, Barón AE, et al. Association of testosterone therapy with mortality, myocardial infarction, and stroke in men with low testosterone levels. JAMA. 2013;310(17):1829–1836. Erratum in: JAMA. 2014;311(9):967.
10. Finkle WD, Greenland S, Ridgeway GK, et al. Increased risk of non-fatal myocardial infarction following testosterone therapy prescription in men. PLoS One. 2014;9(1):e85805.
11. Morgentaler A, Miner MM, Caliber M, Guay AT, Khera M, Traish AM. Testosterone therapy and cardiovascular risk: Advances and controversies. Mayo Clin Proc. 2015;90(2):224–251.
12. U.S. Food and Drug Administration. FDA Drug Safety Communication: FDA cautions about using testosterone products for low testosterone due to aging; requires labeling change to inform of possible increased risk of heart attack and stroke with use [Internet]. 2015 [updated 2018; cited 25.05.2021]. Available from: https://www.fda.gov/drugs/drug-safety-and-availability/fda-drug-safety-communication-fda-cautions-about-using-testosterone-products-low-testosterone-due
13. Corona G, Rastrelli G, Di Pasquale G, Sforza A, Mannucci E, Maggi M. Testosterone and cardiovascular risk: Meta-analysis of interventional studies. J Sex Med. 2018;15(6):820–838.
14. International Society for Sexual Medicine. ISSM Quick reference guide on testosterone deficiency for men [Internet]. 2015 [cited 25.05.2021]. Available from: https://professionals.issm.info/wp-content/uploads/sites/2/2018/05/ISSM-Quick-Reference-Guide-on-TD.pdf
15. Ramachandran S, König CS, Hackett G, Livingston M, Strange RC. Managing clinical heterogeneity: An argument for benefit based action limits. J Med Diagn Ther. 2018;1(3):034701.
16. König CS, Balabani S, Hackett GI, Strange RC, Ramachandran S. Testosterone therapy: An assessment of the clinical consequences of changes in haematocrit and blood flow characteristics. Sex Med Rev. 2019;7(4):650–660.
17. Ohlander SJ, Varghese B, Pastuszak AW. Erythrocytosis following testosterone therapy. Sex Med Rev. 2018;6(1):77–85.
18. Danesh J, Collins R, Peto R & Lowe GD. Haematocrit, viscosity, erythrocyte sedimentation rate: Meta-analyses of prospective studies of coronary heart disease. Eur Heart J. 2000;21(7):515–520.
19. Gagnon DR, Zhang TJ, Brand FN, Kannel WB. Hematocrit and the risk of cardiovascular disease—The Framingham study: A 34-year follow-up. Am Heart J. 1994;127(3):674–682.
20. Lassale C, Curtis A, Abete I, et al. Elements of the complete blood count associated with cardiovascular disease incidence: Findings from the EPIC-NL cohort study. Sci Rep. 2018;8(1):3290.
21. Peters SA, Woodward M, Rumley A, Tunstall-Pedoe HD, Lowe GD. Plasma and blood viscosity in the prediction of cardiovascular disease and mortality in the Scottish Heart Health Extended Cohort Study. Eur J Prev Cardiol. 2017;24(2):161–167.
22. Boffetta P, Islami F, Vedanthan R, et al. A U-shaped relationship between haematocrit and mortality in a large prospective cohort study. Int J Epidemiol. 2013;42(2):601–615.
23. Locatelli F, Conte F & Marcelli D. The impact of haematocrit levels and erythropoietin treatment on overall and cardiovascular mortality and morbidity—The experience of the Lombardy Dialysis Registry. Nephrol Dial Transplant. 1998;13(7):1642–1644.
24. Bhasin S, Cunningham GR, Hayes FJ, et al. Testosterone therapy in adult men with androgen deficiency syndromes: An endocrine society clinical practice guideline. J Clin Endocrinol Metab. 2006;91(6):1995–2010. Erratum in: J Clin Endocrinol Metab. 2006;91(7):2688.
25. Mulhall JP, Trost LW, Brannigan RE, et al. Evaluation and management of testosterone deficiency: AUA guideline. J Urol. 2018;200(2):423–432.
26. Khera M, Adaikan G, Buvat J, et al. Diagnosis and treatment of testosterone deficiency: Recommendations from the Fourth International Consultation for Sexual Medicine (ICSM 2015). J Sex Med. 2016;13(12):1787–1804.
27. Rishpon-Meyerstein N, Kilbridge T, Simone J, Fried W. The effect of testosterone on erythropoietin levels in anemic patients. Blood. 1968;31(4):453–460.
28. Alexanian R. Erythropoietin and erythropoiesis in anemic man following androgens. Blood. 1969;33(4):564–572.
29. Coviello AD, Kaplan B, Lakshman KM, Chen T, Singh AB, Bhasin S. Effects of graded doses of testosterone on erythropoiesis in healthy young and older men. J Clin Endocrinol Metab. 2008;1;93(3):914–919.
30. Dhindsa S, Ghanim H, Batra M, et al. Effect of testosterone on hepcidin, ferroportin, ferritin and iron binding capacity in patients with hypogonadotropic hypogonadism and type 2 diabetes. Clin Endocrinol (Oxf). 2016;85(5):772–780.
31. Shahani S, Braga-Basaria M, Maggio M, Basaria S. Androgens and erythropoiesis: Past and present. J Endocrinol Invest. 2009;32(8):704–716.
32. Bachman E, Feng R, Travison T, et al. Testosterone suppresses hepcidin in men: A potential mechanism for testosterone-induced erythrocytosis. J Clin Endocrinol Metab. 2010;95(10):4743–4747.
33. Beguin Y. Soluble transferrin receptor for the evaluation of erythropoiesis and iron status. Clin Chim Acta. 2003;329(1–2):9–22.
34. Angelova P, Momchilova A, Petkova D, Staneva G, Pankov R, Kamenov Z. Testosterone replacement therapy improves erythrocyte membrane lipid composition in hypogonadal men. Aging Male. 2012;15(3):173–179.
35. Willekens FL, Bosch FH, Roerdinkholder-Stoelwinder B, Groenen-Döpp YA, Werre JM. Quantification of loss of haemoglobin components from the circulating red blood cell in vivo. Eur J Haematol. 1997;58(4):246–250.
36. Leal JK, Adjobo-Hermans MJ, Bosman GJ. Red blood cell homeostasis: Mechanisms and effects of microvesicle generation in health and disease. Front Physiol. 2018;9:703.
37. Al-Ryalat N, AlRyalat SA, Malkawi LW, Abu-Hassan H, Samara O, Hadidy A. The haematocrit to haemoglobin conversion factor: A cross-sectional study of its accuracy and application. N Z Med Lab Sci. 2019;72(1):18–21.
38. Quintó L, Aponte JJ, Menéndez C, et al. Relationship between haemoglobin and haematocrit in the definition of anaemia. Trop Med Int Health. 2006;11(8):1295–1302.
39. Insiripong S, Supattarobol T, Jetsrisuparb A. Comparison of hematocrit/hemoglobin ratios in subjects with alpha-thalassemia, with subjects having chronic kidney disease and normal subjects. Southeast Asian J Trop Med Public Health. 2013;44(4):707–711.
40. Haider KS, Haider A, Doros G, Saad F. Design and conduct of a real-world single-center registry study on testosterone therapy in men with hypogonadism. Androgens Clin Res Ther. 2021:2(1):1–17.
41. Wang C, Cunningham G, Dobs A, et al. Long-term testosterone gel (AndroGel) treatment maintains beneficial effects on sexual function and mood, lean and fat mass, and bone mineral density in hypogonadal men. J Clin Endocrinol Metab. 2004;89(5):2085–2098.
42. Aversa A, Bruzziches R, Francomano D, et al. Effects of testosterone undecanoate on cardiovascular risk factors and atherosclerosis in middle-aged men with late-onset hypogonadism and metabolic syndrome: Results from a 24-month, randomized, double-blind, placebo-controlled study. J Sex Med. 2010;7(10):3495–3503.
43. Lundby C, Thomsen JJ, Boushel R, et al. Erythropoietin treatment elevates haemoglobin concentration by increasing red cell volume and depressing plasma volume. J Physiol. 2007;578(Pt 1):309–314.
44. Stanworth RD, Akhtar S, Channer KS, Jones TH. The role of androgen receptor CAG repeat polymorphism and other factors which affect the clinical response to testosterone replacement in metabolic syndrome and type 2 diabetes: TIMES2 sub-study. Eur J Endocrinol. 2013;170(2):193–200.

45. Arias CF, Arias CF. How do red blood cells know when to die? R Soc Open Sci. 2017;4(4):160850.
46. Rifkind JM, Nagababu E. Hemoglobin redox reactions and red blood cell aging. Antioxid Redox Signal. 2013;18(17):2274–2283.
47. Mohanty JG, Nagababu E, Rifkind JM. Red blood cell oxidative stress impairs oxygen delivery and induces red blood cell aging. Front Physiol. 2014;5:84.
48. Lang F, Qadri SM. Mechanisms and significance of eryptosis, the suicidal death of erythrocytes. Blood Purif. 2012;33(1–3):125–130.
49. Burger P, Hilarius-Stokman P, de Korte D, van den Berg TK, van Bruggen R. CD47 functions as a molecular switch for erythrocyte phagocytosis. Blood. 2012;119(23):5512–5521.
50. Willekens FL, Roerdinkholder-Stoelwinder B, et al. Hemoglobin loss from erythrocytes in vivo results from spleen-facilitated vesiculation. Blood. 2003;101(2):747–751.
51. Willekens FL, Werre JM, Groenen-Döpp YA, et al. Erythrocyte vesiculation: A self-protective mechanism? Br J Haematol. 2008;141(4):549–556.
52. Wittert G, Bracken K, Robledo KP, et al. Testosterone treatment to prevent or revert type 2 diabetes in men enrolled in a lifestyle programme (T4DM): A randomised, double-blind, placebo-controlled, 2-year, phase 3b trial. Lancet Diabetes Endocrinol. 2021;9(1):32–45.
53. Calado RT, Yewdell WT, Wilkerson KL, et al. Sex hormones, acting on the TERT gene, increase telomerase activity in human primary hematopoietic cells. Blood. 2009;114(11):2236–2243.
54. König CS, Atherton M, Cavazzuti M, Gomm C, Ramachandran S. The association of peak systolic velocity in the carotid artery with coronary heart disease: A study based on portable ultrasound. Proc Inst Mech Eng H. 2021;235(6):663–675.

Abbreviations Used

CI = confidence intervals
CVD = cardiovascular disease
HCT = hematocrit
Hb = hemoglobin
RCT = randomized-controlled trial
sTfr = soluble transferrin receptor
T2DM = type 2 diabetes
T4DM = testosterone for diabetes mellitus
TD = testosterone deficiency
TT = total testosterone
TTh = testosterone therapy
TU = testosterone undecanoate

17

Age-Related Testosterone Deficiency Merits Treatment

Abdulmaged M. Traish[1,2,*]

Abstract

The negative effects of testosterone deficiency (TD) on human health and quality of life are well demonstrated, including signs, symptoms, metabolic syndrome, obesity, and increased mortality. Recently, substantial evidence emerged, demonstrating the benefits of testosterone therapy in men with classical and "age-related" hypogonadism. The US Food and Drug Administration (FDA) opposes testosterone therapy in men with age-related hypogonadism but not in men with classical hypogonadism. The FDA acknowledges that TD merits treatment, but the FDA made an artificial distinction between diagnoses where T treatment is warranted and others where the underlying diagnosis is unknown, and treatment is unwarranted. The FDA labeled the unknown category as "age-related." Since the FDA is unable to demonstrate that one group differs in benefits or risks from the other, there are no bases for this distinction. This action by the FDA is not based on scientific or clinical evidence. There is no evidence that the response to testosterone therapy of "age-related" hypogonadism occurs via different physiological or biochemical mechanisms than those historically recognized conditions. Also, there is no evidence that "age-related" hypogonadism responds less well to testosterone therapy than "classical" hypogonadism. More importantly, there is no scientific or clinical evidence to suggest that the risks of testosterone therapy in men with "age-related" hypogonadism are worse or different for men with "classical" hypogonadism. For these reasons, we disagree with the FDA position on testosterone therapy in age-related hypogonadism.

Keywords: testosterone deficiency; classical hypogonadism; age-related hypogonadism, testosterone therapy

Introduction

Hypogonadism (henceforth referred to as "testosterone deficiency") is a clinical syndrome characterized by low serum testosterone (T) and a host of clinical signs/symptoms.[1] T deficiency (TD) occurs as a result of testicular (primary) or pituitary/hypothalamic dysfunction (secondary) and is known historically as "classical" TD, or as a result of unknown underlying pathologies.

Although aging alone does not necessarily cause a significant decline in T levels,[2–9] the predominant form of TD, in aging men, is mixed with primary and secondary hypogonadism components, attributed to varying pathophysiology and comorbidities. Luteinizing hormone (LH) levels can vary in older men based on decreased numbers and function of Leydig cells, decreased sensitivity of the hypothalamus–pituitary gonadal axis to feedback inhibition, and/or decreased LH pulse amplitude despite normal pulse frequency. Decreased LH pulse amplitude may potentially be related to reductions in neuronal cell secretion of gonadotrophic-releasing hormone.[10,11]

"Age-related" hypogonadism (TD) is defined as "a clinical and biochemical syndrome associated with advancing

Departments of [1]Urology and [2]Biochemisty, Boston University School of Medicine, Boston, Massachusetts, USA.

*Address correspondence to: Abdulmaged M. Traish, MBA, PhD, Department of Urology, Boston University School of Medicine, 72 E. Concord Street, A502, Boston, MA 02118, USA, Email: atraish@bu.edu

age, characterized by specific symptoms, and a deficiency in serum testosterone (T)".[12] This syndrome, which often occurs in middle-age and older men, is often referred to as adult-onset hypogonadism.[13] This syndrome does not meet the criteria for either *classical* primary (testicular failure) or secondary (pituitary or hypothalamic failure) hypogonadism. However, it exhibits elements of both presentations.[13] It is noteworthy that the signs and symptoms of TD and the response to treatment are similar, irrespective of the underlying causes (Table 1).[12] It should be noted that "age-related hypogonadism" may be a misnomer since not all healthy men experience decline of T, as they age.[2-9]

"Age-related hypogonadism" was introduced by Nguyen and his colleagues in their perspective published in New England Journal of Medicine (NEJM)[14] stating the position of the US Food and Drug Administration (FDA) on this important clinical issue. In this perspective, the authors strongly expressed concerns on "Testosterone and Age-Related Hypogonadism." Henceforth, in this article, the use of "age-related hypogonadism" is to maintain consistent reference to the FDA original argument against the use of T in older men.

The FDA issued a statement in March 2015 opposing the use of T therapy (*TTh*) in the treatment of hypogonadism attributed to aging, without a defined cause. The FDA position on "age-related" TD is that this condition does not merit treatment.[14] We disagree with the FDA position on this very point. Given next is a summary of the rationale as to why this condition should be treated as any other clinical condition.

On October 1, 2015, an international expert consensus panel convened to discuss the negative impact of TD on human health and quality of life and evaluated the merits of TTh in men with TD. The panel unanimously approved nine resolutions suggesting that: (1) symptoms and signs of TD occur as a result of low T and may benefit from T treatment regardless

of whether there is an identified underlying etiology; (2) there is no scientific basis for any age-specific recommendations against the use of T therapy in men.

Evidence for Benefits of T Treatment in Older Men with TD

TTh in men with TD has been clinically utilized since the 1940s with marked success[15-17] and became FDA approved in the United States in the 1950s. *TTh* for TD has long been considered the standard of care. The main argument advanced by the FDA is that, although *TTh* is indicated for men with "classical" TD, there are insufficient data to support the use of *TTh* in men with "age-related" TD.[14] Nevertheless, nearly all published data involve subjects with "age-related" TD.[18-36]

There are almost no large studies on *TTh* in men with "classical" TD, because such cases are rare. It is unwarranted that the FDA recommendations remain standing despite the recent findings of the T-trials[26] and several meta-analyses of randomized clinical trials,[34-36,] which clearly demonstrated that TD has a negative impact on health and well-being and *TTh* of "age-related" TD improves body composition, glycemic control, and sexual function. Lower T levels are shown to be associated with increased mortality,[37] fracture risk,[38] and cardiovascular disease (CVD).[39,40] The recent T trials have demonstrated that many of these changes attributed to T deficiency are reversible with *TTh* in older men.

The data from the largest National Institutes of Health (NIH)-funded, double blind, placebo-controlled T-trials in the United States, in 790 men with a mean age of 72 years, demonstrated that *TTh* significantly improved symptoms and abnormalities in men >65 years old without "classical" TD.[19-26] *TTh* improved all aspects of sexual function,[19,20] improved walking distance by a small amount,[25] slightly improved mood and depression symptoms,[19] improved hemoglobin and corrected mild and moderate anemia of both known and

Table 1. Signs and Symptoms of Testosterone Deficiency Irrespective of the Underlying Etiology

Signs and symptoms of "classical" hypogonadism	Signs and symptoms of "age-related" hypogonadism	Effects of TTh on the signs and symptoms of hypogonadism, irrespective of etiology
Decreased mobility	Decreased mobility	Improved
Increased sexual dysfunction	Increased sexual dysfunction	Improved
Reduced self-perceived vitality	Reduced self-perceived vitality	Improved
Diminished cognitive abilities	Diminished cognitive abilities,	Improved
Decreased bone mineral density	Decreased bone mineral density	Improved
Reduced glucose tolerance	Reduced glucose tolerance	Improved
Increased anemia	Increased anemia	Improved
Increased coronary artery disease	Increased coronary artery disease	Improved

Reference: Defeudis et al.[137]
TTh, T therapy.

unknown causes,[24] markedly increased volumetric bone mineral density and estimated bone strength,[23] and led to no notable increase in cardiovascular or prostate cancer risk and with fewer hospitalizations.[26]

There is good evidence of benefit in men with metabolic diseases (diabetes, obesity), improving parameters of lean body mass, reduced body fat, waist circumference, and insulin resistance.[14–23–36] The data from the T-trials and other clinical studies (Table 2) are in stark contrast to those reported in the aforementioned clinical studies[41–44] which were significantly flawed and also could not serve as safety trials.[45]

It is critical to highlight that the benefits of *TTh* in men with TD are similar, regardless of age or underlying condition.[18–36] Thus, we conclude that, irrespective of age, the negative effects of TD on human health and quality of life are well demonstrated, including signs, symptoms, metabolic syndrome, obesity, and increased mortality.[45–62] The benefits of *TTh* in men with TD were documented, regardless of age, in clinical trials, registry studies, observational studies, and systematic reviews and meta-analyses (Table 2), and were attributed to restoration of normal T levels.[18–36]

Further, recent advances in endocrinology have uncovered several other etiologies that contribute to TD. These include obesity, diabetes, and opioid use. Interestingly, these etiologies are not encompassed in the indications listed by the FDA for T treatment, demonstrating that clinical science evolves, and the pathophysiological mechanisms of these newly identified idiopathic underpinnings of TD may be recognized and understood in the not-too-distant future.

Does It Really Matter What Causes Low T?

The FDA argues that "age-related" TD does not merit treatment.[14] This argument was borne by the notion that "age-related" TD is a natural consequence of aging and should be left alone. It is illogical to conclude that because a condition is more common with age it does not merit treatment. Clinicians treat numerous "age-related" conditions, including hypertension, type 2 diabetes mellitus, arthritis, cataracts, atherosclerosis, and most cancers.

The FDA believes that if the underlying etiology of low T is classical hypogonadism (primary or secondary) then it merits treatment. However, the FDA believes that if low T is attributed to age-related hypogonadism, then it does not merit treatment, despite lack of any scientific evidence to support such contentions.[19–26]

In addition, the FDA voiced a safety concern regarding *TTh* and risk of CVD based on the following: (1) one

clinical trial halted by the data safety monitoring board and again not designed as a safety trial,[41] in which the authors concluded that the reported evidence may be due to "chance alone"; (2) two observational studies suggesting potential CVD risk associated with *TTh*. Both studies were fraught with methodological and statistical analyses that were not validated at the time[42,43]; (3) one meta-analysis, which included studies that do not meet the criteria for inclusion.[44] These four studies have been rebutted in detail by many published studies and experts in the field.[1,15,27–31,40,45,59,63–66]

Despite all the available evidence to the contrary, and the results of the recent T trials,[19–26] the FDA concluded that, although the limitations and potential confounders or biases in these studies[41–44] preclude a clear conclusion regarding the role of *TTh* in adverse cardiovascular outcomes, a possible association cannot be overlooked.[14] The FDA recommended *TTh* only for "classical" TD but not for "age-related" TD.[14] The FDA's position insists that men afflicted with "age-related" TD should not be treated with T but should be offered behavioral and nutritional life approaches to attain healthier lifestyle. It is important to acknowledge that the FDA position about lifestyle treatment does not exclude the use of *TTh* in older men with TD. More often, such a combined approach may be synergistic and useful.

It is worth emphasizing that the FDA does acknowledge that *TD* is an indication for *TTh*, however limiting such treatments only to men who are diagnosed with "classical" *TD*. This action by the FDA is not based on scientific or clinical evidence and in my view is irrational. We should point out that the listed conditions of "classical" *TD* are largely of a historical nature, representing only those conditions of *TD* recognized by clinicians since the 1940s and 1950s (e.g., testicular failure due to varying pathologies, such as XXY karyotype (Klinefelter syndrome), toxicities (chemotherapy-induced), infectious destruction (mumps orchitis), or radiation-induced damage or physical trauma and injury or pituitary/hypothalamic dysfunction attributed to endocrine disruption or comorbidities).

Advances in science and clinical research have identified new risk factors for *TD*. These include obesity, diabetes, and metabolic syndrome and opioid use, among others.[40,67–80] Therefore, it is irrational to dismiss these newly described conditions and advocate against *TTh* under the guise of "age-related" *TD*. Moreover, in the clinical setting, "age-related" or "idiopathic" *TD* is among the most common etiology noted. There is no evidence that the response to TTh of idiopathic

Table 2. Studies on Benefits of T Therapy in Older Men

Study	Type of study	n	Age (years)	Main outcome
Snyder et al.[19]	RCT	790	65 years or older	TTh produced moderate benefit with respect to sexual function and some benefit with respect to mood and depressive symptoms.
Cunningham et al.[20]	RCT	470	65 years or older	TTh improved sexual desire and activity.
Snyder et al.[23]	RCT	211	65 years or older	TTh for 1 year of older men with low T significantly increased volumetric BMD and estimated bone strength, more in trabecular than peripheral bone and more in the spine than hip.
Snyder et al.[81]	RCT	96	65 years or older	TTh of men older than 65 years of age decreased fat mass, principally in the arms and legs, and increased lean mass, principally in the trunk.
Snyder et al.[82]	RCT	96	65 years or older	TTh of men older than 65 years of age did not increase lumbar spine bone density overall, but increased it in those men with low T.
Srinivas-Shankar et al.[30]	RCT	274	65 years or older	TTh in intermediate-frail and frail elderly men with low to borderline-low T for 6 months may prevent age-associated loss of lower limb muscle strength and improve body composition, quality of life, and physical function.
Cunningham et al.[83]	RCT	790	65 years or older	TTh in older men with normal baseline PSA resulted in 5% increase in PSA of 1.7 ng/mL, and 2.5% increase of 3.4 ng/mL.
Stephens-Shields et al.[84]	RCT	235	65 years or older	TTh resulted in clinically meaningful improvement of sexual desire and is a change of score of ≥0.7 score of Question 1 of PDQ.
Bhasin et al.[25]	RCT	788	65 years or older	TTh consistently improved self-reported walking ability, modestly improved 6MWD in all men participating in the testosterone trials.
Mohler et al.[85]	RCT	788	65 years or older	TTh of 1 year in older men with low testosterone was associated with small reductions in cholesterol and insulin but not with other glucose markers, markers of inflammation or fibrinolysis, or troponin.
Resnick et al.[21]	RCT	493	65 years or older	Among older men with low T and age-associated memory impairment, TTh for 1 year compared with placebo was not associated with improved memory or other cognitive functions.
Roy et al.[24]	RCT	126	65 years or older	TTh significantly increased the hemoglobin levels of those with unexplained anemia as well as those with anemia from known causes.
Benito et al.[86]	Prospective study	10	Median age 51 years (range, 31–78)	TTh in men with TD improved trabecular architecture.
Wang et al.[87]	Prospective study	163	Range 19–68	TTh improved sexual function and mood parameters rapidly and were maintained throughout T treatment. Significant increases in lean body mass and decreased fat mass were noted, and these changes were maintained with TTh.
Snyder et al.[88]	RCT	108	65 years or older	TTh of healthy elderly men for 3 years did not affect any of the lipid or apolipoprotein parameters that we measured.
Wang et al.[89]	RCT	227	Range 51 years	TTh decreased bone reapportion markers, an increased osteoblastic activity marker resulting in a significant increase in BMD.
Wang et al.[90]	RCT	227	Range 19–68	TTh improved sexual function and mood, increased lean mass and muscle strength (principally in the legs), and decreased fat mass.
Traustadottir et al.[9]	RCT	129	65 years or older	The mean 3-year change in $\dot{V}O_2$ peak was significantly smaller in men treated with testosterone than in men receiving placebo and was associated with increases in hemoglobin.
Tapper et al.[91]	RCT	76	Mean 37.3 ± 8.2	Core muscles of the trunk and pelvis are responsive to testosterone administration.
Storer et al.[92]	RCT	156	65 years or older	TTh in older men for 3 years was associated with modest but significantly greater improvements in stair-climbing power, muscle mass, and power.
Storer et al.[93]	RCT	64	Mean 73.6 ± 5.8	TTh in mobility-limited older men increased hemoglobin and attenuated the age-related declines in $\dot{V}O_2$ peak and $\dot{V}O_2\theta$.
Basaria et al.[94]	RCT	308	60 years or older	TTh for 3 years vs. placebo did not result in a significant difference in the rates of change in either common carotid artery intima-media thickness or coronary artery calcium nor did it improve overall sexual function or health-related quality of life.

(continued)

Table 2. (Continued)

Study	Type of study	n	Age (years)	Main outcome
Al Mukaddam et al.[95]	RCT	32	Mean 47.2±4.7 (range 25–70)	TTh significantly increased the structural and mechanical properties of trabecular bone but decreased most of these properties of cortical bone.
Basaaria et al.[96]	RCT	84	Range 18–64	TTh produced greater improvements in pressure and mechanical hyperalgesia, sexual desire, and role limitation due to emotional problems. Testosterone administration was also associated with an improvement in body composition.
Gray et al.[97]	RCT	60	65 years or older	TTh in older men dose dependently improved some components of sexual function, namely, libido and erectile function, as well as one aspect of visuospatial cognition.
Storer et al.[98]	RCT	61		TTh produced specific effects on muscle performance; it increases maximal voluntary strength and leg power but does not affect fatigability or specific tension.
Saad et al.[99]	Registry observational study	411	Mean 59.46±7.05	TTh is an effective approach to achieve sustained WL in obese hypogonadal men irrespective of severity of obesity.
Saad et al.[100]	Registry observational study	255	Mean 58.02±6.30	TTh produced consistent reductions in body weight, waist circumference and body mass index.
Saad et al.[27]	Registry observational study	823	Mean 64.0±4.7	TTh produces reductions in weight, waist circumference, and body mass index.
Haider et al.[28]	Registry observational study	356	Mean 63.7±4.9	TTh in men with type 2 diabetes and TD improves glycemic control and insulin resistance. Remission of diabetes occurred in one-third of the patients.
Behre et al.[101]	RCT	362	Range 50–80	TTh improved body composition and HRQoL in symptomatic men with low to low-normal T, with further improvements over the next 12 months.
Gianatti et al.[102]	RCT	80	Range 35–70	TTh did not substantially improve constitutional or sexual symptoms in obese, aging men with diabetes.
Ho et al.[103]	RCT	120	>40 years old	TTh is effective in improving health-related quality of life, as assessed by the AMS scale in men with TD.
Ng Tang Fui et al.[104]	RCT	100	Median age of 53	TTh improved TD symptoms over and above the improvement associated with weight loss alone, and more severely symptomatic men achieved a greater benefit.
Svartberg et al.[105]	RCT	69	Range 60–80	TTh improved body composition.
Kenny et al.[106]	RCT	67	Mean age 76±4	TTh in men with low T does not impair and may improve cognitive function.
Giltay et al.[107]	RCT	184	Mean 52.1±9.6	TTh may improve depressive symptoms, aging male symptoms, and sexual dysfunction in hypogonadal men with the MetS.
Amory et al.[108]	RCT	70	65 years or older	TTh in older men with low T increases vertebral and hip BMD over 36 months.
Aversa et al.[109]	RCT	52	Mean 57	TTh improved metabolic syndrome components.
Hildreth et al.[110]	RCT	167	Mean 66±5	TTh improved body composition but had no effect on functional performance.
Traish et al.[111]	Registry observational study	255	Mean 58.02±6.30	TTh ameliorates metabolic syndrome components.
Traish et al.[112]	Registry observational study	656	Mean 60.7±7.2	TTh reduced mortality related to CVD.
Rosen et al.[113]	Registry observational study	999	Mean 59.1±10.5	TTh improved major QoL dimensions, including sexual, somatic, and psychological health, which were sustained over 36 months.
Tenover et al.[114]	RCT	13	Range 57–76	TTh increased lean body mass and possibly a decline in bone resorption.
Marin et al.[115]	Observational study	23	Mean 59.9	TTh decreased visceral fat mass without a change in body ass, subcutaneous fat mass, or lean body mass and reduced insulin resistance, improved blood glucose, diastolic blood pressure and reduced serum cholesterol.
Morley et al.[116]	Alternate case control trial	14	Mean 76.5	TTh increased right hand muscle strength and osteocalcin concentration.
Sih et al.[117]	RCT	32	Mean 65±7	TTh improved strength, increased hemoglobin, and it lowered leptin levels in older hypogonadal men.
Ferrando et al.[118]	RCT	12	Mean 68±3	TTh increased net protein balance in the fasted state.
Steidle et al.[119]	RCT	406	Mean 58±10.3	TTh significantly improved spontaneous erections, sexual motivation, sexual desire, and sexual performance.
Casaburi et al.[120]	RCT	53	Mean 67.1	TTh increased lean body mass and increased repetition maximum leg press strength.

(continued)

Table 2. (Continued)

Study	Type of study	n	Age (years)	Main outcome
Page et al.[121]	RCT	70	Mean 71±4	TTh improved physical performance, body composition, and fasting lipid profiles.
Giannoulis et al.[122]	RCT	43	Mean 69.9	TTh has beneficial effects on body composition and cardio-respiratory fitness.
Malkin et al.[123]	RCT	14	Mean 74.1±2.3	TTh fasting insulin sensitivity in men with CHF may also increase lean body mass; these data suggest a favorable effect of testosterone on an important metabolic component of CHF
Allan et al.[124]	RCT	60	Mean 62.1±1.0	TTh selectively lessened visceral fat accumulation without a change in total body FFM and increased total body FFM and total body and thigh skeletal muscle mass.
Sheffield-Moore et al.[125]	RCT	24	Mean 70±2	TTh improved body composition and increased muscle strength.
Frederiksen et al.[126]	RCT	38	Range 68 (62–72)	TTh decreased subcutaneous fat on the abdomen and lower extremities, but visceral fat was unchanged.
Hoyos et al.[127]	RCT	67	Mean age 49±12	TTh improved several important cardio-metabolic parameters.
Kenny et al.[128]	RCT	67	Mean 76±4	TTh prevented bone loss at the femoral neck, decreased body fat, and increased lean body mass in a group of healthy men older than the age of 65 with low bioavailable testosterone levels.
McNicholas et al.[129]	RCT	208	Mean 57.9±10.2	TTh increased lean body mass, produced a significant decrease in percentage body fat, and improved sexual performance, sexual motivation, sexual desire, and spontaneous erections.
Wittert et al.[130]	RCT	76	Mean 68.5±6	TTh in older relatively hypogonadal men results in an increase in muscle mass and a decrease in body fat.
Kapoor et al.[131]	RCT	24	>30 years	TTh reduces insulin resistance and improves glycemic control in hypogonadal men with type 2 diabetes.
Katznelson et al.[132]	RCT	70	Mean 73±5.1	Improved quality of life.
Agledahl et al.[133]	RCT	26	Mean 68.9±5.4	TTh exerted favorable effects on body composition; total fat mass was significantly reduced (pv0.001), whereas fat-free mass was significantly increased (pv0.001) in the testosterone-treated group.
Emmelot-Vonk et al.[134]	RCT	207	Mean 67.1±5.0	TTh increased lean body mass and had mixed metabolic effects.
Mathur et al.[135]	RCT	13	Mean 64.8±7.0	TTh has a protective effect on myocardial ischemia and is maintained throughout treatment without decrement.
O'Connell et al.[136]	RCT	274	Mean 73.9	The effects of TTh seen at 6 months on muscle strength, lean mass, and QoL in frail men are not maintained at 6 months post-treatment discontinuation.

AMS, aging male symptom scale; BMD, bone mineral density; CHF, congestive heart failure; CVD, cardiovascular disease; FFM, fat-free mass; HRQoL, health related quality of life; PDQ, Psychosexual Daily Questionnaire; PSA, prostate specific antigen; RCT, randomized clinical trial; TD, testosterone deficiency; 6MWD, 6-minute walk distance.

(or "age-related") TD occurs via different physiological or biochemical mechanisms than those historically recognized conditions (i.e., *classical TD*). We should point out that clinical guidelines or recommendations from major medical societies failed to make any distinction regarding "age-related" TD and made no mention of differences in treatment approach because of this, including Endo Soc, American Urological Association (AUA), and the International Consultation for Sexual Medicine (ICSM).

We are not aware of any evidence provided by the FDA or to the FDA regarding TTh on CV safety in men with "classical" TD. Thus, to assume that TTh produces adverse effects in men with "age-related" TD but not in men with "classical" TD is simply an illusion. We conclude that the FDA recommendations regarding TTh in men with "age-related" TD are not evidence-based and unwarranted. It is unfortunate that this

particular distinction of TD, based on an historical recognition, was promoted almost entirely by the FDA, without scientific or clinical evidence.[5] We are aware that the FDA, as a regulatory agency, has enormous responsibilities toward the safety of the U.S. public.

Indeed, this differs from the responsibilities of practicing physicians, which are to provide the utmost care for their patients and to relieve pain and suffering and improve quality of life. The FDA is not in the business of dictating the practice of medicine. The practice of medicine is often based on clinical guidelines that are evidence based. It should be emphasized that the T guidelines do not require that patients have classical hypogonadism to be treated. The T guidelines only require low serum T values and signs and symptoms of hypogonadism. The FDA is charged with regulating the pharmaceutical industry, but the FDA is not charged with regulating or providing guidance for the practice of medicine. We, therefore, conclude that *TD* is a pathophysiological condition that merits *T* treatment, irrespective of the underlying causes or the historical terms used to describe it.

Conclusions

The negative effects of *TD* on human health and quality of life are well demonstrated, including signs, symptoms, metabolic syndrome, obesity, and increased mortality. Substantial evidence exists demonstrating benefits of *TTh* in men with "age-related" *TD* (Table 2).[18–36,81–136] More importantly, the T trials demonstrated that *TTh* confers significant and clinically meaningful health benefits in older men with low *T* and this treatment is safe and effective, irrespective of etiology.[18–36] In addition, the T trials provided compelling evidence that T therapy confers significant benefits in the growing population of men with obesity and/or type 2 diabetes.

We are aware that the FDA, as a regulatory agency, has enormous responsibilities toward the safety of the U.S. public. Indeed, this differs from the responsibilities of practicing physicians, which are to provide the utmost care for their patients and to relieve pain and suffering and improve quality of life. The FDA is charged with regulating the pharmaceutical industry, but the FDA is not charged with regulating the practice of medicine. We conclude that TD is a pathophysiological condition that merits T treatment, irrespective of the underlying causes, or the historical terms to define it.

Author Contribution

A.M.T. has conceptualized, drafted, written, and revised the article.

Disclaimer

This article is solely undertaken by the author to contribute to the scientific and clinical community and no resources were sought or obtained from any entity of any kind.

References

1. Morgentaler A, Zitzmann M, Traish AM, et al. Fundamental concepts regarding testosterone deficiency and treatment: International expert consensus resolutions. Mayo Clin Proc. 2016;91(7):881–896.
2. Travison TG, Araujo AB, Kupelian V, O'Donnell AB, McKinlay JB. The relative contributions of aging, health, and lifestyle factors to serum testosterone decline in men. J Clin Endocrinol Metab. 2007;92(2):549–555.
3. Travison TG, Shackelton R, Araujo AB, et al. The natural history of symptomatic androgen deficiency in men: Onset, progression, and spontaneous remission. J Am Geriatr Soc. 2008;56(5):831–839.
4. Liu PY, Beilin J, Meier C, et al. Age-related changes in serum testosterone and sex hormone binding globulin in Australian men: Longitudinal analyses of two geographically separate regional cohorts. J Clin Endocrinol Metab. 2007;92(9):3599–3603.
5. Sartorius G, Spasevska S, Idan A, et al. Serum testosterone, dihydrotestosterone and estradiol concentrations in older men self-reporting very good health: The healthy man study. Clin Endocrinol (Oxf). 2012;77(5):755–763.
6. Handelsman DJ, Yeap B, Flicker L, Martin S, Wittert GA, Ly LP. Age-specific population centiles for androgen status in men. Eur J Endocrinol. 2015;173(6):809–817.
7. Khera M, Broderick GA, Carson CC, et al. Adult-onset hypogonadism. Mayo Clin Proc. 2016;91(7):908–926.
8. Swee DS, Gan EH. Late-onset hypogonadism as primary testicular failure. Front Endocrinol (Lausanne). 2019;10:372.
9. Traustadóttir T, Harman SM, Tsitouras P, et al. Long-term testosterone supplementation in older men attenuates age-related decline in aerobic capacity. J Clin Endocrinol Metab. 2018;103(8):2861–2869.
10. Vermeulen A, Kaufman JM. Ageing of the hypothalamo-pituitary-testicular axis in men. Horm Res. 1995;43(1–3):25–28.
11. Kaufman JM, Vermeulen A. The decline of androgen levels in elderly men and its clinical and therapeutic implications. Endocr Rev. 2005;26(6):833–876.
12. Nieschlag E. Late-onset hypogonadism: A concept comes of age. Andrology. 2020;8(6):1506–1511.
13. Khera M, Broderick GA, Carson CC, et al. Adult-onset hypogonadism. Mayo Clin Proc. 2016;91(7):908–926.
14. Nguyen CP, Hirsch MS, Moeny D, Kaul S, Mohamoud M, Joffe HV. Testosterone and "age-related hypogonadism"—FDA concerns. N Engl J Med. 2015;373:689–691.
15. Aub JC. The use of testosterone. N Engl J Med. 1940; 222:877–881.
16. Aub JC, Kety SS. Recent advances in testosterone therapy. N Engl J Med. 1943;228:338–343.
17. Lesser MA. Testosterone propionate therapy in one hundred cases of angina pectoris. J Clin Endocrinol Metab. 1946; 6:549–557.
18. Wallis CJ, Lo K, Lee Y, et al. Survival and cardiovascular events in men treated with testosterone replacement therapy: An intention-to-treat observational cohort study. Lancet Diabetes Endocrinol. 2016;4(6):498–506.
19. Snyder PJ, Bhasin S, Cunningham GR, et al. Testosterone trials investigators effects of testosterone treatment in older men. N Engl J Med. 2016;374 (7):611–624.
20. Cunningham GR, Stephens-Shields AJ, Rosen RC, et al. Testosterone treatment and sexual function in older men with low testosterone levels. J Clin Endocrinol Metab. 2016;101(8):3096–3104.
21. Resnick SM, Matsumoto AM, Stephens-Shields AJ, et al. Testosterone treatment and cognitive function in older men with low testosterone and age-associated memory impairment. JAMA. 2017;317(7):717–727.
22. Budoff MJ, Ellenberg SS, Lewis CE, et al. Testosterone treatment and coronary artery plaque volume in older men with low testosterone. JAMA. 2017;317(7):708–716.
23. Snyder PJ, Kopperdahl DL, Stephens-Shields AJ, et al. Effect of testosterone treatment on volumetric bone density and strength in older men with low testosterone: A controlled clinical trial. JAMA Intern Med. 2017;177(4):471–479.
24. Roy CN, Snyder PJ, Stephens-Shields AJ, et al. Association of testosterone levels with anemia in older men: A controlled clinical trial. JAMA Intern Med. 2017;177(4):480–490.
25. Bhasin S, Ellenberg SS, Storer TW, et al. Effect of testosterone replacement on measures of mobility in older men with mobility limitation and low testosterone concentrations: Secondary analyses of the Testosterone Trials. Lancet Diabetes Endocrinol. 2018;6(11):879–890.
26. Snyder PJ, Bhasin S, Cunningham GR, et al. Lessons from the testosterone trials. Endocr Rev. 2018;39(3):369–386.
27. Saad F, Doros G, Haider KS, Haider A. Differential effects of 11 years of long-term injectable testosterone undecanoate therapy on

anthropometric and metabolic parameters in hypogonadal men with normal weight, overweight and obesity in comparison with untreated controls: Real-world data from a controlled registry study. Int J Obes. 2020;44:1264–1278.
28. Haider KS, Haider A, Saad, et al. Remission of type 2 diabetes following long-term treatment with injectable testosterone undecanoate in patients with hypogonadism and type 2 diabetes: 11-year data from a real-world registry study. Diabetes Obes Metab. 2020;22(11):2055–2068.
29. Yassin A, Haider A, Haider KS, et al. Diabetes testosterone therapy in men with hypogonadism prevents progression from prediabetes to type 2 diabetes: Eight-year data from a registry study. Diabetic Care. 2019;42(6):1104–1111.
30. Srinivas-Shankar U, Roberts SA, Connolly MJ, et al. Effects of testosterone on muscle strength, physical function, body composition, and quality of life in intermediate-frail and frail elderly men: A randomized, double-blind, placebo-controlled study. J Clin Endocrinol Metab. 2010;95:639–650.
31. Navarro-Peñalver M, Perez-Martinez MT, Gómez-Bueno M, et al. Testosterone replacement therapy in deficient patients with chronic heart failure: A randomized double-blind controlled pilot study. J Cardiovasc Pharmacol Ther. 2018;23(6):543–550.
32. Corona G, Giagulli VA, Maseroli E, et al. Testosterone supplementation and body composition: Results from a meta-analysis of observational studies. J Endocrinol Invest. 2016;39(9):967–981.
33. Corona G, Rastrelli G, Morgentaler A, Sforza A, Mannucci E, Maggi M. Meta-analysis of results of testosterone therapy on sexual function based on international index of erectile function scores. Eur Urol. 2017; 72(6):1000–1011.
34. Cai X, Tian Y, Wu T, Cao CX, Li H, Wang KJ. Metabolic effects of testosterone replacement therapy on hypogonadal men with type 2 diabetes mellitus: A systematic review and meta-analysis of randomized controlled trials. Asian J Androl. 2014;16(1):146–152.
35. Algeffari M, Jayasena CN, MacKeith P, Thapar A, Dhillo WS, Oliver N Testosterone therapy for sexual dysfunction in men with Type 2 diabetes: A systematic review and meta-analysis of randomized controlled trials. Diabet Med. 2018;35(2):195–202.
36. Corona G, Isidori AM, Buvat J, et al. Testosterone supplementation and sexual function: A meta-analysis study. J Sex Med. 2014;11(6):1577–1592.
37. Araujo AB, Dixon JM, Suarez EA, Murad MH, Guey LT, Wittert GA. Clinical review: Endogenous testosterone and mortality in men: A systematic review and meta-analysis. J Clin Endocrinol Metab. 2011;96 (10):3007–3019.
38. Mellström D, Johnell O, Ljunggren O, et al. Free testosterone is an independent predictor of BMD and prevalent fractures in elderly men: MrOS Sweden. J Bone Miner Res. 2006;21(4):529–535.
39. Ohlsson C, Barrett-Connor E, Bhasin S, et al. High serum testosterone is associated with reduced risk of cardiovascular events in elderly men. The MrOS (Osteoporotic Fractures in Men) study in Sweden. J Am Coll Cardiol. 2011;58(16):1674–1681.
40. Boden WE, Miller MG, McBride R, et al. Testosterone concentrations and risk of cardiovascular events in androgen-deficient men with atherosclerotic cardiovascular disease. Am Heart J. 2020;224:65–76.
41. Basaria S, Coviello AD, Travison TG, et al. Adverse events associated with testosterone administration. N Engl J Med. 2010;363:109–122.
42. Vigen R, O'Donnell CI, Barón AE, et al. Association of testosterone therapy with mortality, myocardial infarction, and stroke in men with low testosterone levels. JAMA. 2013;310:1829–1836.
43. Finkle WD, Greenland S, Ridgeway GK, et al. Increased risk of non-fatal myocardial infarction following testosterone therapy prescription in men. PLoS One. 2014;9:e85805.
44. Xu L, Freeman G, Cowling BJ, Schooling CM Testosterone therapy and cardiovascular events among men: A systematic review and meta-analysis of placebo-controlled randomized trials. BMC Med. 2013;11:108.
45. Morgentaler A, Miner MM, Caliber M, Guay AT, Khera M, Traish AM. Testosterone therapy and cardiovascular risk: Advances and controversies. Mayo Clin Proc. 2015;90(2):224–251.
46. Araujo AB, Kupelian V, Page ST, Handelsman DJ, Bremner WJ, McKinlay JB. Arch Sex steroids and all-cause and cause-specific mortality in men. Intern Med. 2007;167(12):1252–1260.
47. Sharma R, Oni OA, Gupta K, et al. Normalization of testosterone level is associated with reduced incidence of myocardial infarction and mortality in men. Eur Heart J. 2015;36(40):2706–2715.
48. Page ST. Testosterone, cardiovascular disease, and mortality in men: Living in the dark. Lancet Diabetes Endocrinol. 2014;2(8):609–611.
49. Shores MM, Matsumoto AM, Sloan KL, Kivlahan DR. Low serum testosterone and mortality in male veterans. Arch Intern Med. 2006;166(15): 1660–1665.
50. Khaw KT, Dowsett M, Folkerd E, et al. Endogenous testosterone and mortality due to all causes, cardiovascular disease, and cancer in men: European prospective investigation into cancer in Norfolk (EPIC-Norfolk) Prospective Population Study. Circulation. 2007;116(23):2694–2701.
51. Yeap BB, Alfonso H, Chubb SA, et al. In older men an optimal plasma testosterone is associated with reduced all-cause mortality and higher dihydrotestosterone with reduced ischemic heart disease mortality, while estradiol levels do not predict mortality. J Clin Endocrinol Metab. 2014;99(1):E9–E18.
52. Shores MM, Moceri VM, Gruenewald DA, Brodkin KI, Matsumoto AM, Kivlahan DR. Low testosterone is associated with decreased function and increased mortality risk: A preliminary study of men in a geriatric rehabilitation unit. J Am Geriatr Soc. 2004;52(12):2077–2081.
53. Tivesten A, Vandenput L, Labrie F, et al. Low serum testosterone and estradiol predict mortality in elderly men. J Clin Endocrinol Metab. 2009; 94(7):2482–2488.
54. Muraleedharan V, Marsh H, Kapoor D, Channer KS, Jones TH. Testosterone deficiency is associated with increased risk of mortality and testosterone replacement improves survival in men with type 2 diabetes. Eur J Endocrinol. 2013;169(6):725–733.
55. Bentmar Holgersson M, Landgren F, Rylander L, Lundberg Giwercman Y. Mortality is linked to low serum testosterone levels in younger and middle-aged men. Eur Urol. 2017;71(6):991–992.
56. Bianchi VE. Testosterone, myocardial function, and mortality. Heart Fail Rev. 2018;23(5):773–788.
57. Muraleedharan V, Jones TH. Testosterone and mortality. Clin Endocrinol (Oxf). 2014;81(4):477–487.
58. Adelborg K, Rasmussen TB, Nørrelund H, Layton JB, Sørensen HT, Christiansen CF. Cardiovascular outcomes and all-cause mortality following measurement of endogenous testosterone levels. Am J Cardiol. 2019;123(11):1757–1764.
59. Morgentaler A. Testosterone deficiency and cardiovascular mortality. Asian J Androl. 2015;17(1):26–31.
60. Shores MM, Biggs ML, Arnold AM, et al. Testosterone, dihydrotestosterone, and incident cardiovascular disease and mortality in the cardiovascular health study. J Clin Endocrinol Metab. 2014;99(6): 2061–2068.
61. Shores MM, Smith NL, Forsberg CW, Anawalt BD, Matsumoto AM. Testosterone treatment and mortality in men with low testosterone levels. J Clin Endocrinol Metab. 2012;97(6):2050–2058.
62. Malkin CJ, Pugh PJ, Morris PD, Asif S, Jones TH, Channer KS. Low serum testosterone and increased mortality in men with coronary heart disease. Heart. 2010;96 (22):1821–1825.
63. Elliott J, Kelly SE, Millar AC, et al. Testosterone therapy in hypogonadal men: A systematic review and network meta-analysis. BMJ Open. 2017; 7(11):e015284.
64. Traish AM, Guay AT, Morgentaler A. Death by testosterone? We think not! J Sex Med. 2014;11(3):624–629.
65. Oni OA, Dehkordi SHH, Jazayeri MA, et al. Relation of testosterone normalization to mortality and myocardial infarction in men with previous myocardial infarction. Am J Cardiol. 2019;124(8):1171–1178.
66. Miner M, Morgentaler A, Khera M, Traish AM. The state of testosterone therapy since the FDA's 2015 labelling changes: Indications and cardiovascular risk. Clin Endocrinol (Oxf). 2018;89(1):3–10.
67. Dhindsa S, Prabhakar S, Sethi M, Bandyopadhyay A, Chaudhuri A, Dandona P. Frequent occurrence of hypogonadotropic hypogonadism in type 2 diabetes. J Clin Endocrinol Metab. 2004;89:5462–5468.
68. Braga PC, Pereira SC, Ribeiro JC, et al. Late-onset hypogonadism and lifestyle-related metabolic disorders. Andrology. 2020; 00: 1–9.
69. Li FP, Wang CZ, Huang JM, et al. Obesity-associated secondary hypogonadism in young and middle-aged men in Guangzhou: A single-centre cross-sectional study. Int J Clin Pract.2020;18:e13513.
70. Dhindsa SS, Irwig MS, Wyne K. Gonadopenia and aging men. Endocr Pract.2018;24(4):375–385.
71. Laaksonen DE, Niskanen L, Punnonen K, et al. Testosterone and sex hormone-binding globulin predict the metabolic syndrome and diabetes in middle-aged men. Diabetes Care. 2004;27(5):1036–1041.

72. Laaksonen DE, Niskanen L, Punnonen K, et al. Sex hormones, inflammation and the metabolic syndrome: A population-based study. Eur J Endocrinol. 2003;149(6):601–608.

73. Giagulli VA, Castellana M, Murro I, et al. The role of diet and weight loss in improving secondary hypogonadism in men with obesity with or without type 2 diabetes mellitus. Nutrients. 2019;11(12):2975.

74. Sarkar M, Yates K, Suzuki A, et al. Low testosterone is associated with nonalcoholic steatohepatitis (NASH) and severity of NASH fibrosis in men with NAFLD. Clin Gastroenterol Hepatol. 2019 [Online ahead of print]; DOI: 10.1016/j.cgh.2019.11.053.

75. Dandona P, Dhindsa S. Update: Hypogonadotropic hypogonadism in type 2 diabetes and obesity. J Clin Endocrinol Metab. 2011;96(9):2643–2651.

76. Dhindsa S, Furlanetto R, Vora M, Ghanim H, Chaudhuri A, Dandona P. Low estradiol concentrations in men with subnormal testosterone concentrations and type 2 diabetes. Diabetes Care. 2011;34(8):1854–1859.

77. Dandona P, Dhindsa S, Chandel A, Chaudhuri A. Hypogonadotropic hypogonadism in men with type 2 diabetes. Postgrad Med. 2009;121(3):45–51.

78. Dandona P, Dhindsa S, Chaudhuri A, Bhatia V, Topiwala S, Mohanty P. Hypogonadotrophic hypogonadism in type 2 diabetes, obesity and the metabolic syndrome. Curr Mol Med. 2008;8(8):816–828.

79. Chandel A, Dhindsa S, Topiwala S, Chaudhuri A, Dandona P. Testosterone concentration in young patients with diabetes. Diabetes Care. 2008;31(10):2013–2017.

80. Tripathy D, Dhindsa S, Garg R, Khaishagi A, Syed T, Dandona P. Hypogonadotropic hypogonadism in erectile dysfunction associated with type 2 diabetes mellitus: A common defect? Metab Syndr Relat Disord. 2003;1(1):75–80.

81. Snyder PJ, Peachey H, Hannoush P, et al. Effect of testosterone treatment on body composition and muscle strength in men over 65 years of age. J Clin Endocrinol Metab. 1999;84:2647–2653.

82. Snyder PJ, Peachey H, Hannoush P, et al. Effect of testosterone treatment on bone mineral density in men over 65 years of age. J Clin Endocrinol Metab. 1999;84:1966–1972.

83. Cunningham GR, Ellenberg SS, Bhasin S, et al. Prostate-specific antigen levels during testosterone treatment of hypogonadal older men: Data from a controlled trial. J Clin Endocrinol Metab. 2019;104(12):6238–6246.

84. Stephens-Shields AJ, Wang C, Preston P, Snyder PJ, Swerdloff RS. Clinically meaningful change in sexual desire in the psychosexual daily questionnaire in older men from the T-trials. J Sex Med. 2019;16(7):951–953.

85. Mohler ER, Ellenberg SS, Lewis CE, et al. The effect of testosterone on cardiovascular biomarkers in the testosterone trials. J Clin Endocrinol Metab. 2018;103(2):681–688.

86. Benito M, Vasilic B, Wehrli FW, et al. Effect of testosterone replacement on trabecular architecture in hypogonadal men. J Bone Miner Res. 2005;20(10):1785–1791.

87. Wang C, Cunningham G, Dobs A, et al. Long-term testosterone gel (AndroGel) treatment maintains beneficial effects on sexual function and mood, lean and fat mass, and bone mineral density in hypogonadal men. J Clin Endocrinol Metab. 2004;89(5):2085–2098.

88. Snyder PJ, Peachey H, Berlin JA, et al. Effect of transdermal testosterone treatment on serum lipid and apolipoprotein levels in men more than 65 years of age. Am J Med. 2001;111(4):255–260.

89. Wang C, Swerdloff RS, Iranmanesh A, et al. Effects of transdermal testosterone gel on bone turnover markers and bone mineral density in hypogonadal men. Clin Endocrinol (Oxf). 2001;54(6):739–750.

90. Wang C, Swerdloff RS, Iranmanesh A, et al. Transdermal testosterone gel improves sexual function, mood, muscle strength, and body composition parameters in hypogonadal men. J Clin Endocrinol Metab. 2000;85(8):2839–2853.

91. Tapper J, Arver S, Pencina KM, et al. Muscles of the trunk and pelvis are responsive to testosterone administration: Data from testosterone dose-response study in young healthy men. Andrology. 2018;6(1):64–73.

92. Storer TW, Basaria S, Traustadottir T, et al. Effects of testosterone supplementation for 3 years on muscle performance and physical function in older men. J Clin Endocrinol Metab. 2017;102(2):583–593.

93. Storer TW, Bhasin S, Travison TG, et al. Testosterone attenuates age-related fall in aerobic function in mobility limited older men with low testosterone. J Clin Endocrinol Metab. 2016;101(6):2562–2569.

94. Basaria S, Harman SM, Travison TG, et al. Effects of testosterone administration for 3 years on subclinical atherosclerosis progression in older men with low or low-normal testosterone levels: A randomized clinical trial. JAMA. 2015;314(6):570–581.

95. Al Mukaddam M, Rajapakse CS, Bhagat YA, et al. Effects of testosterone and growth hormone on the structural and mechanical properties of bone by micro-MRI in the distal tibia of men with hypopituitarism. J Clin Endocrinol Metab. 2014;99(4):1236–1244.

96. Basaria S, Travison TG, Alford D, et al. Effects of testosterone replacement in men with opioid-induced androgen deficiency: A randomized controlled trial. Pain. 2015;156(2):280–288.

97. Gray PB, Singh AB, Woodhouse LJ, et al. Dose-dependent effects of testosterone on sexual function, mood, and visuospatial cognition in older men. J Clin Endocrinol Metab. 2005;90(7):3838–3846.

98. Storer TW, Magliano L, Woodhouse L, et al. Testosterone dose-dependently increases maximal voluntary strength and leg power but does not affect fatigability or specific tension. J Clin Endocrinol Metab. 2003;88(4):1478–1485.

99. Saad F, Yassin A, Doros G, Haider A. Effects of long-term treatment with testosterone on weight and waist size in 411 hypogonadal men with obesity classes I-III: Observational data from two registry studies. Int J Obes (Lond). 2016;40(1):162–170.

100. Saad F, Haider A, Doros G, Traish A. Long-term treatment of hypogonadal men with testosterone produces substantial and sustained weight loss. Obesity (Silver Spring). 2013;21(10):1975–1981.

101. Behre HM, Tammela TL, Arver S, et al.; European Testogel Study Team. A randomized, double-blind, placebo-controlled trial of testosterone gel on body composition and health-related quality-of-life in men with hypogonadal to low-normal levels of serum testosterone and symptoms of androgen deficiency over 6 months with 12 months open-label follow-up. Aging Male. 2012;15:198–207.

102. Gianatti EJ, Dupuis P, Hoermann R, et al. Effect of testosterone treatment on constitutional and sexual symptoms in men with type 2 diabetes in a randomized, placebo-controlled clinical trial. J Clin Endocrinol Metab. 2014;99:3821–3828.

103. Ho CC, Tong SF, Low WY, et al. A randomized, double-blind, placebo-controlled trial on the effect of long-acting testosterone treatment as assessed by the Aging Male Symptoms scale. BJU Int. 2012;110:260–265.

104. Ng Tang Fui M, Hoermann R, Prendergast LA, et al. Symptomatic response to testosterone treatment in dieting obese men with low testosterone levels in a randomized, placebo-controlled clinical trial. Int J Obes (Lond). 2017;41:420–426.

105. Svartberg J, Agledahl I, Figenschau Y, et al. Testosterone treatment in elderly men with subnormal testosterone levels improves body composition and BMD in the hip. Int J Impot Res. 2008;20:378–387.

106. Kenny AM, Bellantonio S, Gruman CA, et al. Effects of transdermal testosterone on cognitive function and health perception in older men with low bioavailable testosterone levels. J Gerontol A Biol Sci Med Sci. 2002;57:M321–M325.

107. Giltay EJ, Tishova YA, Mskhalaya GJ, et al. Effects of testosterone supplementation on depressive symptoms and sexual dysfunction in hypogonadal men with the metabolic syndrome. J Sex Med. 2010;7:2572–2582.

108. Amory JK, Watts NB, Easley KA, et al. Exogenous testosterone or testosterone with finasteride increases bone mineral density in older men with low serum testosterone. J Clin Endocrinol Metab. 2004;89:503–510.

109. Aversa A, Bruzziches R, Francomano D, et al. Efficacy and safety of two different testosterone undecanoate formulations in hypogonadal men with metabolic syndrome. J Endocrinol Invest. 2010;33:776–783.

110. Hildreth KL, Barry DW, Moreau KL, et al. Effects of testosterone and progressive resistance exercise in healthy, highly functioning older men with low-normal testosterone levels. J Clin Endocrinol Metab. 2013;98:1891–1900.

111. Traish AM, Haider A, Doros G, et al. Long-term testosterone: Therapy in hypogonadal men ameliorates elements of the metabolic syndrome: An observational, long-term registry study. Int J Clin Pract. 2014;68:314–329.

112. Traish AM, Haider A, Haider KS, Doros G, Saad F. Long-term testosterone therapy improves cardiometabolic function and reduces risk of cardiovascular disease in men with hypogonadism: A real-life observational registry study setting comparing treated and untreated (control) groups. J Cardiovasc Pharmacol Ther. 2017;22(5):414–433.

113. Rosen RC, Wu F, Behre H, et al. Quality of life and sexual function benefits effects of long-term testosterone treatment: Longitudinal results from the registry of hypogonadism in men (RHYME). J Sex Med. 2017;14: 1104e1115.

114. Tenover JS. Effects of testosterone supplementation in the aging male. J Clin Endocrinol Metab.1992;75:1092–1098.

115. Mårin P, Holmäng S, Jönsson L, et al. The effects of testosterone treatment on body composition and metabolism in middle-aged obese men. Int J Obes Relat Metab Disord. 1992;16:991–997.

116. Morley JE, Perry HM III, Kaiser FE, et al. Effects of testosterone replacement therapy in old hypogonadal males: A preliminary study. J Am Geriatr Soc. 1993;41:149–152.

117. Sih R, Morley JE, Kaiser FE, Perry HM III, Patrick P, Ross C. Testosterone replacement in older hypogonadal men: A 12-month randomized controlled trial. J Clin Endocrinol Metab.1997;82:1661–1667.

118. Ferrando AA, Sheffield-Moore M, Paddon-Jones D, Urban RJ, Wolfe RR. Differential anabolic effects of testosterone and amino acid feeding in older men. J Clin Endocrinol Metab. 2003;88:358–362.

119. Steidle C, Schwartz S, Jacoby K, et al. AA2500 testosterone gel normalizes androgen levels in aging males with improvements in body composition and sexual function. J Clin Endocrinol Metab. 2003;88:2673–2681.

120. Casaburi R, Bhasin S, Cosentino L, et al. Effects of testosterone and resistance training in men with chronic obstructive pulmonary disease. Am J Respir Crit Care Med. 2004;170:870–878.

121. Page ST, Amory JK, Bowman FD, et al. Exogenous testosterone (T) alone or with finasteride increases physical performance, grip strength, and lean body mass in older men with low serum T. J Clin Endocrinol Metab. 2005;90:1502–1510.

122. Giannoulis MG, Sonksen PH, Umpleby M, et al. The effects of growth hormone and/or testosterone in healthy elderly men: A randomized controlled trial. J Clin Endocrinol Metab. 2006;91:477–484.

123. Malkin CJ, Jones TH, Channer KS. The effect of testosterone on insulin sensitivity in men with heart failure. Eur J Heart Failure. 2007;9:44–50.

124. Allan CA, Strauss BJ, Burger HG, Forbes EA, McLachlan RI. Testosterone therapy prevents gain in visceral adipose tissue and loss of skeletal muscle in non-obese aging men. J Clin Endocrinol Metab. 200893:139–146.

125. Sheffield-Moore M, Dillon EL, Casperson SL, et al. A randomized pilot study of monthly cycled testosterone replacement or continuous testosterone replacement versus placebo in older men. J Clin Endocrinol Metab. 2011;96:E1831–E1837.

126. Frederiksen L, Højlund K, Hougaard DM, et al. Testosterone therapy decreases subcutaneous fat and adiponectin in aging men. Eur J Endocrinol. 2012:166:469–476.

127. Hoyos CM, Yee BJ, Phillips CL, Machan EA, Grunstein RR, Liu PY. Body compositional and cardiometabolic effects of testosterone therapy in obese men with severe obstructive sleep apnoea: A randomised placebo-controlled trial. Eur J Endocrinol. 2012;167:531–541.

128. Kenny AM, Prestwood KM, Gruman CA, Marcello KM, Raisz LG. Effects of transdermal testosterone on bone and muscle in older men with low bioavailable testosterone levels. J Gerontol. 2001; 56:M266–M272.

129. McNicholas TA, Dean JD, Mulder H, Carnegie C, Jones NA. novel testosterone gel formulation normalizes androgen levels in hypogonadal men, with improvements in body composition and sexual function. BJU Int. 2003:91:69–74.

130. Wittert GA, Chapman IM, Haren MT, Mackintosh S, Coates P, Morley JE. Oral testosterone supplementation increases muscle and decreases fat mass in healthy elderly males with low-normal gonadal status. J Gerontol. 2003;58:618–625.

131. Kapoor D, Goodwin E, Channer KS, Jones TH. Testosterone replacement therapy improves insulin resistance, glycaemic control, visceral adiposity and hypercholesterolaemia in hypogonadal men with type 2 diabetes. Eur J Endocrinol. 2006;154:899–906.

132. Katznelson L, Robinson MW, Coyle CL, Lee H, Farrell CE. Effects of modest testosterone supplementation and exercise for 12 weeks on body composition and quality of life in elderly men. Eur J Endocrinol. 2006;155:867–875.

133. Agledahl I, Hansen JB, Svartberg J. Impact of testosterone treatment on postprandial triglyceride metabolism in elderly men with subnormal testosterone levels. Scand J Clin Lab Invest. 2008;68:641–648.

134. Emmelot-Vonk MH, Verhaar HJ, Nakhai Pour HR, et al. Effect of testosterone supplementation on functional mobility, cognition, and other parameters in older men: A randomized controlled trial. JAMA. 2008;299: 39–52.

135. Mathur A, Malkin C, Saeed B, Muthusamy R, Jones TH, Channer K. Long-term benefits of testosterone replacement therapy on angina threshold and atheroma in men. Eur J Endocrinol. 2009;161:443–449.

136. O'Connell MD, Roberts SA, Srinivas-Shankar U, et al. Do the effects of testosterone on muscle strength, physical function, body composition, and quality of life persist six months after treatment in intermediate-frail and frail elderly men? J Clin Endocrinol Metab. 2011;9:454–458.

137. Defeudis G, Mazzilli, R, Gianfrilli, D Lenzi A, and Isidori AM. The CATCH checklist to investigate adult-onset hypogonadism. Andrology. 2018;6: 665–679.

Abbreviations Used

AUA = American Urological Association
BMD = bone mineral density
CHF = congestive heart failure
CVD = cardiovascular disease
FDA = US Food and Drug Administration
FFM = fat-free mass
LH = latinizing hormone
HRQoL = health-related quality-of-life
ICSM = International Consultation for Sexual Medicine
NEJM = New England Journal of Medicine
NIH = National Institutes of Health
PDQ = Psychosexual Daily Questionnaire
PSA = prostate specific antigen
RCT = randomized clinical trial
T = testosterone
TD = T deficiency
TTh = T therapy
6MWD = 6-minute walk distance

18

The Effects of Testosterone on the Brain of Transgender Men

Leire Zubiaurre-Elorza,[1] Sebastian Cerdán,[2] Carme Uribe,[3,i] Carmen Pérez-Laso,[4] Alberto Marcos,[4] Mª Cruz Rodríguez del Cerro,[4] Rosa Fernandez,[5] Eduardo Pásaro,[5] and Antonio Guillamon[4,ii,*]

Abstract

Transgender men (TM) experience an incongruence between the female sex assigned when they were born and their self-perceived male identity. Some TM seek for a gender affirming hormone treatment (GAHT) to induce a somatic transition from female to male through continuous administration of testosterone. GAHT seems to be relatively safe. However, testosterone produces structural changes in the brain as detected by quantitative magnetic resonance imaging. Mainly, it induces an increase in cortical volume and thickness and subcortical structural volume probably due to the anabolic effects. Animal models, specifically developed to test the anabolic hypothesis, suggest that testosterone and estradiol, its aromatized metabolite, participate in the control of astrocyte water trafficking, thereby controlling brain volume.

Keywords: transgender men; testosterone; astrocytes; glutamine; androgenic anabolic steroids; MRI

Introduction

Gender identity is one's sense of being a male or a female. The American Psychological Association[1] defines it as "a person's deeply-felt, inherent sense of being a boy, man, or male; a girl, woman, or female; or an alternative gender (e.g., genderqueer, gender nonconforming, gender neutral) that may or may not correspond to a person's sex assigned at birth or to a person's primary or secondary sex characteristics." Transgender men (TM) are persons assigned as female at birth who, however, during childhood, peripuberty, or later in life permanently feel they are male and experience gender incongruence/gender dysphoria. They desire a social transition from female to male and, in some cases, but not all, look for a somatic transition by means of a continuous treatment with testosterone. The European prevalence of TM is 2.6 in 100,000 individuals.[2]

When gender incongruence emerges prepuberally and, depending on the protocol used by the endocrinologist, the transgender boy could receive puberty blockers at the beginning of puberty[3] to stop the growth of secondary sexual characteristics and the discomfort they could cause. This treatment gives the transgender boy time to reach the legal age to decide for himself on receiving continuous testosterone treatment and, perhaps, surgical sex reassignment.

Some TM seek a gender affirming hormone treatment (GAHT) to induce a somatic transition from female to male through the continuous administration of testosterone. The goal of the trans masculine treatment is virilization, which induces the secondary sexual characteristics of a man, and the cessation of menses. TM are treated with doses typically used to treat hypogonadism. Testosterone administration routes include

[1]Department of Methods and Experimental Psychology, Faculty of Psychology and Education, University of Deusto, Bilbao, Spain.
[2]Instituto de Investigaciones Biomédicas Alberto Sols, Consejo Superior de Investigaciones Científicas, Madrid, Spain.
[3]Institute of Neuroscience, University of Barcelona, Barcelona, Spain.
[4]Departamento de Psicobiología, Universidad Nacional de Educación a Distancia, Madrid, Spain.
[5]Departamento de Psicología, Facultade de Ciencias da Educación, Universidade da Coruña, A Coruña, Spain.
[i]ORCID ID (https://orcid.org/0000-0002-1415-687X).
[ii]ORCID ID (https://orcid.org/0000-0001-8821-9688).

*Address correspondence to: Antonio Guillamon, MD, PhD, Departamento de Psicobiología, Universidad Nacional de Educación a Distancia, C/Juan del Rosal 10, Madrid 28040, Spain, Email: aguillamon@psi.uned.es

esters, gels, or patches to keep hormone levels within the male physiological range (300–1000 ng/dL).[4] Since transdermal administration can result in somewhat lower testosterone levels, in those circumstances concomitant progestin administration is needed.[3]

Signs of masculinization appear after ∼3–6 months of treatment. The effects of the virilization treatment in TM have been reviewed. TM experience increased body and facial hair, decreased fat and increased lean mass, a deepening voice, cessation of menstruation, clitoral enlargement, increased sexual desire, and decreased gender dysphoria, anxiety, and depression.[5]

From a clinical perspective, it has been stated that the hormone treatment of TM seems acceptably safe over the short and medium term, but solid clinical data are lacking.[6] The most common gender affirmation surgery in TM is masculine chest reconstruction. A minority undergo oophorectomy or hysterectomy. Less common is genital reconstruction by phalloplasty or metoidioplasty.[4] Psychologically, hormone-treated TM report less social distress, anxiety, and depression.[7]

Testosterone, directly or through its reduced or aromatized metabolites, exerts multiple physiological functions, such as stimulating muscle mass and strength,[8] regulating osteoclastic and osteoblastic activities in the bone,[9] stimulating erythropoiesis,[10] and fat distribution.[11] Moreover, administered in hypogonadal males, testosterone improves sexual desire, depression, and quality of life.[12]

From a molecular-genetic perspective, androgen receptor (AR) and estrogen receptor (ER) polymorphisms have been associated with transgender women[13,14] and estrogen receptor polymorphisms to TM.[15] A recent study in a large and homogeneous sample of adult TM expressing gender incongruence from childhood onward found that the TM population is associated with polymorphisms of the estrogen receptors alpha [(ERα); XbaI-Erα, (rs9340799)] and/or estrogen receptor beta [(Erβ); (CA)n-Erβ, (rs113770630)].[16] It has been hypothesized that subtle changes occurring during brain development underlie the TM brain and behavioral phenotypes.[17,18] The few existing scientific studies that directly address the effects of pharmacological doses of sex steroids on the structure of the TM all note strong effects on the brain structure. Here we briefly address the brain structural characteristics in TM before and after the masculinization treatment. We also provide an explanation that has emerged from changes observed with a recently developed animal model.

The Brain of TM Before the Masculinization Treatment

Brain structural quantitative magnetic resonance imaging (MRI) studies on macroscopic brain structure such as cortical and subcortical volume, cortical thickness, and white matter microstructure show that the brain of TM, before their gender affirming testosterone treatment, shows a mixture of feminine, masculine, and defeminized morphological traits.[17,19]

Several studies have approached the white and gray matter of TM before the masculinizing treatment. At the macroscopic level, volumetric analyses show that the intracranial volume of an adolescent TM is like that of cisgender females. However, regionally, volume decrements have been found in the left superior medial frontal cortex of TM when compared with that of cisgender girls and larger right cerebellum volumes compared with those of cisgender girls.[20] Regarding subcortical structures, the volume of the putamen in TM is like that of cisgender males and larger than in cisgender females.[21] With respect to surface area, cisgender males show a larger surface area than cisgender women in the superior temporal lobe and orbitofrontal regions, whereas cisgender males showed relatively higher brain volume and surface area than cisgender women.[22] A recent study published by the ENIGMA Transgender Working Group[23] points out that TM present lower volumetric values as well as less surface area than cisgender men.

Female and male cisgender subjects show sex differences in cortical thickness, with the four lobes showing a thicker cortex in females than in males.[22,24] Cortical thickness does not differ statistically between TM and cisgender females. Nevertheless, in areas in which male and female cisgender do not differ, like parietal and temporal regions, TM show a thicker cortex than cisgender males. However, unlike cisgender females, TM did not differ from cisgender males in the prefrontal orbital region.[21] This gives them their cortical thickness phenotype.[17]

With respect to the white matter microstructure, it should be remembered that male and female cisgenders differ.[25] Males show greater fractional anisotropy values than cisgender females.[22,26] We confirmed greater fractional anisotropy values in cisgender men than cisgender women. TM, like cisgender men, have greater anisotropy values than cisgender women in the right superior longitudinal fasciculus and the forceps minor, but TM differ from both cisgenders with respect to the corticospinal tract. Consequently, we suggested developmental sex differences between the three groups.[27] Moreover, widespread significant differences were reported in mean diffusivity between groups in almost all white matter tracts. Mean diffusivity describes the magnitude of water diffusion within brain tissue. Cisgender women had the highest mean diffusivities, followed by TM with the next highest.[28] Investigating the structural connectome, it was found that lobar interhemispheric connective was lower in TM than in transgender women or the male and female cisgenders.[29]

The Brain of TM Under Testosterone Treatment

The effects of GAHT on the brain have recently been reviewed in both transgender men and women.[30] In this study, we focus primarily on longitudinal studies investigating the effects of testosterone on gray matter and white matter structure in TM. This is because the explanations provided in the existing literature on the effects of GAHT on the brain come from brain structural studies in TM[31] and an animal model using adult female rat androgenization.[32]

With respect to gray matter, the first study, in a sample of only six TM under testosterone treatment, reported an increase in total brain volume and the hypothalamus.[33] Later, using a longitudinal design, increased cortical volume was found in the cortex and the right thalamus in TM under at least 6-month virilizing treatment with no effect on the ventricular system. In addition, a thicker cortex was also reported in the bilateral postcentral gyrus and unilaterally in the inferior parietal, lingual, pericalcarine, and supramarginal regions of the left hemisphere, and the cuneus and middle frontal region of the right hemisphere. Moreover, serum testosterone changes positively correlated with large clusters of cortical thickness in the lateral occipital, inferior parietal, and fusiform areas. Similarly, a positive correlation was found between the free testosterone index and cortical thickness in the occipital region, inferior and superior parietal, and fusiform areas.[31] Cortical thickening has been confirmed in several regions[34,35] as well as increased volume in subcortical structures.[36]

Regarding white matter microstructure, increases in fractional anisotropy values were first reported in the right superior longitudinal fasciculus and the right corticospinal tract.[27] Interestingly, hierarchical regression analyses showed that increments in fractional anisotropy could be predicted by the prehormonal treatment testosterone index.[37] Similar results have been reported

regarding increases in the left cingulum and decreased mean diffusivity in several corticocortical tracts.[30] Increases in fractional anisotropy were also reported in the fronto-occipital tract.[34] Thus, testosterone treatment in TM increases morphological brain parameters of both gray and white matter.

Testosterone Exerts an Anabolic and Anticatabolic Effect in Brain Tissue of TM Under Treatment

Testosterone androgenic-virilizing and anabolic effects cannot be teased apart. TM feel they are men before receiving testosterone treatment and it should be underscored that their gender feelings are well established before the hormone affirming treatment. The sole objective of the treatment is to virilize their body. Consequently, the effects of testosterone treatment on brain morphology do not affect their firm gender identity as men but relieve their gender incongruence as they meet their bodily gender expectations. Testosterone has effects on those regions in which ARs are expressed and this should focus our attention on ARs and ERs in brain tissue.

Up to the present time, we do not know if the increases in anisotropy, volume and cortical thickness values are mediated through the ARs or the ERs. We cannot discard the participation of either or both kinds of receptors. Cortical and subcortical structures express estrogen[38,39] as well as ARs.[40] Aromatase[41,42] and reductase[43] activities have been detected in the human brain. Testosterone can be aromatized to estradiol, and dihydrotestosterone reduced to 5α-androstane, 3β, 17β-diol that also binds to ERs, particularly ERβ.[44] Therefore, both possibilities remain open. Sex steroids can act through genomic and nongenomic pathways,[45,46] and ARs and ERs can act in a ligand-independent manner.[47,48] Animal studies suggest that testosterone upregulates AR.[49] Thus, we face a myriad of possibilities when a female body receives supraphysiological doses of testosterone to be virilized.

The continuous exposure of TM to pharmacological doses of testosterone might exceed the usual metabolic mechanisms of androgens and their metabolites in the brain. Testosterone and its metabolites stimulate protein synthesis. In men, supraphysiological doses of testosterone, combined with strength training, increase fat-free mass and muscle size and strength[50] as well as increase protein synthesis and net muscle protein balance.[51] In sports, androgens induce performance enhancement in women.[52] In TM, fractional anisotropy increases might reflect a greater richness in axonal microtubules and macromolecules. Consequently, we proposed a process in brain cells that would be like the anabolic one described in the muscle.[31]

An anticatabolic effect has also been hypothesized to explain testosterone effects on muscle. Androgens could exert anticatabolic actions by interfering with glucocorticoid receptor expression.[53] This would induce a positive nitrogen balance. Glucocorticoid receptors have been identified in the human brain.[54] If testosterone influences brain cells as it does muscles, this hypothesis should be taken into consideration.[31]

Testosterone Affects Brain Morphology Changing Astrocyte Size in Adult Female Rats

The fact that testosterone is administered to TM is not the only reason justifying the development of an animal model to study the effects of testosterone on brain tissue. Indeed, testosterone has also been prescribed to treat hypogonadism as well as psychosexual and erectile dysfunctions and fatigue in men.[55–57] Moreover, the anabolic androgenic steroids (AASs), which are synthetic substances derived from testosterone, are widely used by bodybuilders and weightlifters. Although the hormone might be neuroprotective,[58]

chronic administration of AASs is associated with psychiatric disorders in men and women,[59–62] and a neurodegenerative potential has been suggested.[63]

We developed an animal model to test the anabolic hypothesis on the cortical effects of testosterone.[32] We designed a longitudinal study using adult 80-day-old female rats injected weekly with a testosterone dose equivalent to that administered to TM. The anabolic hypothesis predicted increases in fractional anisotropy values, because of increased protein synthesis in brain cells. A response to maintain osmotic homeostasis by the brain cells would be observed as changes in cortical volume. Cortical volume and anisotropy values were measured *in vivo* using T2- and diffusion-weighted images, respectively. Proton magnetic resonance spectroscopy (^{1}H MRS) was used *ex vivo* to assess the metabolic profile of neurochemical metabolites in various brain regions (Fig. 1).

The main hypothesis was verified—although fractional anisotropy values decreased steadily in control female rats over the course of the experiment, no change in their values was observed in androgenized rats (Fig. 2). Decreases in control females could be explained by aging, as is seen in humans.[64–66] This suggests that testosterone prevented age-dependent decreases in fractional anisotropy.

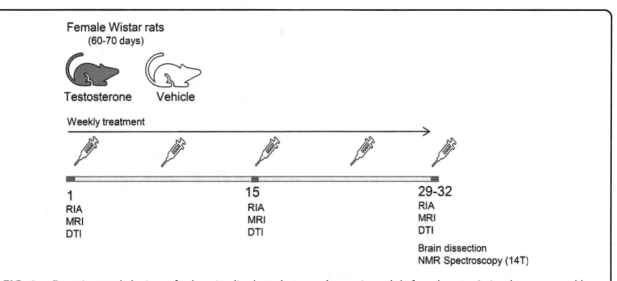

FIG. 1. Experimental design of a longitudinal study to androgenize adult female rats. Animals were weekly injected with testosterone or vehicle. Every 15 days, blood from the tail was collected for immunoassay and MRI was acquired. At the end of the experiment, animals were euthanized and brain was dissected to obtain the metabolic spectrum. DTI, diffusion tensor imaging; MRI, magnetic resonance imaging; NMR, nuclear magnetic resonance; RIA, radioimmunoassay.

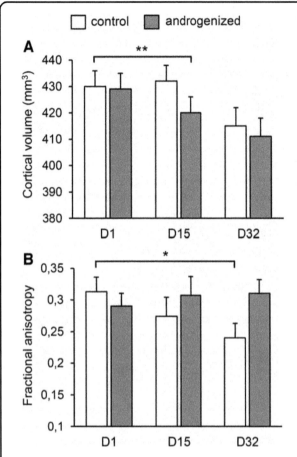

FIG. 2. Effects of testosterone on the cortical volume (**A**) and fractional anisotropy (**B**) in adult androgenized female rats. Androgenized rats showed a sharper decrease in cortical volume while maintaining fractional anisotropy values against/despite aging effect seen in control animals. Data from Perez-Laso et al.[39] *$p < 0.05$; **$p < 0.01$. FA, fractional anisotropy.

Both control and androgenized females showed a decrease in cortical volume that was more pronounced in androgenized females (Fig. 2). Rats achieved their largest cortical volume at 2 months of age, with volume declining from that age[67]; that decline was sharper in androgenized females by day 15 of treatment, and the metabolite profile was also different.

The relative concentrations of some metabolites that function as osmolytes showed different fates in androgenized females than in their controls. Adult androgenized females showed a decrease in *myo*-Inositol (mI), glutamine (Gln), and glycine + Gln (Gly+Gln). Linear

regression analyses indicated that these decreases were due to the increases in testosterone levels. Changes in mI and Gln significantly affected the *N*-acetyl-aspartate/mI ratio, the aspartate/Gln ratio, and the γ-aminobutyric acid (GABA)/aspartate ratio. Since mI and Gln behave as major osmolytes, testosterone levels may alter volume regulation processes, and this may underlie the changes observed in cortical volume. This suggests that the administration of supraphysiological doses of testosterone affects water content in brain cells. It seems that testosterone, or its metabolites, are involved in the osmotic homeostasis of the cell.

mI, as well as being a major osmolyte involved in the regulation of cell volume under osmotic stress conditions,[68] is also an astrocyte marker and the precursor of the phosphatidylinositol second messenger system.[69] In our design,[32] the relative concentration of mI was negatively correlated with the levels of testosterone and associated with a shrinkage of brain cells. The mI- and Gln-driven intracellular water efflux decreased astrocyte volume and hence cortical volume.

In summary, testosterone increases molecular synthesis in astrocytes, inducing increased water intake, which increases cortical volume. To prevent astrocytes from swelling during the hormone treatment and maintain cortical volume constant, it was suggested that mI and Gln would be driven out from the astrocytes into the extracellular space and eliminated through the vascular system. This suggestion is supported by the observation that mI and Gln decreased their relative concentrations in androgenized adult female rats with respect to their controls (Fig. 3).

Decreased Gln levels might have other kinds of consequences. Astrocytes are the only cell type able to synthetize Gln, and Gln is the precursor of inhibitory (γ-amino butyric acid) and excitatory (glutamate [Glu], aspartate) neurotransmitters. When Gln is decreased because of its osmolyte function,[70] the inhibitory and excitatory equilibrium might be affected. This was indicated because the ratios of GABA/aspartate and aspartate/Gln were also decreased.

Decreases in the astrocyte level of Gln should focus our attention on neuron–astrocyte relationships.[71] A decrease in Gln may affect the Gln–Glu cycle.

Concluding Remarks

The animal model already summarized suggests that supraphysiological doses of testosterone exert effects on the brain volume of adult female rats through the astrocytes and, to preserve osmotic homeostasis, the

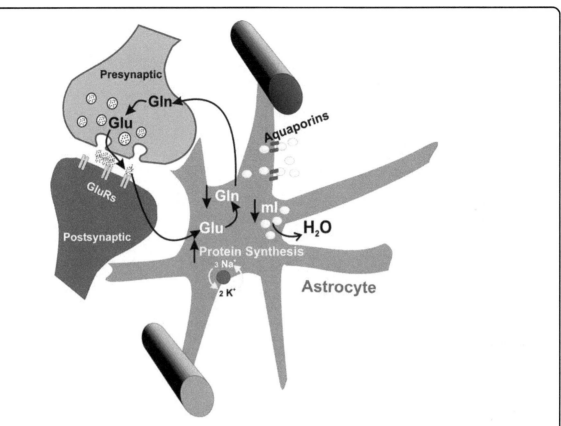

FIG. 3. Suggested mechanism to explain cortical volume decrease in subjects under supraphysiological doses of testosterone. Increased protein synthesis attracts water into the astrocytes. In turn, to maintain the osmotic equilibrium, astrocytes efflux water to the extracellular space by means of osmolytes such as mI and Gln whose relative content decreases. Decreases in the Gln concentration might affect the Gln–Glu cycle. Gln, glutamine; Glu, glutamate; GluRs, glutamate receptors; mI, myo-Inositol.

astrocytes then decrease osmolytes such as Gln and mI. In turn, decreases in Gln would affect the equilibrium of excitatory and inhibitory neurotransmitters (Fig. 3).

What can we learn from the animal model with respect to TM and AAS consumers? The structural brain MRI data we know come from TM during short-medium administration (around a year or less),[31,72] whereas data from AAS consumers are from long-term consumption.[73,74] Over 1-year's consumption of AASs by weightlifters is associated with a thinner cortex and smaller volumes of total gray matter, cerebral cortex, and putamen,[74] but right amygdala enlargement and higher Gln/Glu ratio have also been reported.[73] These reports suggest that the effects of testosterone and other AASs on brain structure depend upon the duration of the administration of these substances.

We do not know whether the effects seen in the brain of TM, weightlifters, and rats are produced by testosterone itself or by its reduced and aromatized metabolites or by all these hormones. In adult male rats, daily estradiol administration produced a decrease in cortical volume associated with increases in the relative concentration of Gln and other metabolites due to water depletion from astrocytes.[75] The fact that both testosterone and estradiol drive a decrease in cortical volume in rats suggests that estradiol plays a role in the effect promoting an active mechanism of neurocellular water extrusion.

We should acknowledge the probable participation of other variables. Specifically, channel proteins such as Aquaporins that regulate water movements across neurocellular membranes.[76] Aquaporin 4 (AQP-4) is located in the astrocytic end feet. This presence provides a link between microvascular blood flow and metabolic coupling between neurons and astrocytes. Testosterone upregulates AQP-4 expression in cultured astrocytes,[77] and estradiol modifies AQP-4 expression. Thus, supporting the relationship between sex steroids and cerebral volume regulation.[78] Moreover, AQP-4 downregulates Glu uptake in astrocytes.[79] Therefore, AQP-4 becomes an excellent candidate for future research into the effect on the brain of the androgenization treatment of transgender men.

Finally, higher or supraphysiological doses of testosterone may increase the risk of psychiatric symptoms in persons with underlying hypomania, mania, or psychotic disorders.[80] Changes in brain cortical volume are observed in both TM and weightlifters. Moreover, the animal model of the treatment indicates that water trafficking is affected in astrocytes and changes in the relative concentrations Gln and Glu are also observed. To contribute to the quality of life of TM, in light of these observations, we would suggest that an MRI scan be taken before receiving testosterone and every to 2 or 3 years during the routine follow-up of the treatment so as to safeguard quality of life.

Authors' Contributions

Conception of the study was done by L.Z.-E., S.C., and A.G.; drafting of the article was done by A.G.; revising and editing of the article were by S.C., M.C.R.d.C., C.P.-L., R.F., E.P., C.U., A.M., and A.G.; funding acquisition was done by A.G., E.P., R.F., and L.Z.-E. All authors have read and agreed to the published version of the article.

References

1. American Psychological Association. Guidelines for psychological practice with transgender and gender nonconforming people. Am Psychol. 2015;70(9):832–864.
2. Arcelus J, Bouman WP, Van Den Noortgate W, Claes L, Witcomb G, Fernandez-Aranda F. Systematic review and meta-analysis of prevalence studies in transsexualism. Eur Psychiatry. 2015;30(6):807–815.
3. Gooren LJ. Clinical practice. Care of transsexual persons. N Engl J Med. 2011;364(13):1251–1257.
4. Safer JD, Tangpricha V. Care of the transgender patient. Ann Intern Med. 2019;171(1):ITC1–ITC16.
5. Irwig MS. Testosterone therapy for transgender men. Lancet Diabetes Endocrinol. 2017;5(4):301–311.
6. Gooren LJ, Giltay EJ, Bunck MC. Long-term treatment of transsexuals with cross-sex hormones: Extensive personal experience. J Clin Endocrinol Metab. 2008;93:19–25.
7. Gómez-Gil E, Zubiaurre-Elorza L, Esteva I, et al. Hormone-treated transsexuals report less social distress, anxiety and depression. Psychoneuroendocrinology. 2012;37(5):662–670.
8. Snyder PJ, Peachey H, Hannoush P, et al. Effect of testosterone treatment on body composition and muscle strength in men over 65 years of age. J Clin Endocrinol Metab. 1999;84(8):2647–2653.
9. Vanderschueren D, Vandenput L, Boonen S, Lindberg MK, Bouillon R, Ohlsson C. Androgens and bone. Endocr Rev. 2004;2(3)5:389–425.
10. Shahani S, Braga-Basaria M, Maggio M, Basaria S. Androgens and erythropoiesis: Past and present. J Endocrinol Invest. 2009;32(8):704–716.
11. O'Reilly MW, House PJ, Tomlinson JW. Understanding androgen action in adipose tissue. J Steroid Biochem Mol Biol. 2014;143:277–284.
12. Elliott J, Kelly SE, Millar AC, et al. Testosterone therapy in hypogonadal men: A systematic review and network meta-analysis. BMJ Open. 2017;7: e015284.
13. Henningsson S, Westberg L, Nilsson S, et al. Sexsteroid-related genes and male-to-female transsexualism. Psychoneuroendocrinology. 2005;30(7): 657–664.
14. Hare L, Bernard P, Sánchez FJ, et al. Androgen receptor repeat length polymorphism associated with male-to-female transsexualism. Biol Psychiatry. 2009;65(1):93–96.
15. Fernández R, Esteva I, Gómez-Gil E, et al. The (CA)n polymorphism of ERβ gene is associated with FtM transsexualism. J Sex Med. 2014;11(3): 720–728.
16. Fernández R, Guillamon A, Cortés-Cortés J, et al. Molecular basis of gender dysphoria: Androgen and estrogen receptor interaction. Psychoneuroendocrinology. 2018;98:161–167.
17. Guillamon A, Junque C, Gómez-Gil E. A review of the status of brain structure research in transsexualism. Arch Sex Behav. 2016;45(7):1615–1648.
18. Uribe C, Junque C, Gómez-Gil E, Abos A, Mueller SC, Guillamon A. Brain network interactions in transgender individuals with gender incongruence. Neuroimage. 2020;211:116613.
19. Kreukels BP, Guillamon A. Neuroimaging studies in people with gender incongruence. Int Rev Psychiatry. 2016;28(1):120–128.
20. Hoekzema E, Schagen SE, Kreukels BP, et al. Regional volumes and spatial volumetric distribution of graymatter in the gender dysphoric brain. Psychoneuroendocrinology. 2015;55:59–71.
21. Zubiaurre-Elorza L, Junque C, Gómez-Gil E, et al. Cortical thickness in untreated transsexuals. Cereb Cortex. 2013;23(12):2855–2862.
22. Ritchie SJ, Cox SR, Shen X, et al. Sex differences in the adult human brain: Evidence from 5216 UK Biobank Participants. Cereb Cortex. 2018;28(8): 2959–2975.
23. Mueller SC, Guillamon A, Zubiaurre-Elorza L, et al. The neuroanatomy of transgender identity: Mega-analytic findings from the ENIGMA Transgender Persons Working Group. J Sex Med. 2021;18(6):1122–1129.
24. Luders E, Narr KL, Thompson PM, et al. Gender effects on cortical thickness and the influence of scaling. Hum Brain Mapp. 2006;27(4): 314–324.
25. Inano S, Takao H, Hayashi N, Abe O, Ohtomo K. Effects of age and gender on white matter integrity. AJNR Am J Neuroradiol. 2011;32:2103–2109.
26. Schneiderman JS, Buchsbaum MS, Haznedar MM, et al. Diffusion tensor anisotropy in adolescents and adults. Neuropsychobiology. 2007;55(2): 96–111.
27. Rametti G, Carrillo B, Gómez-Gil E, et al. White matter microstructure in female to male transsexuals before cross-sex hormonal treatment. A diffusion tensor imaging study. J Psychiatr Res. 2011;45(2):199–204.
28. Kranz GS, Hahn A, Kaufmann U, et al. White matter microstructure in transsexuals and controls investigated by diffusion tensor imaging. J Neurosci. 2014;34(46):15466–15475.
29. Hahn A, Kranz GS, Küblböck M, et al. Structural connectivity networks of transgender people. Cereb Cortex. 2015;25(10):3527–3534.
30. Kranz GS, Seiger R, Kaufmann U, et al. Effects of sex hormone treatment on white matter microstructure in individuals with gender dysphoria. Neuroimage. 2017;150:60–67.
31. Zubiaurre-Elorza L, Junque C, Gómez-Gil E, Guillamon A. Effects of cross-sex hormone treatment on cortical thickness in transsexual individuals. J Sex Med. 2014;11(5):1248–1256.
32. Perez-Laso C, Cerdan S, Junque C, et al. Effects of adult female rat androgenization on brain morphology and metabolomic profile. Cereb Cortex. 2018;28(8):2846–2853.
33. Hulshoff Pol HE, Cohen-Kettenis PT, Van Haren NEM, et al. Changing your sex changes your brain: Influences of testosterone and estrogen on adult human brain structure. Eur J Endocrinol. 2006;55:s107–s114.
34. Burke SM, Manzouri AH, Dhejne C, et al. Testosterone effects on the brain in transgender men. Cereb Cortex. 2018;28(5):1582–1596.
35. Kilpatrick LA, Holmberg M, Manzouri A, Savic I. Cross sex hormone treatment is linked with a reversal of cerebral patterns associated with gender dysphoria to the baseline of cisgender controls. Eur J Neurosci. 2019;50(8):3269–3281.
36. Seiger R, Hahn A, Hummer A, et al. Subcortical gray matter changes in transgender subjects after long-term cross-sex hormone administration. Psychoneuroendocrinology. 2016;74:371–379.
37. Rametti G, Carrillo B, Gómez-Gil E, et al. Effects of androgenization on the white matter microstructure of female-to-male transsexuals. A diffusion

tensor imaging study. Psychoneuroendocrinology. 2012;37(8):1261–1269.

38. Osterlund MK, Gustafsson JA, Keller E, Hurd YL. Estrogen receptor beta (ERbeta) messenger ribonucleic acid (mRNA) expression within the human forebrain: Distinct distribution pattern to ERalpha mRNA. J Clin Endocrinol Metab. 2000;85(10):3840–3846.

39. Gonzalez M, Cabrera-Socorro A, Perez-Garcia CG, et al. Distribution patterns of estrogen receptor alpha and beta in the human cortex and hippocampus during development and adulthood. J Comp Neurol. 2007;503(6):790–802.

40. Beyenburg S, Watzka M, Clusmann H, et al. Androgen receptor mRNA expression in the human hippocampus. Neurosci Lett. 2000;294(1):25–28.

41. Naftolin F, Ryan KJ, Davies IJ, et al. The formation of estrogens by central neuroendocrine tissues. Recent Prog Horm Res. 1975;31:295–319.

42. Moraga-Amaro R, van Waarde A, Doorduin J, de Vries EFJ. Sex steroid hormones and brain function: PET imaging as a tool for research. J Neuroendocrinol. 2018;30(2):e12565.

43. Negri-Cesi P, Poletti A, Celotti F. Metabolism of steroids in the brain: A new insight into role of 5α-reductase and aromatase in brain differentiation and functions. J Steroid Biochem Molec Biol. 1996;58(5–6):455–466.

44. Handa RJ, Pak TR, Kudwa AE, Lund TD, Hinds L. An alternate pathway for androgen regulation of brain function: Activation of estrogen receptor beta by the metabolite of dihydrotestosterone, 5alpha-androstane-3beta,17beta-diol. Horm Behav. 2008;53(5):741–752.

45. Davey RA, Grossmann M. Androgen receptor structure, function and biology: from bench to bedside. Clin Biochem Rev. 2016;37(1):3–15.

46. Fuentes N, Silveyra P. Estrogen receptor signaling mechanisms. Adv Protein Chem Struct Biol. 2019;116:135–170.

47. Olesen KM, Jessen HM, Auger CJ, Auger AP. Dopaminergic activation of estrogen receptors in neonatal brain alters progestin receptor expression and juvenile social play behavior. Endocrinology. 2005;146(9):3705–3712.

48. Ueda T, Mawji NR, Bruchovsky N, Sadar MD. Ligand-independent activation of the androgen receptor by interleukin-6 and the role of steroid receptor coactivator-1 in prostate cancer cells. J Biol Chem. 2002;277(41):38087–38094.

49. Antonio J, Wilson JD, George FW. Effects of castration and androgen treatment on androgen-receptor levels in rat skeletal muscles. J Appl Physiol (1985). 1999;87(2):2016–2019.

50. Bhasin S, Storer TW, Berman N, et al. The effects of supraphysiologic doses of testosterone on muscle size and strength in normal men. N Engl J Med. 1996;335(1):1–7.

51. Griggs RC, Kingston W, Jozefowicz RF, Herr BE, Forbes G, Halliday D. Effect of testosterone on muscle mass and muscle protein synthesis. J Appl Physiol. 1985;66(1):498–503.

52. Kuhn CM. Anabolic steroids. Recent Prog Horm Res. 2002;57:411–434.

53. Kicman AT. Pharmacology of anabolic steroids. Br J Pharmacol. 2008;154(3):502–521.

54. Sarrieau A, Dussaillant M, Agid F, Philibert D, Agid Y, Rostene W. Autoradiographic localization of glucocorticosteroid and progesterone binding sites in the human post-mortem brain. J Steroid Biochem. 1986;25(5B):717–721.

55. Aversa A, Isidori AM, Greco EA, et al. Hormonal supplementation and erectile dysfunction. Eur Urol. 2004;45(5):535–538.

56. Tsujimura A. The relationship between testosterone deficiency and Men's Health. World J Mens Health. 2013;31(2):126–135.

57. Gannon JR, Walsh TJ. Testosterone and sexual function. Urol Clin North Am. 2016;43(2):217–222.

58. Melcangi RC, Giatti S, García-Segura LM. Levels and actions of neuroactive steroids in the nervous system under physiological and pathological conditions: Sex-specific features. Neurosci Biobehav Rev. 2016;67:25–40.

59. Pope HG, Katz DL. Affective and psychotic symptoms associated with anabolic steroid use. Am J Psychiatry. 1988;145(4):487–490.

60. Perry PJ, Yates WR, Andersen KH. Psychiatric symptoms associates with anabolic steroids: A controlled, retrospective study. Ann Clin Psychiatry. 1990;2(1):11–17.

61. Gruber AJ, Pope HG. Psychiatric and medical effects of anabolic androgenic steroid use in women. Psychother Psychosom. 2000;69(1):19–26.

62. Ip EJ, Barnett MJ, Tenerowicz MJ, Kim JA, Wei H, Perry PJ. Women and anabolic steroids: An analysis of a dozen users. Clin J Sport Med. 2010;20(6):475–481.

63. Pomara C, Neri M, Bello S, Fiore C, Riezzo I, Turillazi E. Neurotoxicity by synthetic androgen steroids: Oxidative stress, apoptosis and neuropathology: A review. Curr Neuropharmacol. 2015;13(1):132–145.

64. Bennet IJ, Madden DJ, Vaidya CJ, et al. Age-related differences in multiple measures of white matter integrity: A diffusion tensor imaging study of healthy aging. Hum Brain Mapp. 2010;31(3):378–390.

65. Salami A, Erikson J, Nilson LG, Nyberg L. Age-related white matter microstructural differences partly mediate age-related decline in processing speed but not cognition. Biochim Biophys Acta. 2012;1822(3):408–415.

66. Van Hemmen VJ, Saris IMJ, Cohen-Kettenis PT, Veltman DJ, Pouwels PJW, Bakker J. Sex differences in white matter microstructure in the human brain predominantly reflect differences in sex hormone exposure. Cereb Cortex. 2017;27(5):2994–3001.

67. Mengler L, Khmelinskii A, Diedenhofen M, et al. Brain maturation of the adolescent rat cortex and striatum: Changes in volume and myelination. Neuroimage. 2014;84:35–44.

68. Yancey PH, Clark ME, Hand SC, Bowlus RD, Somero GN. Living with water stress: Evolution of osmolyte systems. Science. 1982;217(4566):1214–1222.

69. Brand A, Richter-Landsberg C, Leibfritz D. Multinuclear NMR studies on the energy metabolism of glial and neuronal cells. Dev Neurosci. 1993;15(3–5):289–298.

70. Zwingman C, Butterword R. Glutamine synthesis and its relation to cell-specific energy metabolism in the hyperammonemic brain: Further studies using NMR spectroscopy. Neurochem Int. 2005;47(1–2):19–30.

71. Magistretti PJ, Pellerin L. Cellular bases of brain energy metabolism and their relevance to functional brain imaging: Evidence for a prominent role of astrocytes. Cereb Cortex. 1996;6(1):50–61.

72. Kranz GS, Zhang BBB, Handschuh P, Ritter V, Lanzenberger R. Gender-affirming hormone treatment—A unique approach to study the effects of sex hormones on brain structure and function. Cortex. 2020;129:68–79.

73. Kaufman MJ, Janes AC, Hudson JI, et al. Brain and cognition abnormalities in long-term anabolic-androgenic steroid users. Drug Alcohol Depend. 2015;152:47–56.

74. Bjørnebekk A, Walhovd KB, Jorstad ML, Due-Tennessen P, Hullstein IR, Fjell AM. Structural brain imaging of longterm anabolic-androgenic steroid users and nonusing weightlifters. Biol Psychiatry. 2017;82(4):294–302.

75. Gómez Á, Cerdán S, Pérez-Laso C, et al. Effects of adult male rat feminization treatments on brain morphology and metabolomic profile. Horm Behav. 2020;125:104839.

76. Nagelhus EA, Ottersen O. Physiological roles of aquaporin-4 in brain. Physiol Rev. 2013;93(4):1543–1562.

77. Gu F, Hata R, Toku K, et al. Testosterone up-regulates aquaporin-4 expression in cultured astrocytes. J Neurosci Res. 2003;72(6):709–715.

78. Rutkowsky JM, Wallace BK, Wise PM, O'Donnell ME. Effects of estradiol on ischemic factor-induced astrocyte swelling and AQP4 protein abundance. Am J Physiol Cell Physiol. 2011;301(1):C204–C212.

79. Zeng X-N, Sun X-L, Gao L, Fan Y, Ding J-H, Hu G. Aquaporin-4 deficiency down-regulates glutamate uptake and GLT-1 expression in astrocytes. Mol Cell Neurosci. 2007;34(1):34–39.

80. World Professional Association for Transgender Health. Standards of care for the health of transsexual, transgender, and gender-conforming people. 2012. https://www.wpath.org/publications/soc (last accessed August 21, 2021).

Abbreviations Used

AASs = anabolic androgenic steroids
AQP-4 = Aquaporin 4
AR = androgen receptor
ER = estrogen receptor
ERα = estrogen receptors alpha
Erβ = estrogen receptor beta
GABA = γ-aminobutyric acid
GAHT = gender affirming hormone treatment
Gln = glutamine
Glu = glutamate
mI = myo-Inositol
MRI = magnetic resonance imaging
TM = transgeder men

19

Mitochondria Dysfunction and Inflammation in Traumatic Brain Injury: Androgens to the Battlefront

Andrew J. McGovern[1] and George E. Barreto[1,2,*,i]

Abstract

The therapeutic response to traumatic brain injury (TBI) still lacks a strategy to treat its acute and chronic phases. Given that TBI affects the lives of 1.5 million people a year, and the management of its early stages has significant effects on outcome, identifying a druggable target to mitigate damage could protect the cognitive and motor function of patients. Given the value of rescuing cells during TBI and of the health of mitochondria in preventing cell death, it is important to explore means of preventing mitochondrial stress. There is a growing body of evidence that identifies a role for androgens (i.e., testosterone and its derivative, dihydrotestosterone) in both this TBI pathology and managing mitochondrial stress. Androgen signaling is involved in regulating gene expression of several proteins that interact with key mitochondrial pathways, and since TBI alters androgen signaling in time-specific stages, it appears to be a promising target for a druggable intervention. In this review, we discuss the physiopathological events underlying TBI pathology, focusing especially on the impact inflammatory cascade has on disrupting cell function and the integrity of mitochondrion. Finally, we propose that the administration of androgens might be considered a promising pharmacological approach to alleviate inflammation and mitochondria impairment post-TBI.

Keywords: androgens; testosterone; dihydrotestosterone; traumatic brain injury; inflammation; mitochondria

Introduction

Traumatic brain injury (TBI) due to traffic accidents and falls is one of the leading causes of death in the world. Currently, it is believed that TBI causes ~ 1.5 million hospitalizations with $\sim 75,000$ deaths per year, the most affected being adults between 19 and 60 years of age. However, an exponential increase has been observed in the elderly population (+65 years old) with some type of brain trauma, whose population is the most vulnerable due to advanced age. The fact TBI affects young people implicates a huge economic and financial impact for a country, as it does not only affect people at productive age but also their relatives who lose their jobs to become full-time lifelong caregivers, which generates an increased financial burden on a country's welfare program. Despite the scientific and technological advances in recent years, there is still no effective therapy to minimize the damage caused by TBI.

TBI is a systemic, heterogeneous, and multifactorial pathology, characterized by acute and chronic phases. First there is an acute abrupt inflammatory response, which involves the destruction of the cerebral vessels leading to hemorrhage, blood–brain barrier (BBB)

[1]Department of Biological Sciences, University of Limerick, Limerick, Ireland.
[2]Health Research Institute, University of Limerick, Limerick, Ireland.
[i]ORCID ID (https://orcid.org/0000-0002-6644-1971).

*Address correspondence to: George E. Barreto, PhD, Department of Biological Sciences, University of Limerick, Limerick, V94 T9PX, Ireland, Email: george.barreto@ul.ie

breakdown with consequent infiltration of neutrophils, leukocytes and monocytes, edema and axonal trauma that produce the massive death of neurons, and glial cells due to mechanical trauma. In response, dying neurons release damage-associated molecular patterns (DAMPs). This promotes microglia to release proinflammatory type 1 interferons,[1,2] IL-1β,[3] IL6,[4,5] TNF-α,[6] CCL2,[7] and chemokines CXCL10, CXCL6,[8] RANTES/CCL5, and MIP-1β or CCL4[9] in the first 24–72 h post-TBI. This continues with an expansion of brain involvement due to the activation of oxidative cascades that not only affect neurons but also astrocytes and microglia, leading to long-term motor and cognitive damage. In the chronic phase of the pathology, generally from day 7 after trauma, there is a latent chronic inflammation, with a sustained activation of microglia that can last for years, affecting the processes of remodeling, recovery, and reorganization of the brain neuronal circuits, leaving the patients with serious motor and cognitive sequelae. At cellular level, during both the acute and chronic phases, there is a severe compromise of mitochondrial integrity, loss of adenosine triphosphate (ATP) production, concomitant with the activation of mitochondrial-dependent cell death cascades such as apoptosis. In dealing with current therapies against TBI, the therapeutic management in each phase is different, and one of the failures in the treatment of this pathology is the lack of complete knowledge of the cellular and molecular processes occurring in each phase to be able to address the problem with more specificity and precision.

An important feature of the pathophysiological mechanism of TBI is the neuroendocrine disruption in the brain. First and the more evident aspect is an altered expression of androgen receptor (AR) TBI.[10] Indeed, not only are the plasma and brain levels of gonadal hormones affected,[11,12] other hormones such as follicle-stimulating hormone, growth hormone, and pituitary hormone[13] are also found to be significantly reduced after a TBI event, for which the magnitude of their levels are inversely correlated with trauma intensity and severity. Considering that the brain is an endocrine organ, it can be speculated that brain-synthetized hormones (i.e., neurosteroidogenesis) are particularly vulnerable and may become a potential complication in chronic post-TBI. It should be noted TBI male patients present lower blood levels of testosterone (T),[14] a similar outcome observed in the brain where its levels reduce up to 72 h but increase by week 2 as opposed to dihydrotestosterone (DHT), a T derivative product of

5α-reductase, whose levels are significantly attenuated.[15] Whether or not these neurosteroid levels are correlated with better prognosis or improved outcome overall, this is still controversial with some studies showing distinct outcome when T levels positively correlate with Glasgow Coma Scale,[14] suggesting that further studies are warranted to precisely link these changes to the degree of protection. Apart from these inconsistencies, the benefits of androgens (T and DHT) to stimulate neuroprotective signaling in TBI is well known by modulating the response of both glial cells and neurons to lesion, including at cellular level the mitochondrial modulation of redox reactions, inflammation, and apoptosis.[16-20] Given the importance of androgens toward mitochondria well-being in this review, we highlight the main aspects of TBI pathology and discuss how T and DHT may have benefits as therapy to counteract inflammation and mitochondria impairment in TBI.

Acute and Chronic Inflammation Post-TBI

Neuroinflammation is a characteristic hallmark of TBI, where several brain cells, namely astrocytes and microglia, work together to control mechanical and pro-oxidative damage at site of injury that may generate an innate immune response that, in most cases, provoke an exaggerated response leading to more severe damage to neurons. Astrocytes bordering the injury become activated, as characterized by an increase in the expression of glial fibrillary protein (GFAP) and vimentin,[21,22] also reflected by an augment in cell body and number of prolongations/ramifications. This early reaction is thought to be an immediate protective mechanism against mechanical damage, with the aim of limiting the expansion of damaged tissue through the formation of a dense glial scar. Glial scarring has long been considered to having a double-edged role that in one side it favors the containment of the lesion but eventually may inhibit axonal regeneration due to the excessive release of proteoglycans and inhibitory proteins that affect the formation of new axonal cones (for full review please see Filous and Silver[23]). Furthermore, the release of cytokines and chemokines by activated astrocytes surrounding the injury likely promotes the activation of neighboring microglia, in addition to contributing to the attraction of immune cells from the periphery, favoring the rise of local inflammation.

The first 48 h postinjury is critical and marked by an exponential increase in the release of proinflammatory molecules, DAMPs, which continue with an initially acute but then chronic activation of glial cells, occurring in parallel with the infiltration of immune cells. On acute onset, both astrocytes and the brain-resident immune cells, microglia, surrounding the lesion wound, release an excessive amount of inflammatory cytokines that, concomitantly with the formation of reactive oxygen species and nitrogen oxygen species (ROS/NOS), can lead to massive death of neurons, which, inevitably, generate motor and cognitive sequelae with time of injury. Of these cytokines, IL6 is significantly upregulated in TBI and considered a biomarker of the severity of the lesion.[24,25] The rapid increase in cytokine levels starts after 1 h post-TBI, with IL6, IL-1β, and TNF-α being the main ones expressed in the first few hours, including lasting up to 12 months after injury.[26] Not only are these cytokines implicated in the pathophysiological mechanism of TBI, but also other chemokines such as CXCL12, CXCL4,[26,27] CXCL10,[25,28] CCL2 and CCR2[8] that can not only increase the local inflammatory process at the site of injury, but also serve as chemical mediators that attract monocytes, neutrophils, T cells, macrophages, and leukocytes. Once reaching the brain tissue due to the loss of permeability of the BBB, these cells release more proinflammatory molecules that cause even more damage to the already injured tissue, leading to a perpetuation of the activation of glial cells.

More recently there is a growing interest in the role played by complement proteins in the secondary injury in TBI. The complement system comprising >30 distinct proteins is part of the innate immune system, and along with adaptive immunity both are responsible for the protection of the brain against pathogens that may eventually enter this organ. Interestingly, M1 microglia, an activated state, express C1q and C3, which seems to participate in or contribute to their reactive morphology. A rise on C1q and C3d and C3b levels has been observed in the area surrounding the injury in TBI patients,[29] which is in accordance with their levels in cerebral spine fluid,[30] suggesting the facilitation of neuroinflammatory signaling with involvement of these proteins. Apart from C1 and C3 anaphylatoxins, C5a has also been a target for further investigation in TBI, with studies showing that genetic deletion of C5 or administration of antagonists against its receptor, C5aR, attenuates secondary damage by reducing the infiltration of immune cells (i.e., leucocytes) and improving behavior outcome in injured animals.[31,32] The fact that the expression of these complement proteins does not occur homogeneously and continues over time

post-TBI, some having a peak in hours while others after days, suggests the importance of identifying the right timing of their levels, whether up or down, for a more precise pharmacological intervention.

Mitochondria response to TBI

Chronically orchestrated inflammation affects cell's ability to maintain its physiological functions. Mitochondria are one of the most affected organelles that lose their integrity and become unable to cope with physiological redox reactions, oxidative phosphorylation for ATP production, and maintaining cellular well-being overall. It is well known and widely accepted that all cells are extremely dependent on mitochondria for their correct functioning, especially considering that the brain has a high energy demand and little capacity to store energy make this organelle vital for pharmacological strategies that can protect them against TBI.

There are pathological events occurring within mitochondria that are pivotal to developing a better understanding of the damaging effects of TBI on a cellular level. Along with the endoplasmic reticulum (ERe), mitochondria play a key role in regulating cytosolic Ca^{+2} levels, which is an essential intracellular mechanism to control the dynamics of mitochondrial metabolism and oxygen consumption,[33] as this ion can be considered as an allosteric activator for some Krebs cycle catabolic enzymes such as pyruvate dehydrogenase and alpha-ketoglutarate dehydrogenase.[34] However, as TBI greatly affects these dynamics by interfering with the ability of the ERe and mitochondria to uptake Ca^{+2}, this ion begins to accumulate intracellularly, leading to the activation of kinases and downstream enzymes capable of degrading membrane phospholipids, and affect kinase proteins regulating cell survival such as extracellular-signal regulated kinase (ERK) and mitogen-activated protein kinase (MAPK).[35] More specifically, this impaired mitochondrial regulation of Ca^{+2} promotes a disruption of the fusion (MFN1/2 and OPA1) and fission (Fis1/Drp1) processes, two critical mechanisms that play an essential role in maintaining mitochondrial homeostasis and quality control. It has been observed, for example, that acute TBI increases fission over mitochondrial fusion,[36] causing mitochondria fragmentation, which may be correlated with mitophagy and a significant decrease in endogenous ATP production. Not only that, but also the massive Ca^{+2} influx to mitochondria[37] causes an uncoupling of the electron transport chain located in the inner mitochondrial membrane (IMM), leading to a reduction in its capacity to accept and donate electrons forming a concentration gradient between the mitochondrial matrix and the mitochondrial intermembrane space. Inevitably, this has three immediate consequences: (1) a major reduction in protonmotive force; (2) this favors a greater production of oxidative stress by increasing free electrons, which are easily trapped by oxygen; and (3) increased levels of ROS are responsible for oxidizing mitochondrial membrane phospholipids such as cardiolipin that are essential to maintain the selectivity and permeability of the IMM.[38] The importance of cardiolipin for mitochondrial integrity is observed when there is a TBI, where this IMM-localized phospholipid is oxidized due to the peroxidase activity of cytochrome C (Cytc).[39] This promotes the cytosolic translocation of Cytc, one of the mitochondria-dependent mechanisms for the activation of apoptosis, programmed cell death, since once in the cytosol Cytc activates caspase proteins (i.e., caspase 3), leading to downstream triggering of the other apoptotic proteins (i.e., caspases 7 and 9).[40]

Neurons and glial cells have developed amazing intracellular mechanisms to counteract, or at least minimize, the secondary damage caused by TBI. A protein expressed by these cells with great involvement in the pathophysiological mechanism of TBI is neuroglobin (Ngb), a protein highly regulated by androgens, especially T[19] (Fig. 1). Belonging to the globin family, similar to myoglobin and its more famous relative, hemoglobin, Ngb with 151 amino acids has a hexacoordinated group in place of the pentacoordinate—as seen with myoglobin and hemoglobin—favoring the union of oxygen with iron groups of the porphyrins. In a slightly different way, in the case of Ngb, His64 and His96 residues form the sixth hem-coordinated link with iron, which when oxygen binds Ngb it causes a displacement of both residues to generate the oxygenated form of this protein. Despite this evidence, the dissociation of Ngb by oxygen seems to be low and, instead of binding O_2 with high affinity, this protein may serve as a sensor for this gas, especially in those hypoxic conditions similar to what occurs in the TBI with destruction of vessels and arteries due to mechanical trauma. Furthermore, Ngb also binds to ROS and NOS,[41] suggesting an antioxidant role, in addition to the fact that it interacts with proteins belonging to mitochondrial complexes III, for example, cytochrome c_1.[42] Indeed, Ngb has the ability to sequester Cytc, with studies showing a physical interaction, avoiding its translocation to the cytosol in case of mitochondrial

damage, thus assuming an antiapoptotic role.[43] It should be noted that Ngb levels reduce post-TBI, meaning that this protein could be considered as a target for future pharmacological strategies with potential clinical interest for the treatment of patients suffering from TBI. Nevertheless, Ngb inability to cross plasma membranes, hence not able to cross the BBB, makes its clinical use of little interest, and some ways to circumvent this is the application of encapsulation methods for its efficient and optimal delivery to the brain.

Involvement of Androgen Signaling in TBI

There are two isoforms of the AR, called AR-A (87 kDa) and AR-B (110 kDa). Isoform A is a minority and is due to a translation of the AR-B messenger from Met188, which produces a protein with the N-terminal region truncated and that could have less transcriptional activity. Isoform B corresponds to the complete coding sequence of the AR.[44–46]

Regulation of gene transcription is the primary mechanism of action of the AR. Upon binding to T or DHT, the AR dimer binds to a specific DNA sequence known as the androgen response element.[47] It has been revealed that the AR, apart from having genomic actions, may also have effects independent of its role as a transcription factor,[48,49] interacting with components of signaling pathways initiated in the plasma membrane that induce, among other effects, rapid modifications in ion transport. Regulation by the AR of signal translation cascades in the cytoplasm can indirectly affect transcriptional activity through phosphorylation of other transcription factors.[50,51] For instance, physical interaction of T with GPRC6A, a membrane AR, has been reported,[52] which may lead to a rapid activation of downstream signaling mediated by ERK and Ca^{+2} as messenger.[53] Being regarded as a zinc transporter, Slc39a9 (or ZIP9) has been predicted to be a target of androgens, in particular T, resulting in a myriad of actions ranging from ERK1/2, CREB, and ATF1 activation, upregulation of apoptotic proteins (i.e., Bax, p53, and caspase 3), and increase in intracellular zinc.[54–59] These mixed effects may rely on cellular type, for example, it has been seen that the activation of ZIP9 in prostate cancer cells is associated with an increase in migration and invasiveness,[60] or perhaps be dependent on the cellular response to the concentration of T administered such as the induction of apoptotic mechanisms in ovarian cancer cells and breast cancer.[56,57]

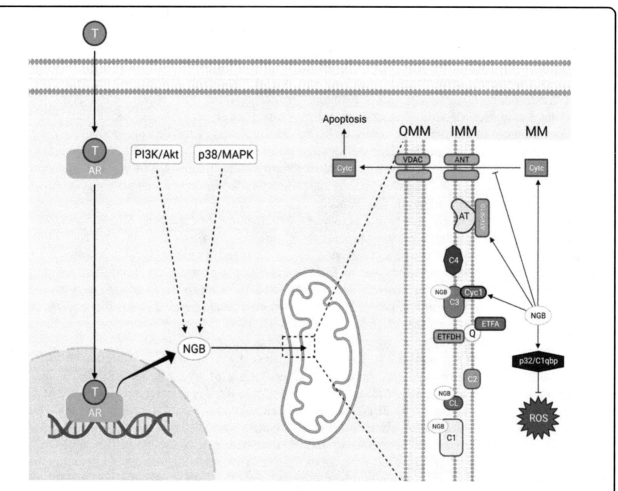

FIG. 1. Androgenic regulation of neuroglobin signaling. Upon binding to testosterone, the AR is internalized to nucleus to stimulate transcriptional regulation of Ngb. Another upstream cascade that may upregulate this protein is through PI3k/AKT and p38/MAPK. Ngb is then transported to mitochondria where it interacts with various complexes of the electron transport chain (C1–C4), stimulating metabolism, oxidative phosphorylation, and regulating ROS-mediated inflammation possibly through the p32/C1qbp complex. Ngb protects CL from oxidation, prevents cytosolic translocation of Cytc, inhibits apoptosis, and also interacts with the mitochondrial transition pore formed by VDAC and ANT. Ngb interacts very intrinsically with cyc1 in complex III, and may also with the ETFDH/Q/ETFA complex, favoring electron transport and promoting ATP synthesis. At ATP synthase (AS), Ngb may bind to ATP5F1D, favoring ATP synthesis. This suggests that Ngb-inducing actions of testosterone are essential to maintain these organelles' stability and integrity under pathological conditions. ANT, adenine nucleotide translocator; AR, androgen receptor; AT, ATP synthase; ATP5F1D, ATP synthase F1 subunit delta; C1, mitochondrial complex I; C2, mitochondrial complex II; C3, mitochondrial complex III; C4, mitochondrial complex IV; CL, cardiolipin; Cytc, cytochrome C; cytc1, cytochrome c1 subunit; ETFA, electron transfer flavoprotein subunit alpha; IMM, inner mitochondrial membrane; MM, mitochondrial matrix; Ngb, neuroglobin; OMM, outer mitochondrial membrane; p32/C1qbp, complement C1q binding protein complexed with p32; p38/MAPK, p38, and mitogen-activated protein kinase; PI3K/AKT, phosphoinositide 3-kinases/protein kinase B; ROS, reactive oxygen species; T, testosterone; VDAC, voltage-dependent anion channel.

Androgen signaling in the brain is severely altered in TBI. For example, AR expression is notably augmented in microglia at 72 h, decreasing afterward by day 28 after lesion.[61] Contrasting results have been observed with proteome data analysis revealing an important reduction of 48% and 42% on the expression of AR at 8 and 24 h, respectively, whereas Slc39a9 is reduced by ~20% at 72 h post-TBI rats.[62] Using zebra finch subjected to unilateral brain injury, Mehos et al. show decreased AR messenger RNA levels at 48 h after damage.[63] Whether AR is up- or downregulated after injury, this indicates that the timing and animal model are two variables to be considered when studying its transient expression in TBI. Because of these discrepancies, one can speculate that due to reduced brain[15] and blood levels of T and DHT as observed in TBI,[64] brain cells may overexpress the AR to compensate the low bioavailability of its substrates or perhaps its reduced expression is coupled to low T, and DHT being not able to trigger a transcriptional regulation of AR. Another possible explanation is that since TBI dysregulates the brain synthesis of neurosteroids, their higher levels might be different and, in some cases, correlated with detrimental rather than protective outcome. Indeed, important to note is that not always the levels of steroids in blood correlate with those in the brain,[65,66] this being a possible confounding factor when analyzing their peripheral versus brain levels. Collectively, these studies suggest three important outcomes: (1) the brain is an endocrine organ severely affected by lower production of local androgens, this impairs the androgenic regulation of mitochondria metabolism, and redox enzymatic reactions due to limited availability of T and DHT; (2) the reduction of T and DHT levels is associated with the development of other diseases (i.e., neurodegenerative diseases), being their levels in some cases inversely correlated with prognosis in TBI; and (3) exogenous supplementation with T might reduce TBI burden, facilitating a faster recovery and better overall outcome.

Actions of Androgens on the Attenuation of TBI Pathology

Mitochondrion is largely an androgen-regulated organelle. The fact that it is considered a converging point between the activation of survival and cell death mechanisms due to inflammatory stimulation demonstrates the importance it has for the post-TBI period. Bearing in mind that endocrine dysfunction occurs in TBI, which can again lead to dysregulation of metabolic

and oxidative processes, the current evidence indicating the presence of ARs within the mitochondria may suggest this organelle as a full target of androgens. Next, we discuss the neuroprotective role of androgens in the setting of a traumatic damage to the brain.

Regulation of gliosis by androgens

One of the first studies to report that T reduces reactive gliosis was described by Garcia-Estrada et al.[67] In this study, they found that GFAP-positive astrocytes located at 0–500 μm from injury are significantly reduced in both cortex and hippocampus when rats are given 250 μg of T at 24, 48, and 72 h after a penetrating brain injury, with this approach also consistent with a significant reduction of proliferating (BrdU-positive) astrocytes close to the wound.[67] These findings were of clinical interest at that time, and many other studies that have tried to further determine how T, or its metabolite DHT, can regulate reactive glia after an injury have been carried out. Confirming the previous evidence, not only T but also DHT at 1 mg/kg was able to reduce reactive microglia in male rats subjected to a penetrating brain lesion,[21] possibly this effect may be directly related to the anti-inflammatory effects of these compounds. In line with this, pretreated BV2 microglial cells with 10 nM of DHT followed by 100 ng/mL of lipopolysaccharide (LPS), an inductor of neuroinflammation, show lower levels of IL6, TNF-α, IL-1β, iNOS, and COX-2, likely by regulating the TLR4/NFκB/MAPK/p38 signaling pathways. These findings are confirmed when studying primary microglia under the same inflammatory stimuli.[68] In the absence of T, animals castrated for 15 days and given 5 mg/kg DHT for 15 days and then injected with LPS have significantly lower levels of reactive microglia and astroglia in both cortex and hippocampus, thus confirming the ability of DHT and T to modulate neuroinflammation and lowering glia activation with LPS.[68]

Since males seem to display more severe brain damage than females after a TBI event,[69,70] to delve into these sex differences over the neuroprotective actions of T and DHT in brain trauma, male and female mice can be used to explore how each sex differentially responds to damage and what mechanisms underlie this. One of the recent attempts was the use of mice subjected to controlled cortical impact (CCI) whose outcome was monitored up to 72 h after lesion.[71] Although there was no significant sex difference with respect to GFAP expression in the ipsilateral hemisphere up to 72 h in TBI animals, there seems to have a sex-dependent effect on the lesion volume. Furthermore, it appears that these effects may be regulated by the endogenous production of hormones in the brain. For example, the animals were treated with either finasteride, an inhibitor of 5α-reductase, the enzyme that converts T to DHT, thus favoring the aromatization of T to estradiol, or letrozole, an aromatase inhibitor, the enzyme converting T to estradiol. Finasteride-treated male mice show a slight rise on the number of GFAP-positive astrocytes, and although this was not observed in the other sex, female mice given letrozole present significant levels of reactive astrocytes compared with vehicle-treated counterparts. It is also possible that the mechanism underlying this could be related to the brain levels of neurotrophins and their receptors, which are found significantly attenuated in TBI. For instance, the lesion itself appears to decrease TrkB and TrkC in both sexes, but the levels of both normal growth factor (NGF) and its receptor, TrkA, are significantly decreased (compared with vehicle) in males treated with finasteride,[71] suggesting that blocking endogenous DHT synthesis causes a disruption of NGF-TrkA as trophic signaling affecting neuronal fate, inflammation, and brain development.[72]

Finally, tibolone, a synthetic steroid with estrogenic, androgenic, and progestogenic properties, may be used for drug repurposing in TBI.[17] For instance, tibolone is prescribed for the treatment of osteoporosis and climacteric symptoms in postmenopausal women.[73] After administration, it is rapidly metabolized in the body into 3α-OH tibolone and 3β-OH-tibolone that mediate their actions through estrogen receptors, whereas δ4-tibolone has preference for androgen and progesterone receptors.[74–76] One of the first studies to show the actions of tibolone in TBI found an important reduction in the number of GFAP-positive astrocytes, and an attenuation of both the number and the reactive phenotype of microglia along with improvement in neuronal survival in animals after a stab wound injury.[77] Although tibolone has anti-inflammatory, antioxidant, and antiapoptotic effects,[78–83] it is still unclear which of its metabolites may be mediating these actions in TBI, and further studies are warranted to explore which enzymes responsible for tibolone metabolism are being regulated in the face of brain injury. If this is confirmed in future studies, it could largely explain whether these benefits of this prodrug are being triggered by its metabolites with estrogenic, progestogenic, or androgenic activity.

Regulation of TBI-induced mitochondria impairment and inflammation by androgens

The mitochondrial network is a critical compartment for cell survival and development, due to its great function such as the proportion of cellular energy. It is a major player in the production of reactive species and regulates apoptotic cell death.[18,84–86] Traumatic brain damage directly affects mitochondrial function[87] by interfering with the electron transport chain and contributing to the loss of mitochondrial membrane potential ($\Delta\Psi$m) and the generation of ATP.

The fact the AR possesses an amino acid sequence for importation into mitochondria[88] suggests an intrinsic relationship between androgens and functions carried out by this organelle. Interestingly, the absence of androgens in male rats due to orchiectomy leads to lower expression of ND1 and ND5, two mitochondrial complex I subunits, leading to an important reduction of this complex's activity, all these cellular processes being ameliorated upon exogenous supplementation of T.[89] Furthermore, T has also been shown to upregulate mitochondrial complex V,[90] boosting ATP production and improving mitochondria integrity and metabolism. In contrast to these previous observations, ectopic expression of AR has some deleterious effects by attenuating the mitochondrial respiratory complexes, whereas an augmented activity of these complexes is noted when the AR is blocked in prostate cells.[88]

Animals treated with T and subjected to CCI show a considerable improvement in $\Delta\Psi$m, O_2 consumption, oxidative phosphorylation, and a reduced level of hydrogen peroxide possibly due to an upregulation of the mitochondrial SOD_2.[16] Similar evidence has been observed in glial cells pretreated with tibolone and subjected to metabolic damage, showing that this compound, in addition to positively stimulating the expression of Ngb, cardiolipin, and $\Delta\Psi$m, is also able to attenuate the expression of 8-hydroxy-2′-deoxyguanosine, a marker of oxidative DNA damage, and 4-hydroxynonenal, a marker of lipid peroxidation.[81,82] Indeed, tibolone reduces 3-nitrotyrosine,[82] a marker of nitrated proteins, in which the incorporation of the nitro group into the phenolic ring of tyrosine produces changes in certain properties of the amino acid.[91] The immediate consequences of tyrosine nitration are (1) no effects on the function of the protein, (2) a loss of function occurs, and (3) a gain of function is observed. An example is the inactivation of MnSOD by nitration of a key tyrosine residue,[92] which could increase the endogenous production of free radicals at the mitochondrial level. Finally, due to the increased production of nitric oxide in TBI,[93] this may inevitably inhibit the antioxidant enzymes glutathione peroxidase[94] and Cytc oxidase within mitochondria,[95] thus altering the mitochondrial respiratory chain, leading to attenuated ATP production.

To better understand how T protects mitochondria in TBI, some proteins known to be targets of this hormone and involved in TBI pathology can be retrieved from public databases for functional assessment. A mitochondrial cluster can be drawn, showing that these proteins are mainly related to the control of apoptosis, neuronal death, and cellular stress response (Fig. 2). For instance, by downregulating caspase 3 and Bax while increasing Bcl-2 family in TBI mice T[16,96] and DHT,[97,98] both are able to negatively regulate mitochondrial-dependent apoptotic signaling. Not only do T and DHT control the expression of proteins responsible for programmed cell death, thus favoring cell survival, but also upregulate AKT1, confirming their prosurvival properties that can be beneficial during post-TBI chronic inflammation. Quite intrigu-

ingly, another protein with possible involvement in the protective mechanism of T is the antiapoptotic member of the BCL2 family, MCL1, which has been sought to be involved in steroidogenesis, its blockade promotes an important reduction in the expression of P450 SCC (Cyp11a1) and steroidogenic acute regulatory protein,[99] and consequently leading to a decrease in precursors for the endogenous synthesis of T. Finally, androgen-deprived animals have higher levels of tumor protein p53,[100] a master regulator of DNA damage and repair with close participation in senescence and apoptosis, suggesting a link between endogenous androgens and processes regulating cell fate applicable to TBI. More recently, our group has discovered that the catalytic subunit of telomerase (TERT) has a key role in not only telomeres maintenance, but also that upon cellular damage it migrates to the cytosol to activate signaling pathways that can be essential for cell survival. It should be noted that its inhibition alters the protective actions of tibolone over astrocytic cells upon metabolic dysfunction,[80] clearly demonstrating TERT participation in neuroprotective mechanisms. Given that tibolone is metabolized into three different metabolites, it is yet to be

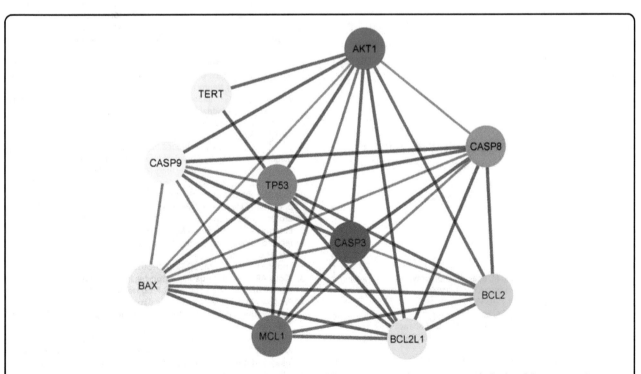

FIG. 2. Mitochondrial subcluster of proteins regulated by testosterone as potential druggable targets in traumatic brain injury pathology.

explored whether these observed effects are due to its conversion to δ4-tibolone, with a potential perspective to regulate the AR.

Conclusions

The therapeutic strategy for TBI still lacks a means to manage the immediate inflammatory response that influences an individual's recovery. This is worrying as early intervention post-TBI has repeatedly been emphasized as critical to outcome, as it can mediate the extent of the damage to the brain and, therefore, protect the faculties of patients. However, although the value of an early intervention is apparent, current treatments are primarily in education, psychological, or rehabilitative assistance for patients and the data have mixed views of the efficacy of these treatments. As such, in this review, we have outlined the importance of considering mitochondrial dysfunction in preventing neuronal cell death as well as identifying important protective agents such as T and DHT by targeting mitochondrial proteins (i.e., Ngb), which have potential as druggable therapeutic targets. TBI also dysregulates the neuroendocrine system, suppressing the action of androgens. This coincides with evidence showing that men have worse outcome to TBI compared with women. We suggest that given the role of androgen signaling in regulating gliosis and protecting mitochondrial function under stress, targeting this system has potential as an early interceptive therapy in the acute stages of TBI.

Authors' Contributions

A.J.M. and G.E.B. wrote the article. Both authors agree with the final article, submission, and publication.

References

1. Karve IP, Zhang M, Habgood M, et al. Ablation of type-1 IFN signaling in hematopoietic cells confers protection following traumatic brain injury. eNeuro. 2016;3(1):ENEURO.0128-15.2016

2. Barrett JP, Henry RJ, Shirey KA, et al. Interferon-beta plays a detrimental role in experimental traumatic brain injury by Enhancing neuroinflammation that drives chronic neurodegeneration. J Neurosci. 2020;40(11): 2357–2370.

3. Clausen F, Hanell A, Israelsson C, et al. Neutralization of interleukin-1beta reduces cerebral edema and tissue loss and improves late cognitive outcome following traumatic brain injury in mice. Eur J Neurosci. 2011; 34(1):110–123.

4. Wang J, Hou Y, Zhang L, et al. Estrogen attenuates traumatic brain injury by inhibiting the activation of microglia and astrocyte-mediated neuroinflammatory responses. Mol Neurobiol. 2021;58(3): 1052–1061.

5. Hergenroeder GW, Moore AN, McCoy JP, Jr., et al. Serum IL-6: A candidate biomarker for intracranial pressure elevation following isolated traumatic brain injury. J Neuroinflammation. 2010;7:19.

6. Scherbel U, Raghupathi R, Nakamura M, et al. Differential acute and chronic responses of tumor necrosis factor-deficient mice to experimental brain injury. Proc Natl Acad Sci U S A. 1999;96(15):8721–8726.

7. Semple BD, Kossmann T, Morganti-Kossmann MC. Role of chemokines in CNS health and pathology: A focus on the CCL2/CCR2 and CXCL8/CXCR2 networks. J Cereb Blood Flow Metab. 2010;30(3):459–473.

8. Israelsson C, Bengtsson H, Kylberg A, et al. Distinct cellular patterns of upregulated chemokine expression supporting a prominent inflammatory role in traumatic brain injury. J Neurotrauma. 2008;25(8): 959–974.

9. Ghirnikar RS, Lee YL, He TR, Eng LF. Chemokine expression in rat stab wound brain injury. J Neurosci Res. 1996;46(6):727–733.

10. Duncan KA, Moon J, Vartosis D, Zee I. Injury-induced expression of glial androgen receptor in the zebra finch brain. J Neurotrauma. 2013;30(22): 1919–1924.

11. Behan LA, Agha A. Endocrine consequences of adult traumatic brain injury. Horm Res. 2007;68(Suppl. 5):18–21.

12. Wagner AK, McCullough EH, Niyonkuru C, et al. Acute serum hormone levels: Characterization and prognosis after severe traumatic brain injury. J Neurotrauma. 2011;28(6):871–888.

13. Leal-Cerro A, Flores JM, Rincon M, et al. Prevalence of hypopituitarism and growth hormone deficiency in adults long-term after severe traumatic brain injury. Clin Endocrinol (Oxf). 2005;62(5):525–532.

14. Agha A, Rogers B, Mylotte D, et al. Neuroendocrine dysfunction in the acute phase of traumatic brain injury. Clin Endocrinol (Oxf). 2004;60(5): 584–591.

15. Lopez-Rodriguez AB, Acaz-Fonseca E, Spezzano R, et al. Profiling neuroactive steroid levels after traumatic brain injury in male mice. Endocrinology. 2016;157(10):3983–3993.

16. Carteri RB, Kopczynski A, Rodolphi MS, et al. Testosterone administration after traumatic brain injury reduces mitochondrial dysfunction and neurodegeneration. J Neurotrauma. 2019;36(14):2246–2259.

17. McGovern AJ, Barreto GE. Network pharmacology identifies IL6 as an important hub and target of tibolone for drug repurposing in traumatic brain injury. Biomed Pharmacother. 2021;140:111769.

18. Mohajeri M, Martin-Jimenez C, Barreto GE, Sahebkar A. Effects of estrogens and androgens on mitochondria under normal and pathological conditions. Prog Neurobiol. 2019;176:54–72.

19. Toro-Urrego N, Garcia-Segura LM, Echeverria V, Barreto GE. Testosterone protects mitochondrial function and regulates neuroglobin expression in astrocytic cells exposed to glucose deprivation. Front Aging Neurosci. 2016;8:152.

20. Acaz-Fonseca E, Avila-Rodriguez M, Garcia-Segura LM, Barreto GE. Regulation of astroglia by gonadal steroid hormones under physiological and pathological conditions. Prog Neurobiol. 2016;144:5–26.

21. Barreto G, Veiga S, Azcoitia I, Garcia-Segura LM, Garcia-Ovejero D. Testosterone decreases reactive astroglia and reactive microglia after brain injury in male rats: Role of its metabolites, oestradiol and dihydrotestosterone. Eur J Neurosci. 2007;25(10):3039–3046.

22. Barreto G, Santos-Galindo M, Diz-Chaves Y, et al. Selective estrogen receptor modulators decrease reactive astrogliosis in the injured brain: Effects of aging and prolonged depletion of ovarian hormones. Endocrinology. 2009;150(11):5010–5015.

23. Filous AR, Silver J. Targeting astrocytes in CNS injury and disease: A translational research approach. Prog Neurobiol. 2016;144:173–187.

24. Penkowa M, Giralt M, Lago N, et al. Astrocyte-targeted expression of IL-6 protects the CNS against a focal brain injury. Exp Neurol. 2003;181(2): 130–148.

25. Woiciechowsky C, Schoning B, Cobanov J, Lanksch WR, Volk HD, Docke WD. Early IL-6 plasma concentrations correlate with severity of brain injury and pneumonia in brain-injured patients. J Trauma. 2002;52(2): 339–345.

26. Helmy A, Carpenter KL, Menon DK, Pickard JD, Hutchinson PJ. The cytokine response to human traumatic brain injury: Temporal profiles and evidence for cerebral parenchymal production. J Cereb Blood Flow Metab. 2011;31(2):658–670.

27. Helmy A, Antoniades CA, Guilfoyle MR, Carpenter KL, Hutchinson PJ. Principal component analysis of the cytokine and chemokine response to human traumatic brain injury. PLoS One. 2012;7(6):e39677.

28. Mukherjee S, Katki K, Arisi GM, Foresti ML, Shapiro LA. Early TBI-induced cytokine alterations are similarly detected by two distinct methods of multiplex assay. Front Mol Neurosci. 2011;4:21.

29. Bellander BM, Singhrao SK, Ohlsson M, Mattsson P, Svensson M. Complement activation in the human brain after traumatic head injury. J Neurotrauma. 2001;18(12):1295–1311.

30. Kossmann T, Stahel PF, Morganti-Kossmann MC, Jones JL, Barnum SR. Elevated levels of the complement components C3 and factor B in ventricular cerebrospinal fluid of patients with traumatic brain injury. J Neuroimmunol. 1997;73(1–2):63–69.

31. Sewell DL, Nacewicz B, Liu F, et al. Complement C3 and C5 play critical roles in traumatic brain cryoinjury: Blocking effects on neutrophil extravasation by C5a receptor antagonist. J Neuroimmunol. 2004;155(1–2): 55–63.

32. Garrett MC, Otten ML, Starke RM, et al. Synergistic neuroprotective effects of C3a and C5a receptor blockade following intracerebral hemorrhage. Brain Res. 2009;1298:171–177.

33. Arundine M, Tymianski M. Molecular mechanisms of glutamate-dependent neurodegeneration in ischemia and traumatic brain injury. Cell Mol Life Sci. 2004;61(6):657–668.

34. Wan B, LaNoue KF, Cheung JY, Scaduto RC, Jr. Regulation of citric acid cycle by calcium. J Biol Chem. 1989;264(23):13430–13439.

35. Jastroch M, Divakaruni AS, Mookerjee S, Treberg JR, Brand MD. Mitochondrial proton and electron leak. Essays Biochem. 2010;47:53–67.

36. Fischer TD, Hylin MJ, Zhao J, Moore AN, Waxham MN, Dash PK. Altered mitochondrial dynamics and TBI pathophysiology. Front Syst Neurosci. 2016;10:29.

37. Bayir H, Kagan VE, Borisenko GG, et al. Enhanced oxidative stress in iNOS-deficient mice after traumatic brain injury: Support for a neuroprotective role of iNOS. J Cereb Blood Flow Metab. 2005;25(6):673–684.

38. Bayir H, Tyurin VA, Tyurina YY, et al. Selective early cardiolipin peroxidation after traumatic brain injury: An oxidative lipidomics analysis. Ann Neurol. 2007;62(2):154–169.

39. Chao H, Lin C, Zuo Q, et al. Cardiolipin-dependent mitophagy guides outcome after traumatic brain injury. J Neurosci. 2019;39(10):1930–1943.

40. Kagan VE, Tyurin VA, Jiang J, et al. Cytochrome c acts as a cardiolipin oxygenase required for release of proapoptotic factors. Nat Chem Biol. 2005;1(4):223–232.

41. Herold S, Fago A, Weber RE, Dewilde S, Moens L. Reactivity studies of the Fe(III) and Fe(II)NO forms of human neuroglobin reveal a potential role against oxidative stress. J Biol Chem. 2004;279(22):22841–22847.

42. Yu Z, Xu J, Liu N, et al. Mitochondrial distribution of neuroglobin and its response to oxygen-glucose deprivation in primary-cultured mouse cortical neurons. Neuroscience. 2012;218:235–242.

43. Fago A, Mathews AJ, Moens L, Dewilde S, Brittain T. The reaction of neuroglobin with potential redox protein partners cytochrome b5 and cytochrome c. FEBS Lett. 2006;580(20):4884–4888.

44. Catalano MG, Pfeffer U, Raineri M, et al. Altered expression of androgen-receptor isoforms in human colon-cancer tissues. Int J Cancer. 2000; 86(3):325–330.

45. Gao T, McPhaul MJ. Functional activities of the A and B forms of the human androgen receptor in response to androgen receptor agonists and antagonists. Mol Endocrinol. 1998;12(5):654–663.

46. Wilson CM, McPhaul MJ. A and B forms of the androgen receptor are present in human genital skin fibroblasts. Proc Natl Acad Sci U S A. 1994; 91(4):1234–1238.

47. Heemers HV, Tindall DJ. Androgen receptor (AR) coregulators: A diversity of functions converging on and regulating the AR transcriptional complex. Endocr Rev. 2007;28(7):778–808.

48. Heinlein CA, Chang C. The roles of androgen receptors and androgen-binding proteins in nongenomic androgen actions. Mol Endocrinol. 2002;16(10):2181–2187.

49. Fix C, Jordan C, Cano P, Walker WH. Testosterone activates mitogen-activated protein kinase and the cAMP response element binding protein transcription factor in Sertoli cells. Proc Natl Acad Sci U S A. 2004; 101(30):10919–10924.

50. Foradori CD, Weiser MJ, Handa RJ. Non-genomic actions of androgens. Front Neuroendocrinol. 2008;29(2):169–181.

51. Michels G, Hoppe UC. Rapid actions of androgens. Front Neuroendocrinol. 2008;29(2):182–198.

52. Pi M, Kapoor K, Wu Y, et al. Structural and functional evidence for testosterone activation of GPRC6A in peripheral tissues. Mol Endocrinol. 2015;29(12):1759–1773.

53. Pi M, Parrill AL, Quarles LD. GPRC6A mediates the non-genomic effects of steroids. J Biol Chem. 2010;285(51):39953–39964.

54. Thomas P, Pang Y, Dong J. Membrane androgen receptor characteristics of human ZIP9 (SLC39A) zinc transporter in prostate cancer cells: Androgen-specific activation and involvement of an inhibitory G protein in zinc and MAP kinase signaling. Mol Cell Endocrinol. 2017;447:23–34.

55. Thomas P. Membrane androgen receptors unrelated to nuclear steroid receptors. Endocrinology. 2019;160(4):772–781.

56. Berg AH, Rice CD, Rahman MS, Dong J, Thomas P. Identification and characterization of membrane androgen receptors in the ZIP9 zinc transporter subfamily: I. Discovery in female atlantic croaker and evidence ZIP9 mediates testosterone-induced apoptosis of ovarian follicle cells. Endocrinology. 2014;155(11):4237–4249.

57. Thomas P, Pang Y, Dong J, Berg AH. Identification and characterization of membrane androgen receptors in the ZIP9 zinc transporter subfamily: II. Role of human ZIP9 in testosterone-induced prostate and breast cancer cell apoptosis. Endocrinology. 2014;155(11):4250–4265.

58. Converse A, Zhang C, Thomas P. Membrane androgen receptor ZIP9 induces croaker ovarian cell apoptosis via stimulatory G protein alpha subunit and MAP kinase signaling. Endocrinology. 2017;158(9):3015–3029.

59. Bulldan A, Dietze R, Shihan M, Scheiner-Bobis G. Non-classical testosterone signaling mediated through ZIP9 stimulates claudin expression and tight junction formation in Sertoli cells. Cell Signal. 2016;28(8):1075–1085.

60. Bulldan A, Bartsch JW, Konrad L, Scheiner-Bobis G. ZIP9 but not the androgen receptor mediates testosterone-induced migratory activity of metastatic prostate cancer cells. Biochim Biophys Acta Mol Cell Res. 2018;1865(12):1857–1868.

61. Garcia-Ovejero D, Veiga S, Garcia-Segura LM, Doncarlos LL. Glial expression of estrogen and androgen receptors after rat brain injury. J Comp Neurol. 2002;450(3):256–271.

62. Natale JE, Ahmed F, Cernak I, Stoica B, Faden AI. Gene expression profile changes are commonly modulated across models and species after traumatic brain injury. J Neurotrauma. 2003;20(10):907–927.

63. Mehos CJ, Nelson LH, Saldanha CJ. A quantification of the injury-induced changes in central aromatase, oestrogenic milieu and steroid receptor expression in the zebra finch. J Neuroendocrinol. 2016;28(2):12348.

64. Hohl A, Zanela FA, Ghisi G, et al. Luteinizing hormone and testosterone levels during acute phase of severe traumatic brain injury: Prognostic implications for adult male patients. Front Endocrinol (Lausanne). 2018; 9:29.

65. Giatti S, D'Intino G, Maschi O, et al. Acute experimental autoimmune encephalomyelitis induces sex dimorphic changes in neuroactive steroid levels. Neurochem Int. 2010;56(1):118–127.

66. Meffre D, Pianos A, Liere P, et al. Steroid profiling in brain and plasma of male and pseudopregnant female rats after traumatic brain injury: Analysis by gas chromatography/mass spectrometry. Endocrinology. 2007;148(5):2505–2517.

67. Garcia-Estrada J, Del Rio JA, Luquin S, Soriano E, Garcia-Segura LM. Gonadal hormones down-regulate reactive gliosis and astrocyte proliferation after a penetrating brain injury. Brain Res. 1993;628(1–2):271–278.

68. Yang L, Zhou R, Tong Y, et al. Neuroprotection by dihydrotestosterone in LPS-induced neuroinflammation. Neurobiol Dis. 2020;140:104814.

69. Ratcliff JJ, Greenspan AI, Goldstein FC, et al. Gender and traumatic brain injury: Do the sexes fare differently? Brain Inj. 2007;21(10):1023–1030.

70. Slewa-Younan S, Green AM, Baguley IJ, Gurka JA, Marosszeky JE. Sex differences in injury severity and outcome measures after traumatic brain injury. Arch Phys Med Rehabil. 2004;85(3):376–379.

71. Golz C, Kirchhoff FP, Westerhorstmann J, et al. Sex hormones modulate pathogenic processes in experimental traumatic brain injury. J Neurochem. 2019;150(2):173–187.

72. Smeyne RJ, Klein R, Schnapp A, et al. Severe sensory and sympathetic neuropathies in mice carrying a disrupted Trk/NGF receptor gene. Nature. 1994;368(6468):246–249.

73. Radowicki S, Arsoba J, Dubrawski W. Tibolon (Livial) w leczeniu dolegliwosci okresu postmenopauzalnego (doniesienie wstepne) [Tibolone (Livial) in the treatment of disorders of the postmenopausal period (preliminary report)]. Ginekol Pol. 1988;59(11):705–708.

74. de Gooyer ME, Kleyn GT, Smits KC, Ederveen AG, Verheul HA, Kloosterboer HJ. Tibolone: A compound with tissue specific inhibitory effects on sulfatase. Mol Cell Endocrinol. 2001;183(1–2):55–62.

75. Escande A, Servant N, Rabenoelina F, et al. Regulation of activities of steroid hormone receptors by tibolone and its primary metabolites. J Steroid Biochem Mol Biol. 2009;116(1–2):8–14.

76. Kloosterboer HJ. Tissue-selective effects of tibolone on the breast. Maturitas. 2004;49(1):S5–S15.

77. Crespo-Castrillo A, Yanguas-Casas N, Arevalo MA, Azcoitia I, Barreto GE, Garcia-Segura LM. The synthetic steroid tibolone decreases reactive gliosis and neuronal death in the cerebral cortex of female mice after a stab wound injury. Mol Neurobiol. 2018;55(11):8651–8667.

78. Martin-Jimenez C, Gonzalez J, Vesga D, Aristizabal A, Barreto GE. Tibolone ameliorates the lipotoxic effect of palmitic acid in normal human astrocytes. Neurotox Res. 2020;38(3):585–595.

79. Del Rio JP, Molina S, Hidalgo-Lanussa O, Garcia-Segura LM, Barreto GE. Tibolone as hormonal therapy and neuroprotective agent. Trends Endocrinol Metab. 2020;31(10):742–759.

80. Gonzalez-Giraldo Y, Garzon-Benitez AV, Forero DA, Barreto GE. TERT inhibition leads to reduction of IL-6 expression induced by palmitic acid and interferes with the protective effects of tibolone in an astrocytic cell model. J Neuroendocrinol. 2019;31(8):e12768.

81. Gonzalez-Giraldo Y, Forero DA, Echeverria V, Garcia-Segura LM, Barreto GE. Tibolone attenuates inflammatory response by palmitic acid and preserves mitochondrial membrane potential in astrocytic cells through estrogen receptor beta. Mol Cell Endocrinol. 2019;486:65–78.

82. Hidalgo-Lanussa O, Avila-Rodriguez M, Baez-Jurado E, et al. Tibolone reduces oxidative damage and inflammation in microglia stimulated with palmitic acid through mechanisms involving estrogen receptor beta. Mol Neurobiol. 2018;55(7):5462–5477.

83. Crespo-Castrillo A, Garcia-Segura LM, Arevalo MA. The synthetic steroid tibolone exerts sex-specific regulation of astrocyte phagocytosis under basal conditions and after an inflammatory challenge. J Neuroinflammation. 2020;17(1):37.

84. Gorabi AM, Aslani S, Barreto GE, et al. The potential of mitochondrial modulation by neuroglobin in treatment of neurological disorders. Free Radic Biol Med. 2021;162:471–477.

85. Giatti S, Garcia-Segura LM, Barreto GE, Melcangi RC. Neuroactive steroids, neurosteroidogenesis and sex. Prog Neurobiol. 2019;176:1–17.

86. Cabezas R, El-Bacha RS, Gonzalez J, Barreto GE. Mitochondrial functions in astrocytes: Neuroprotective implications from oxidative damage by rotenone. Neurosci Res. 2012;74(2):80–90.

87. Lamade AM, Anthonymuthu TS, Hier ZE, Gao Y, Kagan VE, Bayir H. Mitochondrial damage & lipid signaling in traumatic brain injury. Exp Neurol. 2020;329:113307.

88. Bajpai P, Koc E, Sonpavde G, Singh R, Singh KK. Mitochondrial localization, import, and mitochondrial function of the androgen receptor. J Biol Chem. 2019;294(16):6621–6634.

89. Yan W, Kang Y, Ji X, et al. Testosterone upregulates the expression of mitochondrial ND1 and ND4 and alleviates the oxidative damage to the nigrostriatal dopaminergic system in orchiectomized rats. Oxid Med Cell Longev. 2017;2017:1202459.

90. Zhang T, Wang Y, Kang Y, et al. Testosterone enhances mitochondrial complex V function in the substantia nigra of aged male rats. Aging (Albany NY). 2020;12(11):10398–10414.

91. Batthyany C, Bartesaghi S, Mastrogiovanni M, Lima A, Demicheli V, Radi R. Tyrosine-nitrated proteins: proteomic and bioanalytical aspects. Antioxid Redox Signal. 2017;26(7):313–328.

92. Radi R. Peroxynitrite, a stealthy biological oxidant. J Biol Chem. 2013;288(37):26464–26472.

93. Kozlov AV, Bahrami S, Redl H, Szabo C. Alterations in nitric oxide homeostasis during traumatic brain injury. Biochim Biophys Acta Mol Basis Dis. 2017;1863(10 Pt B):2627–2632.

94. Ahmed ME, Selvakumar GP, Kempuraj D, et al. Neuroinflammation mediated by glia maturation factor exacerbates neuronal injury in an in vitro model of traumatic brain injury. J Neurotrauma. 2020;37(14):1645–1655.

95. Huttemann M, Lee I, Kreipke CW, Petrov T. Suppression of the inducible form of nitric oxide synthase prior to traumatic brain injury improves cytochrome c oxidase activity and normalizes cellular energy levels. Neuroscience. 2008;151(1):148–154.

96. Li SS, Xie LL, Li ZZ, Fan YJ, Qi MM, Xi YG. Androgen is responsible for enhanced susceptibility of melatonin against traumatic brain injury in females. Neurosci Lett. 2021;752:135842.

97. Nguyen TV, Jayaraman A, Quaglino A, Pike CJ. Androgens selectively protect against apoptosis in hippocampal neurones. J Neuroendocrinol. 2010;22(9):1013–1022.

98. Yao K, Wu J, Zhang J, Bo J, Hong Z, Zu H. Protective effect of DHT on apoptosis induced by U18666A via PI3K/Akt signaling pathway in C6 glial cell lines. Cell Mol Neurobiol. 2016;36(5):801–809.

99. Guang-Yu L, Hai-Yan L, Ji-Hong L, et al. MCL1 is a key regulator of steroidogenesis in mouse Leydig cells. Mol Reprod Dev. 2016;83(3):226–235.

100. Yawson EO, Akinola OB. Hippocampal cellular changes in androgen deprived insulin resistant rats. Metab Brain Dis. 2021;36(5):1037–1048.

Abbreviations Used

$\Delta\Psi m$ = mitochondrial membrane potential
AKT1 = AKT serine/threonine kinase 1
ANT = adenine nucleotide translocator
AR = androgen receptor
AT = ATP synthase
ATF1 = activating transcription factor 1
ATP = adenosine triphosphate
ATP5F1D = ATP synthase F1 subunit delta
BBB = blood–brain barrier
BCL2 = B cell lymphoma 2
C1 = mitochondrial complex I
C1q = complement C1q
C2 = mitochondrial complex II
C3 = mitochondrial complex III
C3b = complement component 3b
C3d = complement component 3d
C4 = mitochondrial complex IV
C5 = component 5
C5aR = component 5a receptor
CCI = controlled cortical impact
CCL2 = C–C motif ligand 2
CCR2 = C–C chemokine receptor type 2
CL = cardiolipin
COX-2 = cyclooxygenase 2
CREB = CAMP responsive element binding protein
CXCL10 = C–X–C motif chemokine ligand 10
CXCL12 = C–X–C motif chemokine ligand 12
CXCL4 = platelet factor 4
CXCL6 = C–X–C motif chemokine ligand 6
Cyp11a1 = cytochrome P450 family 11 subfamily A member 1
Cytc = cytochrome C
cytc1 = cytochrome c1 subunit
DAMPs = damage-associated molecular patterns
DHT = dihydrotestosterone
Drp1 = dynamin 1 like
ERe = endoplasmic reticulum
ERK = extracellular-signal regulated kinase
ETFA = electron transfer flavoprotein subunit alpha

Abbreviations Used (Cont.)

Fis1 = fission, mitochondrial 1
GFAP = glial fibrillary protein
GPRC6A = G protein-coupled receptor class C
group 6 member A
IL-1β = interleukin 1 beta
IL6 = interleukin 6
IMM = inner mitochondrial membrane
iNOS = inducible nitric oxide synthase
LPS = lipopolysaccharide
MAPK = mitogen-activated protein kinase
MCL1 = myeloid cell leukemia-1
MFN1/2 = Mitofusin 1 and 2
MIP-1β or CCL4 = macrophage inflammatory protein-1β
MM = mitochondrial matrix
NFκB = nuclear factor kappa B
Ngb = neuroglobin
NGF = normal growth factor
NOS = nitrogen oxygen species

OMM = outer mitochondrial membrane
OPA1 = OPA1 mitochondrial dynamin like GTPase
p32/C1qbp = complement C1q binding protein complexed
with p32
p38/MAPK = p38 and mitogen-activated protein kinase
PI3K/AKT = phosphoinositide 3-kinases/protein kinase B
RANTES/CCL5 = C–C motif chemokine ligand
ROS = reactive oxygen species
Slc39a9 (or ZIP9) = solute carrier family 39 member 9
SOD$_2$ (or MnSOD) = manganese superoxide dismutase 2
T = testosterone
TBI = traumatic brain injury
TERT = catalytic subunit of telomerase
TLR4 = toll like receptor 4
TNF-α = tumor necrosis factor alpha
TrkA = tropomyosin receptor kinase A
TrkB = tropomyosin receptor kinase B
TrkC = tropomyosin receptor kinase C
VDAC = voltage-dependent anion channel

20

Klinefelters Syndrome: Change in *T*-Scores with Testosterone, Bisphosphonate and Vitamin D Treatment Over 6 Years

Richard C. Strange,[1] Carola S. König,[2] Amar Puttanna,[3] Abhishek Rao,[3] Geoff Hackett,[4,i] Ahmad Haider,[5] Karim Sultan Haider,[5,ii] Pieter Desnerck,[6] Farid Saad,[7,8,iii] and Sudarshan Ramachandran[1–3,9,*,iv]

Abstract

Background: Klinefelter's syndrome (KS) is characterized by extra X chromosomes and features of primary hypogonadism including osteopenia and osteoporosis. Testosterone therapy (TTh) is widely used to treat men with KS and low serum testosterone/hypogonadal symptoms, though studies on its efficacy in improving bone density show varied outcomes.

Materials and Methods: We studied the effects of TTh, bisphosphonates, and vitamin D/calcium in 38 men with KS and low testosterone, hypogonadal symptoms, and *T*-scores consistent with osteoporosis. Our aim was to investigate at the end of follow-up (median: 87 months, range: 27–147 months), associations between age, baseline total testosterone, and *T*-scores, and change in *T*-scores after treatment.

Results: At final assessment, all men had *T*-score values outside the osteoporotic range (−1.1 standard deviation [SD], −1.8 SD). Baseline age but not median baseline testosterone appeared associated with change in *T*-score and *T*-score at final assessment. All men had dual-energy X-ray absorptiometry every 6 months and demonstrated continued improvement in *T*-scores after 3 months and up to 72 months. Baseline age and *T*-scores (stratified by median) were associated with change in *T*-score at final assessment. Compared with men ≥51 years, those aged <51 years showed significantly greater improvement in *T*-scores between 6 and 30 months. Men with worse *T*-score values (<3.7 SD) showed significantly greater improvement at every time point up to 36 months. Our results indicate that TTh, bisphosphonates, and vitamin D/calcium improve osteoporosis although there is a need to better understand the effects of the individual therapies, age, and baseline *T*-score on treatment efficacy.

Keywords: Klinefelter's syndrome; osteoporosis; testosterone therapy; bisphosphonates; vitamin D; *T*-scores

[1]Institute for Science and Technology in Medicine, Keele University, Staffordshire, United Kingdom.
[2]Department of Mechanical and Aerospace Engineering, Brunel University London, England, United Kingdom.
[3]Department of Diabetes, University Hospitals Birmingham NHS Foundation Trust, West Midlands, United Kingdom.
[4]School of Health and Life Sciences, Aston University, Birmingham, United Kingdom.
[5]Urologische Praxis, Bremerhaven, Germany.
[6]Department of Engineering, University of Cambridge, Cambridge, United Kingdom.
[7]Bayer AG, Medical Affairs Andrology, Berlin, Germany.
[8]Gulf Medical University School of Medicine, Ajman, United Arab Emirates.
[9]Department of Clinical Biochemistry, University Hospitals of North Midlands, Staffordshire, United Kingdom.
[i]ORCID ID (https://orcid.org/0000-0003-2274-111X).
[ii]ORCID ID (https://orcid.org/0000-0003-4396-9324).
[iii]ORCID ID (https://orcid.org/0000-0002-0449-6635).
[iv]ORCID ID (https://orcid.org/0000-0003-2299-4133).

*Address correspondence to: Sudarshan Ramachandran, PhD, FRCPath, Department of Diabetes, University Hospitals Birmingham NHS Foundation Trust, Good Hope Hospital, Rectory Road, West Midlands, B75 7RR, United Kingdom. Email: sud.ramachandran@heartofengland.nhs.uk

Introduction

Klinefelter's syndrome (KS), a condition characterized by extra copies of the X chromosome, is associated with testicular hypotrophy, impaired spermatogenesis, and, even though 40–50% of affected men may have serum testosterone in the normal distribution, features of primary hypogonadism including metabolic syndrome, autoimmune disorders, and osteoporosis.[1-9] Hypogonadism together with age >70 years, body mass index <21 kg/m^2, >10% weight loss, physical inactivity, and prolonged corticosteroid use are recognized risk factors for male osteoporosis.[10-14] Testosterone has direct (through the androgen receptor) and indirect (through aromatization to form estrogens) actions on bone metabolism. These promote periosteal bone formation during puberty and subsequently, decreasing resorption putatively explaining why hypogonadism, characterized by low testosterone levels and accompanying symptoms, is associated with both reduced bone mass and density.[6,15,16]

KS is associated with osteopenia, osteoporosis, and increased fracture risk.[17-20] Reduction of bone density in men with KS is associated with postpubertal testosterone deficiency and although histological change is related to serum testosterone, some individuals with KS develop low bone mineral density even with testosterone levels in the normal distribution.[6,19,21] This suggests a multifactorial etiology[21] with putative contributing factors including androgen receptor insensitivity[16,22,23] and/or hypovitaminosisD.[24]

Guidelines from the National Institute for Health and Care Excellence (https://bnf.nice.org.uk/treatment-summary/osteoporosis.html) and National Osteoporosis Guideline Group support lifestyle measures including increasing weight bearing activity and body mass index between 20 and 25 kg/m^2 together with therapeutic interventions to prevent fractures in osteoporotic individuals.[25] Oral bisphosphonates inhibit bone resorption and are front-line agents in osteoporotic males with denosumab and teriparatide used in individuals intolerant to bisphosphonates.[25] Daily cholecalciferol supplements of 800 IU are recommended in men aged >50 years with confirmed osteoporosis.[25]

There is debate whether men with serum testosterone in the normal distribution without hypogonadal symptoms benefit from testosterone therapy (TTh) and currently no international guidelines regarding TTh use in men with KS exists.[20] The clinical consensus appears to be that men with KS and low serum testosterone/hypogonadal symptoms require TTh.

Ferlin et al. suggested a diagnostic and therapeutic flow pathway for KS patients based on bone mineral density and serum testosterone.[6] In men with low bone mineral density and low serum testosterone, TTh and bisphosphonates with possible vitamin D/calcium supplements and repeat dual-energy X ray absorptiometry (DEXA) monitoring at 24 monthly intervals are recommended.[6] Longitudinal studies on the efficacy of TTh in improving bone mineral density in men with hypogonadism show varied outcomes, possibly because of heterogeneity.[20,26] A study of 72 hypogonadal patients (21 men with KS) showed TTh was associated with increased bone mineral density[27] whereas Ferlin et al. showed that bone mineral density improvement was associated with concurrent TTh and vitamin D supplementation in 14 men but with no improvement in 12 men given only TTh.[24] Haider et al. showed significant improvement in bone mineral density in 45 men with hypogonadism and osteoporosis given testosterone undecanoate (TU).[28]

We describe further study of the impact of TTh on bone density (T-score) in an expanded version of the registry data base described by Haider et al.[28] The study group comprised 38 men with KS and osteoporosis with focus on those presenting with back pain and osteoporosis and on combination treatment with TTh, bisphosphonates, and vitamin D/calcium. Our aim was to document T-scores at the end of follow-up (median: 87 months, IQR: 57–117, range: 27–147 months) and T-score change at 3–6 monthly intervals up to 72 months. We examined the data for associations between age, baseline total testosterone, and T-scores, and change in T-scores after combination treatment.

Materials and Methods

We used the database from an ongoing observational, prospective, and cumulative registry study that included data from 47 men with KS confirmed by karyotyping. DEXA identified osteoporosis in 39 men with KS and this study presents data from the 38 men treated with TU, bisphosphonates (all the men were on oral alendronate 70 mg once weekly), and vitamin D (colecalciferol 20,000 IU per week)/calcium during the entire or part of follow-up. Alendronate was discontinued in 4, 19, 22, 23, 24, and 26 men (cumulative numbers) by 12, 24, 36, 48, 60, and 72 months of follow-up, respectively, whereas 12 men continued with the treatment after 72 months. The one man treated only with TTh was excluded. The complete registry database currently comprises 823 men who presented with urological symptoms and low testosterone levels (≤12.1 nmol/L) and hypogonadal symptoms; 737 and 39 men were diagnosed with adult onset testosterone deficiency and non-KS primary hypogonadism, respectively. Gonadotropin and estrogen levels were not measured either at baseline or during follow-up. The median age of the cohort was 51 (IQR: 44/55) years at presentation and TTh commencement. Some of the 38 men in the study cohort were on antihypertensive agents (2 men), oral hypoglycamic agents (1 man), statins (3 men), and phosphodiesterase-5 inhibitors (7 men); the dates of initiation of these agents were not available.

Osteoporosis was identified using DEXA to measure bone mineral density in the spine and/or hip.[10] Results were compared with those of a healthy young adult and a T-score provided as standard deviations (SD); T-scores between +1 and −1 SD, −1 SD and −2.5 SD, and <2.5 SD indicate normal bone density, osteopenia, and osteoporosis, respectively.[11–13] After diagnosis of osteoporosis, TTh (1000 mg TU, interval between first and second administration: 6 weeks, thereafter: 12 weekly) was initiated. Of this cohort, 35 men were commenced on bisphosphonates at baseline (1 man was started at 6 months and the remaining 2 men after 9 months) and all were on vitamin D/calcium supplements at baseline. Data including DEXA were entered into the database at least 6 monthly (many had 3 monthly DEXA) during follow-up. As the study is longitudinal, number of patients decreased with follow-up; data were available on 36, 35, 35, 29, 23, and 16 (of the 38) men at 12, 24, 36, 48, 60, and 72 months, respectively. None of the men suffered from fractures during the follow-up period. The German Medical Association's ethical guidelines for observational studies were followed and each participant consented to be included in the register and their data were analyzed after being provided study details. Ethics committees (Germany and England) reviewed the study and stated that formal approval was not required. Keele University Staffordshire and University Hospitals Birmingham NHS Foundation Trust reviewed the manuscript/study and provided Institutional Review Board Statements.

Study Measurements

Serum testosterone was measured using the Abbott Architect immunoassay. Bone mineral density was measured by using a whole body dual-energy X-ray densitometer (Norland XR-800), with calculations performed in line with the standardized procedures issued by the manufacturer. The daily quality assurance calibration procedures were in accordance with the manufacturer's recommendation using a QA Calibration Standard and a QC Spine Phantom. The accuracy of AP spine scans and hip scans was within 1.0% of industry standard. The *in vivo* precision of AP spine scan and hip scan is 0.84% (bone mineral density lumbar vertebra 2–4 coefficient of variation) and 1.4% (bone mineral density femoral neck coefficient of variation), respectively. Bone mineral density is expressed in gram per square centimeter. The individual bone mineral density variation was expressed as T-score measurements of the spine (lumbar vertebra 2–4) and femoral neck.

Statistical analysis

Nonparametric tests were carried out to compare between- (rank-sum) and within-(sign-rank) cohort changes in T-scores during the follow-up. All analyses were performed on Stata 14 (StataCorp LLC, TX).

Results

Table 1 gives median age, total testosterone, and T-score values at baseline that were 51 years, 9.7 nmol/L, and −3.7 SD, respectively, in the 38 men with KS treated with TTh, bisphosphonates, and vitamin D/calcium. The footnote of Table 1 shows other baseline characteristics. One man had type 2 diabetes at baseline with no further cases diagnosed during follow-up. Three men were prescribed statins. At baseline, all the men had T-score values consistent with osteoporosis (between −2.6 and −4.2 SD). At final assessment, all the men had T-scores outside the osteoporotic range (between −1.1 and −1.8 SD), the difference between baseline and final assessment values was significant ($p < 0.0001$). Median trough total testosterone levels increased from 9.7 to 18.4 nmol/L after TTh.

Table 1 also gives the effects of TTh, bisphosphonates, and vitamin D/calcium in subgroups stratified by median values of age, baseline testosterone, and baseline T-scores. T-scores and follow-up values together with within- (sign-rank tests) and between (rank-sum)-group differences are presented for each subgroup. Regardless of stratification, all subgroups showed significantly (within-group sign-rank test) improved T-scores at the end of follow-up. Age and baseline total testosterone levels (stratified by median) were not associated with baseline T-scores or duration of follow-up. However, baseline age appeared associated with change in T-score and T-score at final assessment

Table 1. *T*-Score at Baseline and Final Assessment in the Total Cohort and Subgroups Stratified by Median Age, Total Testosterone Concentrations, and *T*-Score at Baseline

	Baseline	Follow-up (months)	Final assesssment	Δ (Final assessment— baseline)	Within-group difference (sign-rank)
Patients on TTh, biphosphonates, and vitamin D (*n* = 38)		87 (57–117)			
Age (years): median (IQR)	51 (44/55)				NA
Total testosterone (nmol/L): median (IQR)	9.7 (8.3/10.1)		18.4 (17.7/19.8)	9.0 (8.0/11.1)	*p* < 0.0001
T-score: median (IQR)	−3.7 (−3.8/−2.9)		−1.2 (−1.8/−1.1)	1.85 (1.6/2.4)	*p* < 0.0001
Subgroups (stratified by baseline values)					
Age <median (51 years), *n* = 18		88.5 (81/111)			
T-score: median (IQR)	−3.55 (−3.8/−2.9)		−1.2 (−1.2/−1.1)	2 (1.8/2.5)	*p* = 0.0002
Age ≥median (51 years), *n* = 20		81 (43.5/124.5)			
T-score: median (IQR)	−3.75 (−3.8/−2.85)		−1.4 (−2.15/−1.2)	1.65 (1.45/2.4)	*p* = 0.0001
Between-group difference (rank-sum)	*p* = 0.81	*p* = 0.30	*p* = 0.0069	*p* = 0.023	
Total testosterone <median (9.7 nmol/L), *n* = 18					
T-score: median (IQR)	−3.75 (−3.8/−2.9)	87 (60/123)	−1.2 (−1.8/−1.2)	1.85 (1.5/2.5)	*p* = 0.0002
Total testosterone ≥median (9.7 nmol/L), *n* = 20					
T-score: median (IQR)	−3.65 (−3.8/−2.9)	85.5 (55.5/111)	−1.2 (−1.85/−1.15)	1.85 (1.7/2.4)	*p* = 0.0001
Between-group difference (rank-sum)	*p* = 0.84	*p* = 0.90	*p* = 0.63	*p* = 0.83	
T-score <median (−3.7 SD), *n* = 21					
T-score: median (IQR)	−3.8 (−3.9/−3.8)	60 (45/87)	−1.8 (−2.1/−1.2)	2.1 (1.7/2.5)	*p* = 0.0001
T-score ≥median (−3.7 SD), *n* = 17					
T-score: median (IQR)	−2.9 (−3.1/−2.8)	117 (105/126)	−1.2 (−1.2/−1.1)	1.8 (1.6/1.9)	*p* = 0.0003
Between-group difference (rank-sum)	NA	*p* < 0.0001	*p* < 0.0001	*p* = 0.096	

Demography [Median (IQR) for continuous variables, % for discrete variables].

Baseline—waist circumference: 100 (98/105) cm, weight: 91.5 (85/103) kg, Hb: 14.8 (14.5/15.2) g/dL, hematocrit: 46 (45/46), PSA: 0.35 (0.12/0.69), HbA1c: 5.4 (5.1/5.7)%, systolic blood pressure: 132.5 (128/136) mmHg, diastolic blood pressure: 77 (74/82) mmHg, IIEF-EF score: 15.5 (11/22), cholesterol: 7.2 (6.8/7.5) mmol/L, triglycerides: 2.6 (2.5/2.9) mmol/L, HDL-cholesterol: 0.93 (0.70/1.11) mmol/L, diabetes: 2.6%, smoking: 47.4%, statin treatment: 7.9%, vitamin D treatment: 100%, bisphosphonates treatment: 92.1%. Final assessment—diabetes: 2.6%, smoking: 47.4%, statin treatment: 7.9%, vitamin D and bisphosphonate treatment: 100%, mortality: 0%, cardiovascular disease: 0%.

SD, standard deviation; TTh, testosterone therapy.

after treatment, whereas no difference was observed between the men when stratified by median baseline total testosterone. Table 1 also gives data for the men stratified by median baseline *T*-score; follow-up significantly varied (*p* < 0.0001) between the two groups. Despite that men with a baseline *T*-score <−3.7 SD demonstrated greater improvement, although not statistically significant (*p* = 0.096).

Change in T-scores at 3 monthly time points for 72 months

Table 2 and Figure 1 show median *T*-score values at 3 monthly intervals, all men having had DEXA every 6 months and many every 3 months. Using fixed time points removed impact of treatment duration (follow-up) as a confounder. Table 2 presents the number of men showing improvement, no change or deterioration in *T*-score values, compared with values obtained at baseline and the DEXA scan carried out 3 months previously. Table 2 demonstrates continued improvement up to 72 months with *T*-scores significantly better than baseline values after only 3 months

treatment (no man had a *T*-score worse than his baseline value at any time point). The *T*-score range at each time is presented and this shows that after 9 months treatment, every man had improved values. After 45 months treatment, every man (30/36 men had follow-up ≥45 months) had a *T*-score above the osteoporosis cutoff of −2.5 SD. A worsening of *T*-scores compared with that obtained 3 months previously was evident in only one individual between 36 and 39 months and another between 60 and 63 months.

Change in T-score at 3 monthly time points for 36 weeks in groups stratified by baseline median age and T-scores

Data in Table 1 indicate baseline age and *T*-scores (stratified by median) are associated with change in *T*-score at final assessment after treatment. Age (stratified by median) was not associated with *T*-scores at baseline (Table 1, *p* = 0.81) or baseline total testosterone (*p* = 0.64). We now studied the associations between age, baseline *T*-score (both stratified by median), and change in *T*-scores (compared with

Table 2. Median *T*-Score Values at 3 Monthly Intervals in the Total Cohort and the Number of Men Showing Improvement, No Change, and Deterioration in *T*-Score Values Compared with Baseline and DEXA 3 Months Previously

Time of DEXA during follow-up (No. of men)	*T*-score	*T*-score change from baseline: No. of men	*T*-score change over past 3 months: No. of men
TTh/biphosphonate/vitamin D treatment	Median/(range)	Benefit/no change/worsening (sign-rank)	Benefit/no change/worsening (sign-rank)
Baseline (*n* = 38)	−3.7/(−4.2/−2.6)		
3 months (*n* = 38)	−3.4/(−4.1/−2.6)	23/15/0 (*p* < 0.0001)	23/15/0 (*p* < 0.0001)
6 months (*n* = 36)	−3.1/(−3.9/−2.4)	34/2/0 (*p* < 0.0001)	33/3/0 (*p* < 0.0001)
9 months (*n* = 38)	−2.85/(−3.7/−2.3)	38/0/0 (*p* < 0.0001)	24/12/0 (*p* < 0.0001)
12 months (*n* = 36)	−2.7/(−3.6/−2.1)	36/0/0 (*p* < 0.0001)	29/7/0 (*p* < 0.0001)
15 months (*n* = 36)	−2.6/(−3.5/−1.9)	36/0/0 (*p* < 0.0001)	26/8/0 (*p* < 0.0001)
18 months (*n* = 36)	−2.5/(−3.3/−1.8)	36/0/0 (*p* < 0.0001)	27/7/0 (*p* < 0.0001)
21 months (*n* = 35)	−2.3/(−3.4/−1.8)	35/0/0 (*p* < 0.0001)	24/9/0 (*p* < 0.0001)
24 months (*n* = 35)	−2.3/(−3.1/−1.7)	35/0/0 (*p* < 0.0001)	24/8/0 (*p* < 0.0001)
27 months (*n* = 35)	−2.2/(−3.1/−1.6)	35/0/0 (*p* < 0.0001)	19/13/0 (*p* < 0.0001)
30 months (*n* = 35)	−2.1/(−3.0/−1.6)	35/0/0 (*p* < 0.0001)	19/13/0 (*p* < 0.0001)
33 months (*n* = 31)	−2.0/(−2.5/−1.4)	31/0/0 (*p* < 0.0001)	20/10/0 (*p* < 0.0001)
36 months (*n* = 35)	−1.9/(−2.8/−1.2)	35/0/0 (*p* < 0.0001)	19/11/0 (*p* < 0.0001)
39 months (*n* = 30)	−1.85/(−2.3/−1.3)	30/0/0 (*p* < 0.0001)	17/11/1 (*p* = 0.0002)
42 months (*n* = 32)	−1.75/(−2.5/−1.3)	32/0/0 (*p* < 0.0001)	16/12/0 (*p* = 0.0006)
45 months (*n* = 30)	−1.7/(−2.1/−1.2)	30/0/0 (*p* < 0.0001)	16/12/0 (*p* = 0.0001)
48 months (*n* = 29)	−1.7/(−2.4/−1.2)	29/0/0 (*p* < 0.0001)	7/19/0 (*p* = 0.0083)
51 months (*n* = 29)	−1.6/(−2.1/−1.2)	29/0/0 (*p* < 0.0001)	10/16/0 (*p* = 0.0017)
54 months (*n* = 29)	−1.5/(−2.2/−1.2)	29/0/0 (*p* < 0.0001)	10/16/0 (*p* = 0.0017)
57 months (*n* = 28)	−1.4/(−2.0/−1.2)	28/0/0 (*p* < 0.0001)	9/17/0 (*p* = 0.0029)
60 months (*n* = 23)	−1.3/(−1.8/−1.2)	23/0/0 (*p* < 0.0001)	9/13/0 (*p* = 0.0029)
63 months (*n* = 26)	−1.3/(−1.8/−1.2)	26/0/0 (*p* < 0.0001)	4/16/1 (*p* = 0.19)
66 months (*n* = 17)	−1.3/(−1.6/−1.2)	17/0/0 (*p* = 0.0003)	7/9/0 (*p* = 0.0086)
69 months (*n* = 25)	−1.3/(−1.7/−1.2)	25/0/0 (*p* < 0.0001)	5/10/0 (*p* = 0.026)
72 months (*n* = 16)	−1.2/(−1.5/−1.2)	16/0/0 (*p* = 0.0004)	5/9/0 (*p* = 0.026)

DEXA, dual-energy X ray absorptiometry.

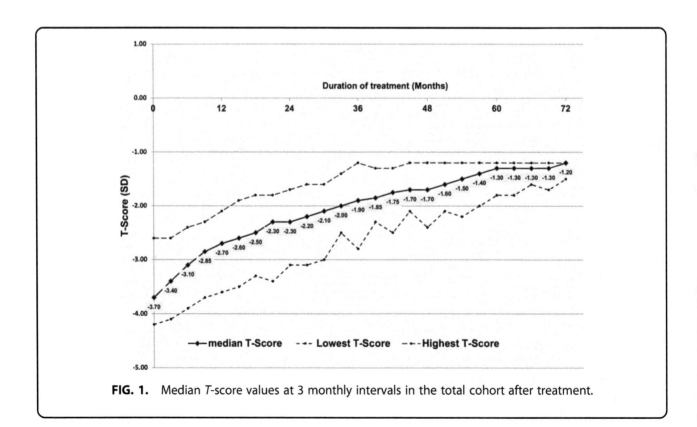

FIG. 1. Median *T*-score values at 3 monthly intervals in the total cohort after treatment.

Table 3. Median *T*-Score Change After Treatment in the Cohort Stratified by Median Age and *T*-Scores at Baseline

Time of DEXA during follow-up (No. of men)	Median *T*-score change from baseline		Between-group difference (rank-sum)
Cohort stratified by median age (51 years)	Baseline age <51 years	Baseline age ≥51 years	
0 (*n* = 38)			
3 (*n* = 38)	0.1	0.1	*p* = 0.18
6 (*n* = 36)	0.3	0.2	*p* = 0.029
9 (*n* = 38)	0.5	0.3	*p* = 0.0060
12 (*n* = 36)	0.7	0.4	*p* = 0.017
15 (*n* = 36)	0.8	0.45	*p* = 0.0049
18 (*n* = 36)	0.95	0.6	*p* = 0.011
21 (*n* = 35)	1.25	0.6	*p* = 0.0027
24 (*n* = 35)	1.4	0.8	*p* = 0.0066
27 (*n* = 35)	1.45	0.7	*p* = 0.0041
30 (*n* = 35)	1.55	1.0	*p* = 0.026
33 (*n* = 31)	1.65	1.3	*p* = 0.091
36 (*n* = 35)	1.65	1.3	*p* = 0.074
Cohort stratified by median *T*-score (−3.7 SD)	Baseline *T*-score < −3.7	Baseline *T*-score ≥ −3.7	
3 (*n* = 38)	0.1	0.0	*p* = 0.0001
6 (*n* = 36)	0.3	0.2	*p* = 0.0194
9 (*n* = 38)	0.4	0.2	*p* = 0.0038
12 (*n* = 36)	0.6	0.3	*p* = 0.0083
15 (*n* = 36)	0.7	0.5	*p* = 0.0297
18 (*n* = 36)	0.9	0.5	*p* = 0.0043
21 (*n* = 35)	1.2	0.6	*p* = 0.0434
24 (*n* = 35)	1.4	0.8	*p* = 0.0072
27 (*n* = 35)	1.4	0.8	*p* = 0.0114
30 (*n* = 35)	1.6	0.9	*p* = 0.0032
33 (*n* = 31)	1.8	1.0	*p* = 0.0004
36 (*n* = 35)	1.7	1.0	*p* < 0.0001

baseline) at 3 monthly time points up to 36 months (number of patients decreased with follow-up). Compared with men aged ≥51 years, those aged <51 years showed significantly greater improvement in *T*-scores between 6 and 30 months (Table 3 and Fig. 2). Between-group difference in the change in *T*-score was maximal at 27 months (0.75 SD) and then decreased (30 months: 0.55, 36 months: 0.35, values from the same 35 men). Table 3 and Figure 3 show that men with worse *T*-score values (<3.7 SD) showed significantly greater improvement at every time point up to 36 months. There did not appear to be any convergence in the *T*-score change.

Discussion

We studied changes in *T*-scores in 38 men with KS after treatment with TTh, bisphosphonates, and vitamin D/calcium and then determined whether baseline age, testosterone, and *T*-scores predicted change in *T*-scores. Baseline *T*-scores of <−2.5 SD (range: −4.2/−2.6) indicated all 38 men had osteoporosis. Improvement in *T*-scores was noted in some after 3 months treatment and in all men after 9 months. After 45 weeks, no patient had a *T*-score in the osteo-

porotic range. Treatment in men <51 years or with a baseline *T*-score <−3.7 effected significantly greater improvement in score after 6–30 months and 3–36 months, respectively.

Currently there appears consensus that TTh is beneficial for most men and adolescents with KS with elevated serum luteinizing hormone and low (or low-normal) testosterone levels.[20] As the men we studied had total testosterone <12.1 nmol/L and symptoms of hypogonadism, TTh was appropriate treatment and every man in our cohort demonstrated improved *T*-scores after 9 months. Indeed, a previous study showed that although combined TTh and vitamin D treatment improved bone mineral density in KS, TTh without vitamin D supplementation was not beneficial.[24] Furthermore, Stepan et al. studied the effects of intravenous ibandronate on bone density and biochemical bone markers in 14 men with KS (mean aged 55.2 years, 5.9 years follow-up) and found hypovitaminosis D adversely affected the efficacy of bisphosphonate therapy.[19]

Our analyses for 36 months of treatment showed men <51 years enjoyed greater benefit (statistically significant during 6–30 months treatment) than their

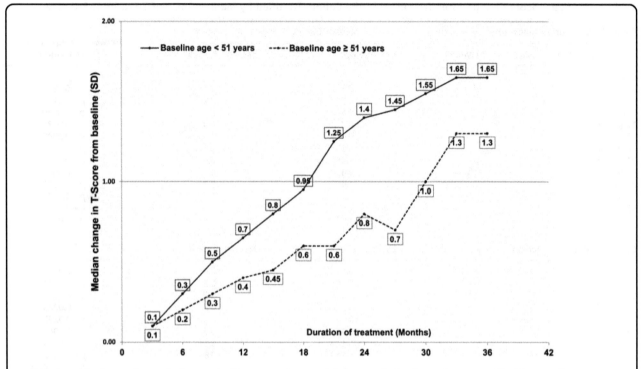

FIG. 2. Median values of change in *T*-score at 3 monthly intervals in the cohort stratified by median age at baseline (51 years).

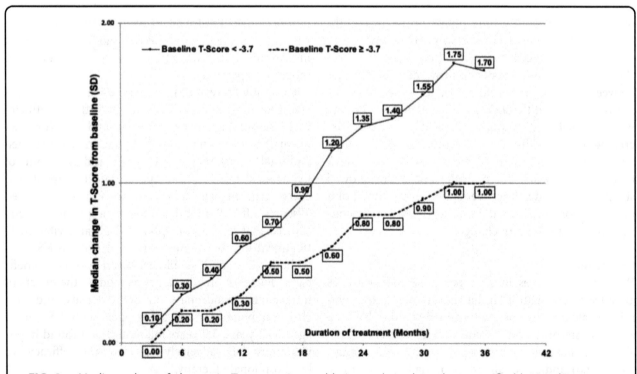

FIG. 3. Median values of change in *T*-score at 3 monthly intervals in the cohort stratified by median baseline *T*-score (−3.7 SD). SD, standard deviation.

older counterparts. Men with T-score <3.7 SD also demonstrated greater benefit during the entire 36 weeks studied than men with T-scores between −3.6 and −2.6 SD. Limited number of patients did not allow study of interactions between these predictive baseline factors, though importantly age was not related to baseline T-score and, therefore, does not appear related to the etiology of osteoporosis in KS. If our findings are validated, treatment with one or more of the therapeutic agents we used may be more efficacious in younger men. The relationship between baseline T-score and change in values after treatment is in accordance with the Wilder principle that states that the "direction of response of body function to any agent depends to a large degree on the initial value of that function."[29] The lack of a significant association between baseline testosterone and T-scores perhaps does not suggest that TTh alone reverses the low T-scores associated with hypogonadism. This suggests that there may be other factors that we have not identified that could be part of a multifactorial etiology. Furthermore, as all the men had serum total testosterone levels <12.1 nmol/L at baseline, a possible association with T-scores could have been lost due to compression of the baseline serum testosterone level. However, the observed association is reassuring as men with the lowest T-scores gained greatest benefit, enabling each man to have a T-score above the osteoporosis threshold at final assessment. Currently repeat DEXA is recommended after a minimum of 2 years though we found benefit after 9 months of treatment, suggesting the time period for repeating DEXA could be less frequent for men given TTh, bisphosphonates, and vitamin D/calcium.[6]

Bone mineral density (spine and hip) measurements were significantly improved in the 211 men (≥65 years) participating in the bone trial arm of the T-trials randomized to either testosterone or placebo gel for 12 months.[30] Ng Tang Fui et al. recently reported that 2 years of TU treatment of 92 men with hypogonadism, compared with 85 men on placebo, was associated with increased tibial and spinal bone mineral density in a double-blind RCT (T4Bone substudy).[31] Porcelli et al. reviewed the trials of male osteoporosis treatment with bisphosphonates, denosumab, and teriparatide, and suggested that earlier diagnosis of the condition and secondary causes together with improved treatment were essential.[32] Thus, it is our intention to carry out a similar analysis of the combination of TTh, bisphonates, and vitamin D treatments as well as the effects

of the individual treatments, data permitting, on men with adult onset TD treated similarly to study T-score changes and predictors of change. We avoided pooling both cohorts in view of the varying etiologies.

This longitudinal registry study has strengths and weaknesses. As TU was injected in clinic, compliance was absolute. Follow-up was long and we had a complete data set for all men at 6 monthly and most at 3 monthly intervals. Although clinical guidelines do not advocate 3 monthly DEXA, this was in accordance with the local orthopedic scientific practice with an interest in short-term changes in bone density and performed at no additional cost to the patient.[28] We recognize that this frequency of testing is neither needed nor feasible in routine clinical practice, but the availability of the data allowed us to define the change in bone density over time with confidence. The number of patients was limited and hence, we could not study interactions between age, baseline T-scores, and effect of treatment. The declining number of patients during follow-up is not due to drop-out rates, but a result of cumulative ongoing recruitment (there was follow-up data in 35 of the 38 men at 36 weeks). As the 38 men were on TTh, bisphosphonates, and vitamin D, study outcomes are only applicable to this combination therapy as opposed to single agents. Interestingly, although the action of bisphosphonates is mainly antiosteoclastic,[25] TTh has been demonstrated to increase osteocalcin levels, suggestive of osteoblastic stimulation.[33] Furthermore, we did not have serum vitamin D levels at baseline or during follow-up. The German Health Interview and Examination Survey for Adults analyzed vitamin D status (serum vitamin D concentration ≤50 nmol/L considered low and suitable for supplementation) in German adults and found the mean serum vitamin D levels to be 45.6 nmol/L (61.6% and 30.2% of the individuals had levels <50 and <30 nmol/L, respectively) with no gender differences.[34] Subgroup analysis showed that the 759 men residing in northern Germany at a latitude between 52° and 54° (Bremerhaven is situated at an approximate latitude of 53.5°) had a mean vitamin D concentration of 45.1 nmol/L.[34]

Conclusions

We studied 38 men with KS and low total testosterone, hypogonadal symptoms, and T-scores consistent with osteoporosis who were treated with TTh, bisphosphonates, and vitamin D/calcium supplements. Beneficial change in T-scores was seen in all patients after only

9 months. Men with the lowest *T*-scores improved most. Our results indicate the need to better understand the effects of the individual therapies and the effects of age and baseline *T*-score on treatment efficacy. Defining patient subgroups and studying their outcomes should improve therapeutic efficacy. A further factor in considerations of TTh use are studies showing improvements in muscle mass preservation in healthy men and preserved knee extensor muscle mechanical function in men with T2DM.[35,36] Thus, TTh may in at least some men offer improvements to both bone density and muscle function.

Authors' Contributions

R.C.S. contributed to design of study, data analysis, and preparation of article; C.S.K. contributed to design of study and preparation of article; A.P. contributed to design of study and preparation of article; A.R. contributed to data analysis and preparation of article; G.H. contributed to design of study and preparation of article; A.H. and K.S.H. contributed to patient recruitment, data collection, and preparation of article; P.D. contributed to transposing the data, data analysis, and maintaining the database; F.S. contributed to maintaining the database, design of study, and preparation of article; S.R. contributed to design of study, data analysis, and preparation of article.

References

1. Rocca MS, Pecile V, Cleva L, et al. The Klinefelter syndrome is associated with high recurrence of copy number variations on the X chromosome with a potential role in the clinical phenotype. Andrology. 2016;4(2):328–334.
2. Berglund A, Viuff MH, Skakkebæk A, Chang S, Stochholm K, Gravholt CH. Changes in the cohort composition of turner syndrome and severe non-diagnosis of Klinefelter, 47, XXX and 47, XYY syndrome: A nationwide cohort study. Orphanet J Rare Dis. 2019;14(1):16.
3. van Rijn S, de Sonneville L, Swaab H. The nature of social cognitive deficits in children and adults with Klinefelter syndrome (47,XXY). Genes Brain Behav. 2018;17(6):e12465.
4. Salzano A, D'Assante R, Heaney LM, et al. Klinefelter syndrome, insulin resistance, metabolic syndrome, and diabetes: Review of literature and clinical perspectives. Endocrine. 2018;61(2):194–203.
5. Seminog OO, Seminog AB, Yeates D, Goldacre MJ. Associations between Klinefelter's syndrome and autoimmune diseases: English national record linkage studies. Autoimmunity. 2015;48(2):125–128.
6. Ferlin A, Schipilliti M, Di Mambro A, Vinanzi C, Foresta C. Osteoporosis in Klinefelter's syndrome. Mol Hum Reprod. 2010;16(6):402–410.
7. Lanfranco F, Kamischke A, Zitzmann M, Nieschlag E. Klinefelter's syndrome. Lancet. 2004;364(9430):273–283.
8. Bonomi M, Rochira V, Pasquali D, et al. Klinefelter syndrome (KS): Genetics, clinical phenotype and hypogonadism. J Endocrinol Invest. 2017;40(2):123–134.
9. Bhartia M, Ramachandran S. Klinefelter's syndrome—A diagnosis mislaid for 46 years. BMJ. 2012;345:e6938.
10. Blake GM, Fogelman I. The role of DXA bone density scans in the diagnosis and treatment of osteoporosis. Postgrad Med J. 2007;83(982):509–517.
11. Sözen T, Özışık L, Başaran NÇ. An overview and management of osteoporosis. Eur J Rheumatol. 2017;4(1):46–56.
12. Tu KN, Lie JD, Wan CKV, et al. Osteoporosis: A review of treatment options. P T. 2018;43(2):92–104.
13. Choksi P, Jepsen KJ, Clines GA. The challenges of diagnosing osteoporosis and the limitations of currently available tools. Clin Diabetes Endocrinol. 2018;4:12.
14. Shapses SA, Sukumar D. Bone metabolism in obesity and weight loss. Annu Rev Nutr. 2012;32:287–309.
15. Golds G, Houdek D, Arnason T. Male hypogonadism and osteoporosis: The effects, clinical consequences, and treatment of testosterone deficiency in bone health. Int J Endocrinol. 2017;2017:4602129.
16. Chen JF, Lin PW, Tsai YR, Yang YC, Kang HY. Androgens and androgen receptor actions on bone health and disease: From androgen deficiency to androgen therapy. Cells. 2019;8(11):1318.
17. Bojesen A, Gravholt CH. Klinefelter syndrome in clinical practice. Nat Clin Pract Urol. 2007;4(4):192–204.
18. Aksglaede L, Molgaard C, Skakkebaek NE, Juul A. Normal bone mineral content but unfavourable muscle/fat ratio in Klinefelter syndrome. Arch Dis Child. 2008;93(1):30–34.
19. Stepan JJ, Burckhardt P, Hána V. The effects of three-month intravenous ibandronate on bone mineral density and bone remodeling in Klinefelter's syndrome: The influence of vitamin D deficiency and hormonal status. Bone. 2003;33(4):589–596.
20. Chang S, Skakkebaek A, Davis SM, Gravholt CH. Morbidity in Klinefelter syndrome and the effect of testosterone treatment. Am J Med Genet C Semin Med Genet. 2020;184(2):344–355.
21. Seo JT, Lee JS, Oh TH, Joo KJ. The clinical significance of bone mineral density and testosterone levels in Korean men with non-mosaic Klinefelter's syndrome. BJU Int. 2007;99(1):141–146.
22. Ferlin A, Schipilliti M, Vinanzi C, et al. Bone mass in subjects with Klinefelter syndrome: Role of testosterone levels and androgen receptor gene CAG polymorphism. J Clin Endocrinol Metab. 2011;96(4):E739-E745.
23. Zitzmann M, Depenbusch M, Gromoll J, Nieschlag E. X-chromosome inactivation patterns and androgen receptor functionality influence phenotype and social characteristics as well as pharmacogenetics of testosterone therapy in Klinefelter patients. J Clin Endocrinol Metab. 2004;89(12):6208–6217.
24. Ferlin A, Selice R, Di Mambro A, et al. Role of vitamin D levels and vitamin D supplementation on bone mineral density in Klinefelter syndrome. Osteoporos Int. 2015;26(8):2193–2202.
25. Compston J, Cooper A, Cooper C, et al. UK clinical guideline for the prevention and treatment of osteoporosis. Arch Osteoporos. 2017;12(1):43.
26. Ramachandran S, Konig CS, Hackett G, Livingston M, Strange RC. Managing clinical heterogeneity: An argument for benefit based action limits. J Med Diagn Ther 2018;1(3):034701.
27. Behre HM, Kliesch S, Leifke E, Link TM, Nieschlag E. Long-term effect of testosterone therapy on bone mineral density in hypogonadal men. J Clin Endocrinol Metab. 1997;82(8):2386–2390.
28. Haider A, Meergans U, Traish A, et al. Progressive improvement of T-scores in men with osteoporosis and subnormal serum testosterone levels upon treatment with testosterone over six years. Int J Endocrinol. 2014;2014:496948.
29. Messerli FH, Bangalore S, Schmieder RE. Wilder's principle: Pre-treatment value determines post-treatment response. Eur Heart J. 2015;36(9):576–579.
30. Snyder PJ, Kopperdahl DL, Stephens-Shields AJ, et al. Effect of testosterone treatment on volumetric bone density and strength in older men with low testosterone: A controlled clinical trial. JAMA Intern Med. 2017; 177 (4):471–479.
31. Ng Tang Fui M, Hoermann R, Bracken K, et al. Effect of Testosterone treatment on bone microarchitecture and bone mineral density in men: A two-year RCT. J Clin Endocrinol Metab. 2021. [Epub ahead of print]; DOI: 10.1210/clinem/dgab149/6162862.
32. Porcelli T, Maffezzoni F, Pezzaioli LC, Delbarba A, Cappelli C, Ferlin A. Management of endocrine disease: Male osteoporosis: Diagnosis and management—Should the treatment and the target be the same as for female osteoporosis? Eur J Endocrinol. 2020;183(3):R75–R93.

33. Ghanim H, Dhindsa S, Green K, et al. Increase in osteocalcin following testosterone therapy in men with type 2 diabetes and subnormal free testosterone. J Endocr Soc. 2019;3(8):1617–1630.
34. Rabenberg M, Scheidt-Nave C, Busch MA, Rieckmann N, Hintzpeter B, Mensink GB. Vitamin D status among adults in Germany—Results from the German Health Interview and Examination Survey for Adults (DEGS1). BMC Public Health. 2015;15:641.
35. Storer TW, Basaria S, Traustadottir T, et al. Effects of testosterone supplementation for 3 years on muscle performance and physical function in older men. J Clin Endocrinol Metab. 2017;102(2):583–593.
36. Magnussen LV, Hvid LG, Hermann AP, et al. Testosterone therapy preserves muscle strength and power in aging men with type 2 diabetes-a randomized controlled trial. Andrology. 2017;5(5):946–953.

Abbreviations Used

DEXA = dual-energy X ray absorptiometry
KS = Klinefelter's syndrome
NICE = National Institute for Health and Care Excellence
SD = standard deviations
TTh = testosterone therapy
TU = testosterone undecanoate

21

The Prevalence of Late-Onset Hypogonadism in Middle-Aged Men and Cardiovascular Risk Factors

Nataliya B. Lebedeva[1,*] and Vladimir V. Gofman[2]

Abstract

Background: Life expectancy has increased dramatically worldwide, resulting in a sharp rise of age-associated diseases, including late-onset hypogonadism (LOH) in men.

Aim: To assess the prevalence of LOH and to determine its relationships with cardiovascular risk factors in healthy middle-aged men.

Material and Methods: A total of 200 men aged 44–55 (median 48.44, interquartile range 45.02–52.50) undergoing regular medical examinations were enrolled in a study. All participants were asked to complete the International Index of Erectile Dysfunction, Aging Male's Symptoms, and Beck Depression Inventory questionnaires. Sex and gonadotropin hormones were measured in all participants. Cardiovascular diseases (CVD) risk was assessed in all participants by using the Systematic Coronary Risk Evaluation scale, and additional risk factors were recommended in the 2019 European Society of Cardiology and European Atherosclerosis Society guidelines for the management of dyslipidemias: lipid modification to reduce cardiovascular risk.

Results: Ninety-eight (49%) men suffered from LOH. Men with total testosterone (TT) of <12 nmol/L were considered testosterone-deficient. The mean TT level was 8.9±2.4 nmol/L in the LOH group. Clinical signs and symptoms of LOH were associated with lower TT levels: 7.78±2.49 and 10.15±1.32 in the groups with and without LOH, respectively ($p = 0.004$). The prevalence of obesity, metabolic syndrome, and depression was significantly higher among men with LOH, compared with men without it. High cardiovascular risk was found only in those participants present with LOH ($p = 0.003$). After collecting other risk factors, we found that 94.9% of participants assigned to the LOH group had high cardiovascular risk.

Conclusion: The prevalence of LOH is high among healthy middle-aged men. Moreover, it is associated with an increased cardiovascular risk. Early measurement of TT levels in this population group may predict the development of CVD and allow the introduction of timely primary prevention measures to reduce cardiovascular morbidity and mortality.

Keywords: late-onset hypogonadism; erectile dysfunction; cardiovascular risk

Introduction

Life expectancy has increased dramatically among the global population, resulting in a sharp rise of age-related diseases, including late-onset hypogonadism (LOH). LOH, being commonly an overlooked condition, has been recently associated with a higher risk of cardiovas-cular diseases (CVD) among men.[1] Despite the decline of testosterone levels in aging men being rather common, androgen deficiency is often associated with diabetes, abdominal obesity, and other related diseases.[1] The Massachusetts Male Aging Study has reported a 1.2% per year decline in testosterone levels in different

[1]Department of Clinical Cardiology, Research Institute for Complex Issues of Cardiovascular Diseases, Kemerovo, Russia.
[2]Clinical Department, State Budgetary Health Care Institution "Berezovskaya Central City Hospital," Kemerovo, Russia.

*Address correspondence to: Nataliya B. Lebedeva, MD, DSc, Department of Clinical Cardiology, Research Institute for Complex Issues of Cardiovascular Diseases, Kemerovo 650002, Russia, Email: lebenb@mail.ru

age groups in the general population starting from 1987.[2] However, this trend cannot be explained by an increase in the incidence of obesity and metabolic syndrome, as well as a decrease in smoking in the population.

The LOH in men has been recognized as a growing clinical problem among aging men.[3,4] The LOH is defined as a clinical and biochemical syndrome in middle-aged men with normal pubertal development and is primarily associated with a decrease in testosterone levels. Men with total testosterone (TT) levels of <12 nmol/L are considered testosterone-deficient, and TT levels of <8 nmol/L require hormone replacement therapy.[5,6] Many patients with LOH are believed to go unrecognized, since the symptoms are nonspecific and can occur even at normal androgen levels. Moreover, diagnostic criteria for LOH remain controversial (e.g., erectile dysfunction [ED]), being a key criterion for LOH, and they can be associated with other diseases, such as early atherosclerosis.[6]

In addition, men may present with primary testosterone deficiency without any clinical manifestations: This could be considered as asymptomatic low testosterone.[7] The prevalence of LOH in men aged 40–70 years varies from 30% to 40%, whereas subclinical LOH occurs in 23–38% of patients.[7–9] The incidence of androgen deficiency is significantly higher among men with CVD, obesity, diabetes, osteoporosis, and metabolic syndrome.[10–13] Low testosterone level (>10 nmol/L) in older men has been reported to be associated with a higher risk of mortality, whereas TT level of >12 nmol/L may increase the life expectancy and improve the quality of life.[14] The relationship between low testosterone levels and the development of depression, hypertension, obesity, lipid metabolism disorders, insulin resistance, and diabetes mellitus is of particular concern for middle-aged men, as LOH may contribute to the early onset of atherosclerosis and a high risk of adverse events.[10,15–17]

The LOH can be considered as a marker and even an independent CVD risk factor.[11,18] Testosterone plays an important role in lipid, carbohydrate, and protein metabolism. It has been reported to produce a significant impact on the cardiovascular system, thereby becoming a clinical concern for biomedical society.[10,11,14,19,20] The LOH is commonly accompanied by abdominal obesity, elevated triglyceride levels, and elevated cholesterol and glucose levels, leading to the development of insulin resistance and diabetes. The LOH is associated with arterial hypertension, which is generally considered as the leading CVD, contributing to high cardiovascular mor-

bidity and mortality.[20–22]Thus, LOH has similar components than that of metabolic syndrome. A few researchers have considered metabolic syndrome as a main cause of testosterone deficiency and an independent CVD risk factor.[8,23] Metabolic syndrome has been reported to increase the risk of thromboembolism due to the hemostatic alterations related to increased circulating levels of plasminogen activation inhibitor-1 (PAI-1).[24] Insulin resistance may cause an imbalance between the production of nitric oxide, a physiological vasodilator, and the production of endothelin-1 (ET-1), a physiological vasoconstrictor. Nitric oxide production decreases, whereas ET-1 production increases.[25] On the other hand, a higher risk of thromboembolism in men with hypogonadism may be associated with hypofibrinolysis caused by androgen deficiency. Thromboembolism and myocardial infarction in men with hypogonadism have been recently reported to be mediated by low fibrinolytic activity at baseline. Hypogonadism in men has been associated with increased fibrinolytic inhibition due to increased synthesis of the plasminogen activator inhibitor PAI-1.[26] The effects of testosterone replacement therapy in LOH on cardiovascular risk appear to be associated with secondary polycythemia and a higher risk of thromboembolism.[27]

Our study is aimed at assessing the prevalence of LOH and determining the relationships with cardiovascular risk factors in healthy middle-aged men.

Methods

The study was conducted in accordance with the principles of the Declaration of Helsinki. The Local Ethics Committee approved the study design, protocol, and the form of the informed consent. All participants provided the written informed consent before being recruited to the study. A total of 200 participants aged 44–60 years (the median age 48.44 [45.02–52.5]) referred to the general medical examination at the Federal State Healthcare Institution "Kemerovo Region Primary Healthcare Unit of the Ministry of the Internal Affairs of the Russian Federation" were enrolled in the study.

All participants underwent electrocardiography (The Schiller Cardiovit AT-1 G2 ECG machine), fluoroscopy (X-ray diagnostic complex MRC—"OKO"), blood tests (Mindray Hematology Analyzer), urine protein test (Uni-Test-BM), lipid profiling, and glucose testing (automatic biochemical analyzer ABX Pentra). All participants were examined by neurologists, otorhinolaryngologists, ophthalmologists, surgeons, dentists, psychiatrists, and general physicians. Anthropometric measurements, including the height, weight, and waist circumference, were collected from each participant. We calculated body mass index by using a weight-to-height ratio and the World Health Organization classification.[1] All participants were stratified by CVD risk, received the recommendations on lifestyle changes and nutrition, and were prescribed medical therapy.

Levels of TT were measured with enzyme-linked immunosorbent assay (ELISA) by using the automatic Evolis Twin Plus System analyzer. Reference values 12.1 nmol/L are higher. The average values of the optical density of the calibration samples were 1, 3, 1, 30, and 60 nmol/L. The laboratory normal range was 4.5–35.4 nmol/L for men. If TT level was <12.1 nmol/L, the measurement was repeated. Free testosterone (FT) was calculated by using an open-access software (www.csm4you.ru/kalkuljatory) according to the Vermuelen Formula. To calculate FT, sex hormone-binding globulin (SHBG) was measured at a fixed albumin of 4.3 g/dL. Serum levels of follicle-stimulating hormone (FSH) and luteinizing hormone (LH) were measured with ELISA by using the automatic Evolis Twin Plus System analyzer. A cut-off of 12.1 nmol/L for TT and 0.243 nmol/L for FT was used as laboratory criteria for LOH.[5,7]

All participants were asked to complete the Aging Male's Symptoms (AMS) questionnaire to measure health-related quality of life and symptoms in aging males.[7,28] The AMS rating scale consists of 17 symptoms evaluated on a 5-score scale. The LOH symptom severity was defined as "no/little" (17–26 scores), "mild" (27–36 scores), "moderate" (37–49 scores), and "severe" (≥50 scores). The ED was assessed by the International Index of Erectile Dysfunction (IIEF-5). IIEF-5 ranges from 5 to 25 points, classifying ED into severe (5–7 points), moderate (8–11), mild to moderate (12–16), mild (17–21), and absence of ED (22–25).[29] Participants with a total AMS or ED score of at least 27 were considered to have LOH symptoms. The Beck Depression Inventory was used to evaluate depression and its severity. An index score of ≤9 is considered to be within normal range, whereas a score of 10 suggests the presence of depressive symptomatology from minimal to severe.

The LOH symptoms without a laboratory confirmed reduction in TT or FT were considered as manifestations of general somatic pathology.

All subjects were examined by a urologist to confirm LOH. We used the cut-off of 12.1 nmol/L for TT in diagnosing male hypogonadism. The LOH was diagnosed in case of positive laboratory criteria combined with associated clinical symptoms after excluding other causes. Asymptomatic low testosterone was diagnosed in the absence of clinical symptoms.[6]

Statistical analysis was performed by using the commercially available IBM SPSS Statistics 25 software. The Shapiro–Wilk test was used to examine the data distribution. If variables were normally distributed, the Student's t-test was used to compare two sets of quantitative data. One-way analysis of variance was used to compare three or more independent groups. The Scheffé method was used to perform a one-step multiple comparison procedure. The Mann–Whitney U test was used to compare differences between two independent groups when the variables were not normally distributed. The Kruskal–Wallis test was used to compare three or more groups. In case statistically significant differences were detected, the Mann–Whitney U test was used for pairwise comparison. Contingency tables were used to compare qualitative variables in two independent groups. The Fisher's exact test was used for 2×2 tables, whereas the likelihood ratio was used for multiple columns. In both cases, the Cramer's V criterion was used to assess the strength of the relationship between the selected variables. The interpretation of the obtained values of statistical criteria was performed in accordance with the recommendations of Rea and Parker.[30] A p-value of 0.05 was considered statistically significant. Quantitative variables are presented as the mean and standard deviation ($M \pm \sigma$).

Results

Ninety-eight participants (49%) reported TT levels below 12.1 nmol/L. After being consulted with an endocrinologist and excluding other causes of androgen deficiency, participants with confirmed LOH were assigned to the LOH group. Of them, 72 (73.5%) cases reported decreased levels of TT and FT. Twenty-six (26,5%) participants had an isolated reduction of TT levels, but FT levels were within the reference range. There were no cases of isolated reduction of FT levels. The mean TT level was significantly lower in the LOH group than in the group without LOH (8.9 ± 2.4 nmol/L vs. 22.5 ± 2.8 nmol/L, $p = 0.000$).

One hundred ten participants (55%) in the study population more often had ED and other symptoms measured with the AMS questionnaire than a decrease in testosterone levels. The LOH and asymptomatic low testosterone was confirmed by signs and symptoms, laboratory tests, and specialists' examinations in 42 (21%) and 56 participants (28%), respectively.

Table 1. Mean Levels of Sex and Gonadotropin Hormones in the Study Subgroups

Parameter	Group 1 (n = 102)			p
	Group 1 (n = 102)	Subgroup 1 (n = 42)	Subgroup 2 (n = 56)	
TT (nmol/L)	22.95 ± 9.40	7.78 ± 2.49	10.15 ± 1.32	$p = 0.000$ $p_{I-1} = 0.000$ $p_{I-2} = 0.000$ $p_{1-2} = 0.004$
FT (nmol/L)	0.520 ± 0.243	0.180 ± 0.049	0.261 ± 0.047	$p_{total} = 0.000$ $p_{I-1} = 0.000$ $p_{I-2} = 0.000$ $p_{1-2} = 0.000$
FSH (mIU/mL)	4.224 ± 1.347	4.683 ± 1.545	3.855 ± 1.077	$p = 0.211$
Luteinizing hormone (mIU/mL)	4.338 ± 1.329	4.289 ± 1.520	4.436 ± 1.737	$p = 0.930$

FSH, follicle-stimulating hormone; FT, free testosterone; TT, total testosterone.

We divided the study population into two groups depending on the presence and absence of LOH. One hundred two men with a mean age of 46.43 ± 1.7 years with normal testosterone levels were assigned to Group 1 (non-LOH group). Ninety-eight men with a mean age of 46.26 ± 2.44 years and confirmed LOH were assigned to Group 2 (LOH group). Group 2 was then divided into Subgroup 1 with 42 enrolled partici-pants presenting with LOH and clinical signs, and Sub-group 2 with 56 enrolled participants and confirmed asymptomatic low testosterone.

Clinical signs of LOH were associated with lower TT levels (Group 2 TT level of 7.78 ± 2.49 nmol/L vs. Group 1 TT level of 10.15 ± 1.32 nmol/L, $p = 0.004$).

Both groups reported significant differences in the mean levels of TT and FT. However, no differences were found in the mean levels of FSH and LH. Clinical signs of LOH were associated with the lowest mean lev-els of TT and FT according to the pairwise comparison in the subgroups (Table 1).

Figure 1 reports the results of the AMS scale depend-ing on the presence of LOH. The major proportion of participants in Group 1 reported no clinical symp-toms or had mild to moderate symptoms. Alternatively, more than half of the participants in Group 2 suffered from LOH of varying severity. A relationship of good strength between the severity of clinical signs of LOH and reduced TT levels had been reported (Cramer's V criterion 0.301; $p < 0.05$).

Table 2 demonstrates the prevalence of ED and its severity among the study population. The mean IIEF-5 score was lower in the LOH group as compared with the non-LOH group (19.8 ± 2.4 vs. 21.5 ± 1.9, $p = 0.012$, respectively).

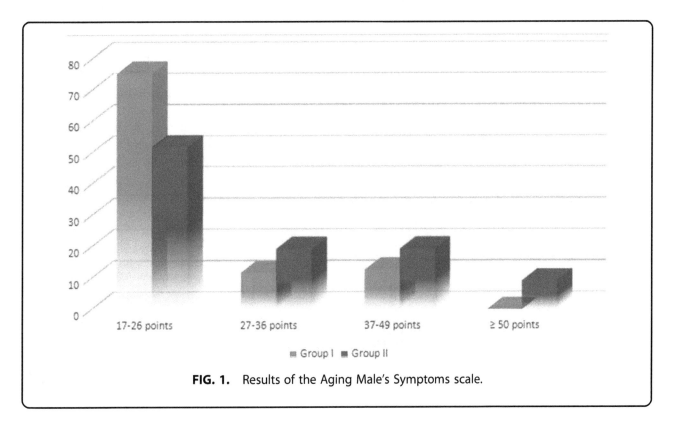

FIG. 1. Results of the Aging Male's Symptoms scale.

Table 2. Results of the International Index of Erectile Dysfunction

Parameter	Group 1 (n = 102) (100%)	Group 2 (n = 98) (100%)	p
Average score IIEF-5	21.5 ± 1.9	19.8 ± 2.4	0.012
21–25 points, n (%)	73 (71.6%)	36 (36.7%)	0.001
16–20 points, n (%)	29 (28.4%)	59 (60.2%)	
11–15 points, n (%)	0 (0.0%)	3 (3.1%)	
5–10 points, n (%)	0 (0.0%)	0 (0.0%)	

IIEF-5, International Index of Erectile Dysfunction.

The highest proportion of participants in the non-LOH group had either no symptoms of ED, or mild ones. However, most of the participants enrolled in the LOH group had symptoms of ED, including moderate ones. There were no cases of severe ED in both groups. A relationship of moderate strength between the severity of ED and low testosterone levels had been reported (Cramer's V criterion 0.352; $p < 0.05$).

Thus, participants with ED and other symptoms measured by the AMS scale prevailed in Group 2. Men with either ED, or other AMS symptoms were less commonly found in Group 2. There were cases of asymptomatic low testosterone among men enrolled in Group 2.

To estimate the relationships between LOH with CVD risk, we analyzed the prevalence of CVD risk factors in Groups 1 and 2. Table 3 demonstrates the prevalence of CVD risk factors among the study population.

We found a high proportion of participants without positive CVD history who had high prevalence of CVD risk factors. Among these factors, lipid metabolism disorders and markers of subclinical lesions prevailed.

Table 3. Prevalence of Cardiovascular Risk Factors in the Study Population

Cardiovascular risk factors	n = 200 (100%), n (%)
Smoking	65 (32.5)
Abdominal obesity	87 (43.5)
High cholesterol	153 (76.5)
Dyslipidemia	165 (82.5)
High triglyceride	75 (37.5)
Glucose intolerance	51 (25.5)
Arterial hypertension	113 (56.5)
Metabolic syndrome	77 (38.5)
GFR below 60 mL/min/1.72 m² (MDRD formula)	3 (1.5)
Atherosclerotic plaques	2 (1.5)
IMT >0.9	20 (10.0)
ABI <0.9	23 (11.5)
MAU	76 (38.0)
LVH	31 (15.5)

ABI, ankle-brachial index; GFR, glomerular filtration rate; IMT, intima-media thickness measured by duplex scanning of brachiocephalic arteries; LVH, left ventricular hypertrophy; MAU, microalbuminuria; MDRD, Modification of Diet in Renal Disease.

To estimate the relationships between LOH and CVD risk, the prevalence of CVD risk factors was assessed in both groups, with and without LOH (Table 4).

Both groups had a similar prevalence of dyslipidemia and hypertension. Obesity, metabolic syndrome, and depression prevailed in Group 2 (Table 4). Relationships of good strength had been found between LOH and obesity, LOH and metabolic syndrome, and LOH and depression (Cramer's V criterion 0.269, $p = 0.005$; 0.316, $p = 0.001$ and 0.348, $p = 0.0001$, respectively).

In the present study, the study of insulin concentrations in blood plasma was not performed; however, when analyzing the level of fasting glycemia in Groups 1 and 2, no differences were found: 6.05 ± 1.53 versus 5.95 ± 1.39 mmol/L, $p = 0.982$.

Depression was commonly found in the LOH group and had the strongest relationship despite the severity of androgen deficiency (15.2% of severe depression cases in the LOH group vs. 0.0% of cases in the non-LOH group, $p = 0.000$). The relationship of good strength had been found between LOH and depression severity (Cramer's V criterion 0.518, $p = 0.000$).

CVD risk was assessed in all participants by using the Systematic Coronary Risk Evaluation (SCORE) scale to determine the associations between a decline in TT level and total CVD risk. Participants with moderate to high risk prevailed in the study population. There were a few high-risk participants; however, very high-risk participants were not reported. Importantly, high-risk participants were found only among men with LOH ($p = 0.003$; Fig. 2).

However, recent evidence has suggested that the SCORE model does not fully predict CVD risk, since the impact of certain risk factors may be underestimated. These factors include high cholesterol, high blood pressure, obesity, metabolic syndrome, and markers of subclinical organ damage (decreased glomerular filtration rate [GFR], left ventricular hypertrophy, microalbuminuria, and signs of peripheral atherosclerosis).[31]

Table 4. Prevalence of Cardiovascular Risk Factors in the Non-Late-Onset Hypogonadism (LOH) Group and LOH Group

Risk factors	Group 1 (n = 102) (100%), n (%)	Group 2 (n = 98) (100%), n (%)	p
Dyslipidemia	81 (79.4)	85 (86.7)	0.444
Arterial hypertension	55 (53.9)	59 (60.2)	0.558
Obesity	32 (31.4)	58 (59.1)	0.006
Metabolic syndrome	26 (25.5)	55 (56.1)	0.001
Depression	13 (12.7)	23 (23.4)	0.000

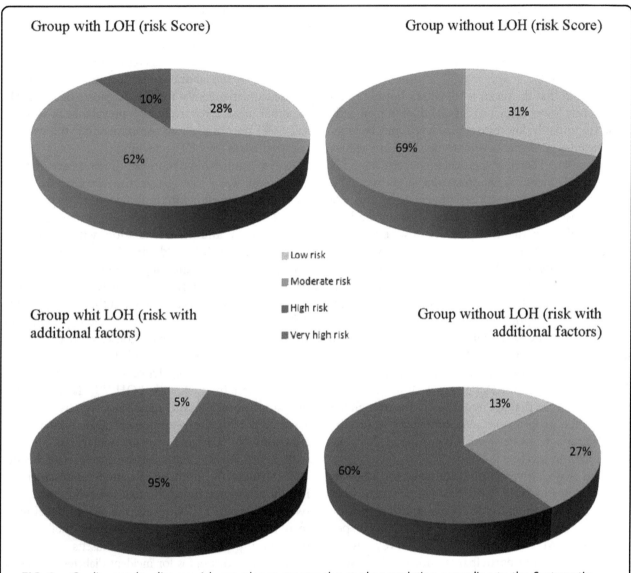

FIG. 2. Cardiovascular disease risk prevalence among the study population according to the Systematic Coronary Risk Evaluation model and after the adjustment to additional risk factors ($p = 0.001$). LOH, late-onset hypogonadism.

After adjusting the resultant model to additional CVD risk factors, risk stratification in both groups changed toward men with high risk. Differences found between the groups became more pronounced in the LOH group, where the highest proportion of participants (94.9%) had a high risk of CVD (Fig. 2).

Discussion

The study on hypogonadism in males reported a prevalence of hypogonadism of 38% in men aged ≥45 years.[9] Recent studies have demonstrated a similar prevalence of LOH of varying severity in men aged 40–70 years, ranging from 30% to 40%. Our results have confirmed a high prevalence of LOH among healthy middle-aged men, which is generally consistent with the medical literature.[8,9,15] Therefore, diagnosis and treatment of LOH remain an issue of concern for middle-aged men. Due to its multifactorial etiology, the clinical symptoms of androgen deficiency are nonspecific and can be even found in men with normal testosterone levels.[5] It seems reasonable that the diagnostic process should rely on the laboratory measurements of testosterone levels and require the exclusion of other possible causes of hypogonadism.[5,7]

We found that the mean levels of sex hormones are significantly lower in men with LOH than in men without it. Importantly, low testosterone levels may be found even in those participants who do not have any clinical signs of LOH.[7] Therefore, particular concern should be paid to timely identify low testosterone levels in middle-aged men even in the absence of clinical symptoms. The mean testosterone level that is even lower in the LOH subgroup than in the asymptomatic low testosterone subgroup has stated the relationship between the clinical severity of LOH and sex hormone levels. The etiopathogenesis of LOH includes the mechanisms underlying the development of both, primary and secondary hypogonadism.[7-9] The absence of significant differences in gonadotropin levels in the study population has suggested the mixed etiopathogenesis of LOH. In addition, compensated androgen deficiency in the non-LOH group with normal levels of sex hormones that are maintained due to high levels of gonadotropins may also contribute to leveling the differences out between the groups in the mean gonadotropin levels.

There is no universal questionnaire for assessing the symptoms of LOH. The AMS questionnaire, being a widely used method for detecting clinical manifestations of LOH, has a sensitivity of 50–54% and a specificity of 40–41.2%.[32] However, this survey allowed us to detect 63% of participants with LOH. In addition, the relationship of good strength between the severity of symptoms and the presence of LOH was reliable.

One of the most specific symptoms of LOH is ED.[4,5,33] However, we found that in some cases LOH was manifested only by ED, determined by the IIEF-5. The prevalence of ED in the LOH group was significantly higher, suggesting a significant contribution of decreased testosterone levels to the onset of ED. The detection of ED in both groups allows us to assume the presence of other causes, in addition to androgen deficiency. Psychological, neurological, vascular, and endocrine diseases as well as certain medications can cause ED. This argument may explain its detection among men who did not suffer from LOH.[34] Since ED has been recently considered as a marker of atherosclerosis, we may suggest that there are

common pathogenetic mechanisms underlying the development of ED and LOH.

As ED and other clinical symptoms of LOH can be detected even without the decreased testosterone levels confirmed by the laboratory testing, none of them can be used independently for the diagnosis of LOH. On the other hand, a relatively high prevalence of subclinical LOH does not allow recommending the existing questionnaires for LOH screening.

Recent studies have reported the presence of associations between low testosterone levels and CVD, including hypertension and coronary artery disease. The effects of testosterone on heart and vascular functions and its association with CVD risk factors such as lipid and carbohydrate metabolism disorders, obesity, and depression have been also reported.[10-12,14] We found rather weak and moderate signs of LOH that may explain the absence of the differences between the groups in lipid parameters. However, the literature data have stated the negative effects of LOH on lipid profile.[22] In addition, we have not found higher prevalence of dyslipidemia and hypertension in men with LOH.[11,15] However, depression, obesity, and metabolic syndrome were associated with the presence of LOH, which could contribute to a higher cardiovascular risk in men with LOH. We did not measure the level of insulin and calculate the homeostasis model assessment of insulin resistance index, though the relationship between FT levels, SHBG levels, the risk of developing insulin resistance, and type 2 diabetes mellitus has been already reported. The Massachusetts Male Aging Study found odds ratios for incident diabetes of 1.58 for a 1 standard deviation decrease in free (ubound) T (4 ng/dL) and 1.89 for SHBG (16 nmol/L).[2] Thus, androgen deficiency in men is closely correlated with insulin resistance and hyperinsulinemia, and the administration of testosterone may improve it.

Whether low testosterone level may be considered as a risk factor or a marker for developing diseases associated with androgen deficiency remains unknown.[11,18,22] The reported relationships between LOH and CVD risk factors may suggest their mutual potentiation with the formation of a so-called "vicious circle," which requires active detection of LOH, as well as strict control of these factors in men with androgen deficiency.

The prospective cycle of this study will be devoted to the analysis of major adverse cardiac events in the study population after a 3-year follow-up.

Conclusion

The relevance of early diagnosis and management of LOH in middle-aged men may ensure the improvement of the quality of life, an increase of work capacity, and the ability to manage risk factors, resulting in a more efficient reduction of CVD morbidity and mortality. Therefore, timely diagnosis of testosterone deficiency by using TT levels is preferable, especially when patients suffer from ED, obesity, metabolic syndrome, and depression. If LOH is diagnosed, it will require medical therapy and a more aggressive approach to the modification of CVD risk factors should be adopted.

Authors' Contributions

N.B.L. has conceptualized, written, and revised the article. V.V.G. has performed data acquisition and analysis.

References

1. World Health Organization. World Health Statistics 2018: Monitoring health for the SDGs. World Health Organization, 2018. https://apps.who.int/iris/handle/10665/272596 (accessed on May 17, 2021).
2. O'Donnell AB, Araujo AB, McKinlay JB. The health of normally aging men: The Massachusetts Male Aging Study (1987–2004). Exp Gerontol. 2004;39(7):975–984.
3. Sieminska L, Wojciechowska C, Swietochowska E, et al. Serum free testosterone in men with coronary artery atherosclerosis. Med SeiMonit. 2003;9(5):214–218.
4. Corona G, Rastrelli G, Monami M, et al. Hypogonadism as a risk factor for cardiovascular mortality in men: A meta-analytic study. Eur J Endocrinol. 2011;165(5):687–701.
5. Morden NE, Woloshin S, Brooks CG, Schwartz LM. Trends in testosterone prescribing for late-onset hypogonadism in men with and without heart disease. JAMA Intern Med. 2019;179(3):446–448.
6. Herring MJ, Oskui PM, Hale SL, Kloner RA. Testosterone and the cardiovascular system: A comprehensive review of the basic science literature. J Am Heart Assoc. 2013;2(4):e000271.
7. Lunenfeld B, Saad F, Hoesl CE. ISA, ISSAM and EAU recommendations for the investigation, treatment and monitoring of late-onset hypogonadism in males: Scientific background and rationale. Aging Male. 2005;8(2):59–74.
8. Wang C, Nieschlag E, Swerdloff R, et al. Investigation, treatment and monitoring of late-onset hypogonadism in males: ISA, ISSAM, EAU, EAA and ASA recommendations. Eur J Endocrinol. 2008;159(5):507–514.
9. Hirokawa K, Taniguchi T, Fujii Y, Takaki J, Tsutsumi A. Job demands as a potential modifier of the association between testosterone deficiency and andropause symptoms in Japanese middle-aged workers: A cross-sectional study. Maturitas. 2012;73(3):225–229.
10. Giannetta E, Gianfrilli D, Barbagallo F, Isidori AM, Lenzi A. Subclinical male hypogonadism. Best Pract Res Clin Endocrinol Metab. 2012;26(4):539–550.
11. Tajar A, Huhtaniemi IT, O'Neill TW, et al. Characteristics of androgen deficiency in late-onset hypogonadism: Results from the European Male Aging Study (EMAS). J Clin Endocrinol Metab. 2012;97(5):1508–1516.
12. Mulligan T, Frick M, Zuraw Q, Stemhagen A, McWhirter C. Prevalence of hypogonadism in males aged at least 45 years: The HIM study. Int J Clin Pract 2006;60(7):762–769.
13. Liu Q, Zhao Y, Gu Y, et al. The association of age-related differences in serum total testosterone and sex hormone-binding globulin levels with the prevalence of diabetes. Arch Gerontol Geriatr. 2020;88:104040.
14. Misiorowski W. Osteoporosis in men. Prz Menopauzalny. 2017;16(2):70–73.
15. Svartberg J, von Mühlen D, Schirmer H, Barrett-Connor E, Sundfjord J, Jorde R Association of endogenous testosterone with blood pressure and left ventricular mass in men. The Tromso Study. Eur J Endocrinol. 2004;150(1):65–71.
16. Lakshman KM, Bhasin S, Araujo AB. Sex hormone-binding globulin as an independent predictor of incident type 2 diabetes mellitus in men. J Gerontol A Biol Sci Med Sci. 2010;65(5):503–509.
17. Brand JS, van der Tweel I, Grobbee DE, Emmelot-Vonk MH, vander Schouw YT. Testosterone, sex hormone-binding globulin and the metabolic syndrome: A systematic review and meta-analysis of observational studies. Int J Epidemiol. 2011;40:189–207.
18. Cattabiani C, Basaria S, Ceda GP, et al. Relationship between testosterone deficiency and cardiovascular risk and mortality in adult men. J Endocrinol Invest. 2012;35(1):104–120.
19. Matsumoto AM. Fundamental aspects of hypogonadism in the aging male. Rev Urol. 2003;5(Suppl. 1):3–10.
20. Goodale T, Sadhu A, Petak S, Robbins R. Testosterone and the heart. Methodist Debakey Cardiovasc J. 2017;13(2):68–72.
21. Ahern T, Wu FC. New horizons in testosterone and the ageing male. Age Ageing. 2015;44(2):188–195.
22. Zhang K, Chen Y, Liu L, et al. The Triglycerides and Glucose Index rather than HOMA-IR is more associated with Hypogonadism in Chinese men. Sci Rep. 2017;7(1):15874.
23. Corona G, Rastrelli G, Morelli A, et al. Treatment of functional hypogonadism besides pharmacological substitution. World J Mens Health. 2020;38(3):256–270.
24. Kostapanos MS, Florentin M, Elisaf MS, Mikhailidis DP. Hemostatic factors and the metabolic syndrome. Curr Vasc Pharmacol. 2013;11(6):880–905.
25. Quon MJ. Reciprocal relationships between insulin resistance and endothelial dysfunction: Insights from therapeutic interventions. Zhong Nan Da Xue Xue Bao Yi Xue Ban. 2006;31(3):305–312.
26. Gencer B, Bonomi M, Adorni MP, Sirtori CR, Mach F, Ruscica M. Cardiovascular risk and testosterone—From subclinical atherosclerosis to lipoprotein function to heart failure. Rev Endocr Metab Disord. 2021;22(2):257–274.
27. Tsametis CP, Isidori AM. Testosterone replacement therapy: For whom, when and how? Metabolism. 2018;86:69–78.
28. Chueh KS, Huang SP, Lee YC, et al. The comparison of the aging male symptoms (AMS) scale and androgen deficiency in the aging male (ADAM) questionnaire to detect androgen deficiency in middle-aged men. J Androl. 2012;33(5):817–823.
29. Rhoden EL, Telöken C, Sogari PR, Vargas Souto CA. The use of the simplified International Index of Erectile Function (IIEF-5) as a diagnostic tool to study the prevalence of erectile dysfunction. Int J Impot Res. 2002;14(4):245–250.
30. Rea LM, Parker RA. Designing and Conducting Survey Research: A Comprehensive Guide, 4th Edition. San Francisco, CA: Jossey-Bass 2014.
31. Mach F, Baigent C, Catapano AL, et al. ESC Scientific Document Group 2019 ESC/EAS Guidelines for the management of dyslipidaemias: Lipid modification to reduce cardiovascular risk: The Task Force for the management of dyslipidaemias of the European Society of Cardiology (ESC) and European Atherosclerosis Society (EAS). Eur Heart J. 2020;14(1):111–188.
32. Chueh KS, Huang SP, Lee YC, et al. The comparison of the aging male symptoms (AMS) scale and androgen deficiency in the aging male (ADAM) questionnaire to detect androgen deficiency in middle-aged men. J Androl. 2012;33(5):817–823.
33. Wu FC, Tajar A, Beynon JM, et al. EMAS Group Identification of late-onset hypogonadism in middle-aged and elderly men. N Engl J Med. 2010;363(2):123–135.
34. Yafi FA, Jenkins L, Albersen M, et al. Erectile dysfunction. Nat Rev Dis Primers. 2016;2:16003.

Abbreviations Used

ABI = ankle-brachial index
AMS = Aging Male's Symptoms
CVD = cardiovascular diseases
ET-1 = endothelin-1
ED = erectile dysfunction

ELISA = enzyme-linked immunosorbent assay
FT = free testosterone
FSH = follicle-stimulating hormone
GFR = glomerular filtration rate
IIEF = International Index of Erectile Dysfunction
IMT = intima-media thickness measured by duplex scanning of brachiocephalic arteries
LOH = late-onset hypogonadism
LH = luteinizing hormone
LVH = left ventricular hypertrophy
MAU = microalbuminuria
MDRD = Modification of Diet in Renal Disease
PAI-1 = plasminogen activation inhibitor-1
SCORE = Systematic Coronary Risk Evaluation
SHBG = sex hormone-binding globulin
TT = total testosterone

Permissions

All chapters in this book were first published by Mary Ann Liebert; hereby published with permission under the Creative Commons Attribution License or equivalent. Every chapter published in this book has been scrutinized by our experts. Their significance has been extensively debated. The topics covered herein carry significant findings which will fuel the growth of the discipline. They may even be implemented as practical applications or may be referred to as a beginning point for another development.

The contributors of this book come from diverse backgrounds, making this book a truly international effort. This book will bring forth new frontiers with its revolutionizing research information and detailed analysis of the nascent developments around the world.

We would like to thank all the contributing authors for lending their expertise to make the book truly unique. They have played a crucial role in the development of this book. Without their invaluable contributions this book wouldn't have been possible. They have made vital efforts to compile up to date information on the varied aspects of this subject to make this book a valuable addition to the collection of many professionals and students.

This book was conceptualized with the vision of imparting up-to-date information and advanced data in this field. To ensure the same, a matchless editorial board was set up. Every individual on the board went through rigorous rounds of assessment to prove their worth. After which they invested a large part of their time researching and compiling the most relevant data for our readers.

The editorial board has been involved in producing this book since its inception. They have spent rigorous hours researching and exploring the diverse topics which have resulted in the successful publishing of this book. They have passed on their knowledge of decades through this book. To expedite this challenging task, the publisher supported the team at every step. A small team of assistant editors was also appointed to further simplify the editing procedure and attain best results for the readers.

Apart from the editorial board, the designing team has also invested a significant amount of their time in understanding the subject and creating the most relevant covers. They scrutinized every image to scout for the most suitable representation of the subject and create an appropriate cover for the book.

The publishing team has been an ardent support to the editorial, designing and production team. Their endless efforts to recruit the best for this project, has resulted in the accomplishment of this book. They are a veteran in the field of academics and their pool of knowledge is as vast as their experience in printing. Their expertise and guidance has proved useful at every step. Their uncompromising quality standards have made this book an exceptional effort. Their encouragement from time to time has been an inspiration for everyone.

The publisher and the editorial board hope that this book will prove to be a valuable piece of knowledge for researchers, students, practitioners and scholars across the globe.

List of Contributors

Nariko Kuwahara, Kate Nicholson, Lauren Isaacs and Neil J. MacLusky
Department of Biomedical Sciences, University of Guelph, Guelph, Ontario N1G 2W1, Canada

Mélanie Bourque
Centre de Recherche du CHU de Québec-Université Laval, Axe Neurosciences, Québec, Canada

Denis Soulet and Thérése Di Paolo
Centre de Recherche du CHU de Québec-Université Laval, Axe Neurosciences, Qué bec, Canada
Facultéde pharmacie, Pavillon Ferdinand-Vandry, Université Laval, Québec, Canada

Julietta A. Sheng, Sarah M.L. Tan and Robert J. Handa
Department of Biomedical Sciences, Colorado State University, Fort Collins, Colorado, USA

Taben M. Hale
Department of Basic Medical Science, University of Arizona College of Medicine - Phoenix, Arizona, USA

Samantha A. Blankers
Graduate Program in Neuroscience, The University of British Columbia, Vancouver, Canada
Djavad Mowafaghian Centre for Brain Health, The University of British Columbia, Vancouver, Canada

Liisa A.M. Galea
Graduate Program in Neuroscience, The University of British Columbia, Vancouver, Canada
Department of Psychology, The University of British Columbia, Vancouver, Canada

Sandro La Vignera, Aldo E. Calogero, Rossella Cannarella, Rosita A. Condorelli and Cristina Magagnini
Department of Clinical and Experimental Medicine, University of Catania, Catania, Italy

Antonio Aversa
Department of Experimental and Clinical Medicine, Magna Graecia University, Catanzaro, Italy

Michael Polchert, Igor Voznesensky, Ayman Soubra and Wayne J.G. Hellstrom
Department of Urology, Tulane University School of Medicine, New Orleans, Louisiana, USA

Rebecca Glaser
Millennium Wellness Center, Dayton, Ohio, USA
Department of Surgery, Wright State University Boonshoft School of Medicine, Dayton, Ohio, USA

Constantine Dimitrakakis
First Department of Ob-Gyn, Athens University Medical School, Athens, Greece
NICHD, National Institutes of Health, Bethesda, Maryland, USA

Adeeba Ahmed
Department of Diabetes, University Hospitals Birmingham NHS Foundation Trust, West Midlands, England, United Kingdom

Karim S. Haider
Praxis Dr. Haider, Bremerhaven, Germany

Sudarshan Ramachandran
Institute for Science and Technology in Medicine, Keele University, Staffordshire, United Kingdom
Department of Mechanical and Aerospace Engineering, Brunel University London, United Kingdom
Department of Clinical Biochemistry, University Hospitals Birmingham, United Kingdom
Department of Clinical Biochemistry, University Hospitals of North Midlands, Staffordshire, United Kingdom

Nadezhda Shlykova
Men's Health Boston, Chestnut Hill, Massachusetts, USA
Beth Israel Deaconess Medical Center, Harvard Medical School, Boston, Massachusetts, USA

Kristina Groti Antonič
Department of Endocrinology, Diabetes and Metabolic Diseases, University Medical Center Ljubljana, Ljubljana, Slovenia
Faculty of Medicine, University of Ljubljana, Ljubljana, Slovenia

Marija Pfeifer
Faculty of Medicine, University of Ljubljana, Ljubljana, Slovenia

Blaž Antonič
Blaž Antonič s.p, Ljubljana, Slovenia

Abraham Morgentaler
Men's Health Boston, Division of Urology, Department of Surgery, Beth Israel Deaconess Medical Center, Harvard Medical School, Chestnut Hill, Massachusetts, USA

Monica Caliber
Medical Writer, Fort Lauderdale, Florida, USA
American Medical Writers Association (AMWA), Rockville, Maryland, USA
International Society for Medical Publication Professionals (ISMPP), Tarrytown, New York, USA

Farid Saad
Medical Affairs Consultant, Hamburg, Germany
Research Department, Gulf Medical University, Ajman, United Arab Emirates
Dresden International University, Center of Medicine and Health Sciences, Dresden, Germany

Karim Sultan Haider
Private Urology Practice, Bremerhaven, Germany

Gheorghe Doros
Department of Epidemiology and Biostatistics, Boston University School of Public Health, Boston, Massachusetts, USA

Xiao Zhang, Karim and Xiaohui Xu
Department of Epidemiology and Biostatistics, School of Public Health, Texas A&M University, College Station, Texas, USA

Ke Huang
Department of Statistics, Texas A&M University, College Station, Texas, USA
Department of Statistics, University of California, Riverside, California, USA

Sultan Haider and Ahmad Haider
Private Urology Practice, Bremerhaven, Germany

Alejandro Abello
Division of Urology, Department of Surgery, Beth Israel Deaconess Medical Center, Harvard Medical School, Boston, Massachusetts, USA

Glenn Bubley
Division of Hematology and Oncology, Department of Medicine, Beth Israel Deaconess Medical Center, Harvard Medical School, Boston, Massachusetts, USA

Nathan Lorde and Amro Maarouf
Department of Clinical Biochemistry, University Hospitals Birmingham NHS Foundation Trust, West Midlands, England, United Kingdom

Geoff Hackett
School of Health and Life Sciences, Aston University, Birmingham, United Kingdom

Abdulmaged M. Traish
Departments of Urology, Boston University School of Medicine, Boston, Massachusetts, USA
Departments of Biochemisty, Boston University School of Medicine, Boston, Massachusetts, USA

Leire Zubiaurre-Elorza
Department of Methods and Experimental Psychology, Faculty of Psychology and Education, University of Deusto, Bilbao, Spain

Sebastian Cerdán
Instituto de Investigaciones Biomédicas Alberto Sols, Consejo Superior de Investigaciones Científicas, Madrid, Spain

Carme Uribe
Institute of Neuroscience, University of Barcelona, Barcelona, Spain

Carmen Pérez-Laso, Alberto Marcos, Ma Cruz Rodríguez del Cerro and Antonio Guillamon
Departamento de Psicobiología, Universidad Nacional de Educación a Distancia, Madrid, Spain

Rosa Fernandez and Eduardo Pásaro
Departamento de Psicología, Facultade de Ciencias da Educación, Universidade da Coruña, A Coruña, Spain

Andrew J. McGovern
Department of Biological Sciences, University of Limerick, Limerick, Ireland

George E. Barreto
Department of Biological Sciences, University of Limerick, Limerick, Ireland
Health Research Intitute, University of Limerick, Limerick, Ireland

Richard C. Strange
Institute for Science and Technology in Medicine, Keele University, Staffordshire, United Kingdom

Carola S. König
Department of Mechanical and Aerospace Engineering, Brunel University London, England, United Kingdom

Amar Puttanna and Abhishek Rao
Department of Diabetes, University Hospitals Birmingham NHS Foundation Trust, West Midlands, United Kingdom

Karim Sultan Haider
Urologische Praxis, Bremerhaven, Germany

Pieter Desnerck
Department of Engineering, University of Cambridge, Cambridge, United Kingdom

Nataliya B. Lebedeva
Department of Clinical Cardiology, Research Institute for Complex Issues of Cardiovascular Diseases, Kemerovo, Russia

Vladimir V. Gofman
Clinical Department, State Budgetary Health Care Institution' Berezovskaya Central City Hospital," Kemerovo, Russia

Index

Printed in the USA
CPSIA information can be obtained
at www.ICGtesting.com
JSHW051405091023
49903JS00006B/281